T0355571

THE GEORGE GUND FOUNDATION
IMPRINT IN AFRICAN AMERICAN STUDIES

The George Gund Foundation has endowed
this imprint to advance understanding of
the history, culture, and current issues
of African Americans.

The publisher and the University of California Press
Foundation gratefully acknowledge the generous support
of the George Gund Foundation Imprint in
African American Studies.

Support for this research was provided by the University of
Wisconsin–Madison Office of the Vice Chancellor for
Research with funding from the Wisconsin Alumni
Research Foundation.

Fatal Denial

Reproductive Justice: A New Vision for the Twenty-First Century

EDITED BY RICKIE SOLINGER (SENIOR EDITOR),

KHIARA M. BRIDGES, LAURA BRIGGS, KRYSTALE

E. LITTLEJOH, RUBY TAPIA, AND CARLY THOMSEN

1. *Reproductive Justice: An Introduction,* by Loretta J. Ross and Rickie Solinger
2. *How All Politics Became Reproductive Politics: From Welfare Reform to Foreclosure to Trump,* by Laura Briggs
3. *Distributing Condoms and Hope: The Racialized Politics of Youth Sexual Health,* by Chris A. Barcelos
4. *Just Get on the Pill: The Uneven Burden of Reproductive Politics,* by Krystale E. Littlejohn
5. *Reproduction Reconceived: Family Making and the Limits of Choice after Roe v. Wade,* by Sara Matthiesen
6. *Laboratory of Deficiency: Sterilization and Confinement in California, 1900–1950s,* by Natalie Lira
7. *Abortion Pills Go Global: Reproductive Freedom across Borders,* by Sydney Calkin
8. *Fighting Mad: Resisting the End of Roe v. Wade,* edited by Krystale E. Littlejohn and Rickie Solinger
9. *Fatal Denial: Racism and the Political Life of Black Infant Mortality,* by Annie Menzel
10. *The Pregnancy Police: Conceiving Crime, Arresting Personhood,* by Grace E. Howard

Fatal Denial

RACISM AND THE POLITICAL LIFE OF BLACK INFANT MORTALITY

Annie Menzel

UNIVERSITY OF CALIFORNIA PRESS

University of California Press
Oakland, California

Library of Congress Cataloging-in-Publication Data
Names: Menzel, Annie, author.
Title: Fatal denial : racism and the political life of black infant
    mortality / Annie Menzel.
Other titles: Reproductive justice ; 9.
Description: Oakland, California : University of California Press,
    [2024] | Series: Reproductive justice : a new vision for the 21st
    century ; 9 | Includes bibliographical references and index.
Identifiers: LCCN 2023048955 (print) | LCCN 2023048956 (ebook) |
    ISBN 9780520297197 (hardback) | ISBN 9780520297203
    (paperback) | ISBN 9780520969650 (ebook)
Subjects: LCSH: African American infants—Mortality—United
    States. | Biopolitics—United States. | Race discrimination—
    United States.
Classification: LCC HB1323.I42 U663 2024 (print) | LCC HB1323.I42
    (ebook) | DDC 304.6/40832—dc23/eng/20231229
LC record available at https://lccn.loc.gov/2023048955
LC ebook record available at https://lccn.loc.gov/2023048956

32 31 30 29 28 27 26 25 24
10 9 8 7 6 5 4 3 2 1

Contents

List of Illustrations *vii*

Preface *ix*

Acknowledgments *xvii*

Introduction: Fatal Deflections *1*

1. The Cult of True Babyhood: Innocence and Infant Mortality *43*

2. Three Forms of Innocence in W.E.B. Du Bois's "Of the Passing of the First-Born" *100*

3. Innocence and Inheritance: Mary Church Terrell and the Reproduction of the White World *136*

4. The Midwife's Bag *183*

5. From Infants in Crisis to Maternal Health Crisis: Birth Justice against Racial Innocence *215*

Notes *259*

Bibliography *311*

Index *339*

Illustrations

1. Midwives in Canton County, Mississippi, 1920s *187*
2. Florida Midwife Institute *188*
3. Midwife bag tag *189*
4. *All My Babies:* Midwife Mary Coley *204*
5. Midwife bag contents *204*
6. Midwife meeting *205*
7. Black bag and laundry bundle *206*
8. Midwife Coley *207*
9. "A Healthy Baby Begins with You" brochure front *219*
10. "Healthy Baby" brochure back *219*

Preface

This project began in a very different moment. In 2023 the notion that medical and societal racism, compounded with sexism and class oppression, are physiologically harmful and potentially fatal for Black infants, mothers, and birthing people sounds intuitive. It is shaping policy and interventions from the federal level, as in the Black Maternal Health Momnibus Act and the 2022 White House Blueprint for Addressing the Maternal Health Crisis, to transformative community-based work at the state and local scales led by Black midwives, doulas, and birth justice organizers and advocates. The 2012–14 period, when this book was beginning to take shape in dissertation form, was a more paradoxical moment.

On the one hand, a substantive body of research demonstrating these links was well-established by that time.[1] Black-led birthwork practices, including Kathryn Hall-Trujillo's Birthing Project USA and Jennie Joseph's JJ Way/Easy Access midwifery model, had long been making these links.[2] Media coverage and public health reports were bringing increasing attention to this research. On occupied Ho-Chunk land, in the place called Teejop in the Ho-Chunk language, where I live, work, parent, and make community in the white-majority city of Madison, Wisconsin, reports on racism in education and policing, as well as vastly inequitable infant survival rates, countered the city's self-congratulatory progressive self-image.[3] On the other hand, prevailing interventions nevertheless tended to deflect blame onto Black mothers and communities themselves—a recurring pattern stretching back more than a century, bringing into view the kinds of measurement and analysis that aligned with that story. Moreover, the benignity of medical care itself was presumed; there was as yet little reckoning with the routinized protocols of violence and neglect toward Black mothers and pregnant people and their infants that medical anthropologist Dána-Ain Davis calls "obstetric racism."[4]

Before graduate school, I trained as a midwife and was licensed from 2003 through 2015. In a 2012 letter of resignation from a national midwifery organization after decades of institutional racism, a group of leading Black midwives and midwives of color foregrounded the violence of preventable Black infant mortality. In that document and elsewhere, these birthworkers illuminated fatal patterns of denial and disavowal—within pregnancy and birth care, within health policy and campaigns, and within the broader polity— that allowed these harms to persist. They called for the white-dominant midwifery organizations to which I belonged to confront this violence as well.[5] Studying Black political thought as a graduate student during those same years, I found James Baldwin's formulations of US whites' innocence—our willful denials of the founding violences of genocide and slavery that continue to structure the US polity—powerfully diagnostic. Baldwin's insights, alongside Audre Lorde's rigorous invitations to white feminists to see and renounce their replications of race, class, sexuality, and gender hierarchies, and Dorothy Roberts's and Angela Davis's accounts of reproductive racism and Black women's struggles for reproductive freedom, illuminated so much at once. These illuminations spanned the defensiveness of white midwifery around the profession's racism and colonial appropriations, the whitewashing and erasure of the histories of Black midwifery, the everyday anti-Black racism and sexism in reproductive medicine, and the status quo–preserving interventions at the federal and state levels.[6] As part of a group that formed in the wake of the resignation, Anti-Racism and Anti-Oppression in Midwifery, we wrote that "white midwives' failure to acknowledge this history while laying claim to 'traditional knowledge' from the 1970s onward is an act of violence, erasing midwives of color from the past and creating an 'innocent' present for white-dominant midwifery."[7] While midwifery is the primary focus of only one chapter here, that moment was a key part of seeding this book's framework.

There is a long lineage of white scholars writing about Black infant mortality, presuming a politics of knowledge that situates the former as objective (and normative) diagnosticians separate from and above their (deviant/damaged) object of analysis.[8] Throughout this book I have attempted to reverse this diagnostic lens. I aim to diagnose the political mechanisms of denial and deflection within that lineage that have functioned—often alongside attestations to the contrary—to endanger Black pregnant people and infants, while preserving white dominance, along with misogyny, ableism, and class oppression, within health care and the broader polity alike. I call this the biopolitics of racial innocence. Where my analysis nevertheless colludes in any way with the systemic violence that it hopes to offer some small conceptual tools toward dismantling, I am ready to hear and, if possible, to repair.

Dominant US medical and public health approaches to Black infant mortality have maintained the status quo presumption of American innocence—the nonculpability and even benignity of US racial capitalism, colonization, and imperialism—and thus deflected attention from the actual infanticidal policies and practices at work. Historian Richard Meckel dates public health concern about infant mortality—even as the parameters of that category were still jelling—in US cities from the 1850s.[9] This concern thus emerged in the mid-nineteenth-century context of enslavement; the legal and dominant cultural negation of Black maternity, parenthood, and kinship; the commodification and sale of Black children and destruction of Black families for profit; and the mass killing and stealing of children from Native Nations as an explicit strategy of genocide.[10] The public clamor for baby-saving in its foundational decades focused solely on US-born white and European immigrant babies. This call to save infant life thus not only excluded Black and Indigenous babies, but comprised a set of public feelings and political demands integrated within a polity that was actively killing and stealing them, as well as justifying those deaths and thefts as legal, right, and inevitable. Governmental attention shifted to an attitude of concern for Black infants, as well as infants of Native Nations and among US colonial occupations like the Philippines, in the second decade of the twentieth century. This new official concern, however, erased the historical and ongoing violence threatening infant life, and maternal and cultural deficiency took center stage as the alleged main obstacles to infant thriving. As I show, the terms of these fatal denials have shifted over time, but the deflections of racial innocence have persisted.

While findings about racism's specific physiological harms and routinized medical violence are relatively new, the outlines of this analysis are not. Historian Wangui Muigai shows that by the 1940s the US Black press was representing infant death "as embodying society's indifference to black children."[11] Communist leader Claudia Jones's 1949 "An End to the Neglect of the Problems of the Negro Woman" makes the connections between infant and maternal mortality and racial, gender, and class domination crystal clear, citing numbers and conditions that remain strikingly and shamefully relevant today.[12] Insofar as the discourse, politics, and practices have turned in recent years toward addressing the actual root causes of Black infant mortality, it has primarily been because of the work of Black practitioners, organizers, and scholars. Especially crucial has been the movement, theory, and analytical framework of Reproductive Justice, an approach forged by a group of Black women health organizers in 1994: Dr. Toni M. Bond Leonard, Reverend Alma Crawford, Evelyn S. Field, Terri James, Bisola Marignay, Cassandra McConnell, Cynthia Newbille, Loretta Ross, Elizabeth Terry, "Able" Mable Thomas, Winnette P. Willis, and Kim Youngblood. Reproductive justice comprises the core human rights to bodily and reproductive autonomy—to have a child, not to have a child, to raise children in safe and healthy environments, and, more recently, gender and sexual freedom.[13] From these visionary Black feminist roots, reproductive justice as framework and movement extends across many fronts of resistance and transformation. Characterized by cofounder Ross and Rickie Solinger as "open-source code" designed to be taken up in ways that best serve specific communities' particular struggles, reproductive justice spans climate change activism, decolonization, land and water defense, abortion access, gender justice, abolition, and much more, illuminating the connection points between organizing and praxes for a livable world.[14]

Organizations and forwarding justice in pregnancy and birth—including Black Women Birthing Justice, the Southern Birth Justice Network, the National Birth Equity Collaborative, Ancient Song Doula Services, SisterSong, HealthConnect One, Birth Detroit, the National Association to Advance Black Birth, the Black Mamas Matter Alliance, Elephant Circle, Tewa Women United, Bold Futures, the National Perinatal Task Force, Birthing Cultural Rigor, Bronx (Re) Birth and Progress Collective, Restoring Our Own Through Transformation, Uzazi Village, and, here in Teejop/Madison and nearby Milwaukee, Harambee Village Doulas, The Foundation for Black Women's Wellness, Roots4Change, and Maroon Calabash (just a few among the many, many organizations nationwide whom I do not yet have the honor to know) have further extended the reproductive justice framework into the realms of pregnancy and birth, centering prenatal, birth, and postpartum care rooted in birthing people and their babies' own communities. These Black, Indigenous, and/or Latine-led organizations name and refuse long-standing forms of obstetric racism and violence, and work to create policies, infrastructures, and spaces of safety and connection that truly support the dignity and bodily autonomy of all birthing people.[15]

Birth justice organizers, scholars, and practitioners confront a highly uneven geography of birth care and experiences, stratified by colonial, white supremacist, anti-Black, class, ability, gender, citizenship, and sexuality hierarchies; a carceral system that cages mothers and pregnant people, still shackles many birthing people, and separates them from their children; a legal landscape where pregnancy and abortion alike are increasingly criminalized, especially for Black and Indigenous people, undocumented people, people of color, and poor people; wage, housing, and food injustices; and the long-standing colonial racial capitalist ecological violence whose horrors and harms extend further each season.[16] White gestation and birth and infancy—including my grandmothers', my mother's, my own, and my daughter's lives—have been unjustly insulated from the acute impacts of these harms, in no small part through the biopolitics of racial innocence. Yet the reproductive justice framework makes clear that, though at vastly different timescales and horrifically unjust distributions, the systems that cause harm to Black infants, mothers, and gestating and birthing people are the systems that endanger all beings on earth.[17] White supremacy, reproductive violence, extraction, property, and profit threaten all of the relations and care that makes life possible.

In this moment of truth-telling about these systems of violence and their impacts on Black infants' life chances, this book examines the foundations of the biopolitics of American racial innocence that for so long has functioned to foreclose such a reckoning. It articulates key moments of contestation in the work of two key Black political thinkers who experienced infant loss as parents themselves: W.E.B.

Du Bois and Mary Church Terrell. It situates the key Black community praxes of Jim Crow–era midwifery in relation to these thinkers, in naming the forces actually at work in structural infanticide and stripping bare the ruses of Southern health officials' innocence. The book closes by querying how and where, even in this moment of confrontation and avowal of structural racism, these older patterns may yet shape policies and practices—and by uplifting the transformative work that refuses these patterns; that remembers, honors, and reinvigorates lineages of lifegiving care; and that is already making justice in pregnancy and birth a reality.

Acknowledgments

The political visions, analyses, and care practices of midwives, doulas, birth workers, physicians, and organizers working for justice in birth set the coordinates for this book. For my understanding of birth justice as well as its breadth and power, I am particularly indebted to the work of Black Women Birthing Justice, the Southern Birth Justice Network, Tewa Women United, the Black Mamas Matter Alliance, Ancient Song Doula Services, visionary midwife Jennie Joseph, Elephant Circle, Racha Tahani Lawler Queen, Tehmina Islam, Tia Murray, Tamara Thompson Moore, Micaela Berry-Smith, Hakima Tafunzi Payne, Marinah Farrell, Kathryn Hall-Trujillo, Claudia Booker (in beloved memory and enduring power), Alexis Pauline Gumbs, Carmen Mojica, Indra Lusero Esq., Paula X. Rojas, Micaela Cadena, Liam Kali, Jaqxun Darling, Wendy Gordon, Marijke Van Roojen, Kristin Effland, Jeannette McCulloch, Vivian Gutierrez, Wičáŋȟpi Iyótaŋ Wiŋ, Monica McLemore, Karen Scott, Monica Basile, Cheré Suzette Bergeron, Sarah Davis, Heather Sinclair, Devorah Herman, Ruth Kauffman, Ashley Hartman Annis, Natalie Lake, Deb Kaley, and Gretchen Spicer.

Profound thanks to Keisha Goode, whose work on racism in US midwifery and Black midwives' relation to reproductive justice is crucial—I am so excited to read and teach *Birthing, Blackness and the*

Body: *Black Midwives and the Pursuit of Reproductive Justice,* forthcoming from Columbia University Press. It has been an honor to witness some of the local organizations in Teejop/Madison and nearby doing powerful work in support of equity and justice in birth, including Harambee Village Doulas, Maroon Calabash, Roots4Change, the Foundation for Black Women's Wellness, the Black Maternal and Child Health Alliance of Dane County, and the Wisconsin Doulas of Color Collective. I know that my knowledge is partial and that there are many more organizations engaged in this work.

So many people have supported, encouraged, and inspired me during the very, very long process of writing and revising this book. Deepest gratitude to Dána-Ain Davis for your generous encouragement, intellectual exchange, insights, critical eye, friendship—and for your visionary work for birth justice. Enormous thanks to my beloved friend, mentor, and kindred spirit George Shulman, for constant and heartful accompaniment during this long process. I am so grateful to and for you, George. Thank you so much to Monica Casper, who graciously and generously read an early draft of the manuscript and offered such generative and helpful feedback. I am particularly indebted to Juliet Hooker, whose generous and incisive review of the first draft helped to anchor fundamental reorientations of the project. Appreciation also to the anonymous reviewer for helpful comments. Shannon Sullivan and Lawrie Balfour have been careful and generatively critical readers at both the beginning stages and final push of the project—deep appreciation and thanks. Many thanks to Laura Briggs for an early vote of confidence. Thank you so much to Monique Allewaert for your sustained support, pulling me back from many cliff edges, and friendship. Christine Di Stefano, Chip Turner, Naomi Murakawa, and Bob Mugerauer (in beloved memory) were a deeply supportive dissertation committee and wonderful mentors.

I learned from so many conversations about parts of this project with beloved friends and brilliant comrades in political theory and beyond, inside and outside the academy. For your radiant queer Black feminist abolitionist theorizing and praxis, calling lifegiving horizons into being, thank you, Jasmine Syedullah. For companionship and beautiful queer and kinful thinking, Lisa Beard, love and thanks. For the power of the captive maternal and the unsparing truth always, deep gratitude to visionary Joy James. I am grateful beyond words for connection and conversation with Cristina Beltrán, Jimmy Casas Klausen, Tiffany Willoughby Herard, Lori Marso, Stephen Marshall, Kirstine Taylor, Shatema Threadcraft, Heather Pool, Anand Commissiong, Randa Jarrar, Rachel Sanders, Kevin Bruyneel, Daniel Ho-Sang, Rob Nichols, Joe Lowndes, Ainsley LeSure, M. Shadee Malaklou, Lawrie Balfour, Libby Anker, Jakeet Singh, Lester Spence, Andrew Dilts, Sina Jo Kramer, Ella Myers, Kathy Ferguson, Neil Roberts, Marcela Garcia-Castañon, James Martel, Charles Mills (in dear memory and enduring inspiration), Nikhil Pal Singh, Patchen Markell, Melvin Rogers, Chad Shomura, Desmond Jagmohan, Robyn Marasco, Deva Woodly, Andrés Fabián Henao, Elva Orozco, Kennan Ferguson, Chris Barcelos, Ron Watson, Christa Craven, Jina Kim, Maged Zaher, Tish Lopez, Heather Sinclair, Natalí Valdez, Susan Raffo, Sophie Lewis, Rajni Shah, Sameena Mulla, M Murphy, and Kaden Paulsen-Smith.

In the Department of Gender and Women's Studies at the University of Wisconsin–Madison, I am beyond fortunate to count some of the most stellar humans that I know as colleagues: Sami Schalk, Jess Waggoner, Kelly Ward, Pernille Ipsen, Keisha Lindsay, Jill Casid, Anna Campbell, Finn Enke, Aurora Santiago Ortiz, Ruth Goldstein, Jamie Priti Gratrix, Lyddia Ruch-Doll, Nina Valeo Cooke, Joslyn Mink, Chris Garlough, Ellen Samuels, Judy Houck, Kai Pyle, Kong Pheng Pha, Sara Chadwick, Maria Lepowsky, Kate Walsh, and Leigh Senderowitz. LiLi Johnson and James McMaster, you are sorely missed! I am grateful to be affiliated with the Collaborative for Reproductive Equity: many thanks to Zakiyyah Sorensen, Jenny Higgins, and Amy Williamson.

Gratitude to fantastic UW colleagues—current and some very much missed former—Kasey Keeler, Tiffany Green, Nadia Chana, Cherene Sherrard-Johnson, Amadi Ozier, Steph Tai, Timothy Yu, Keith Woodward, Christy Clark-Pujara, Larissa Duncan, Frederic Neyrat, Megan Massino, Steve Kantrowitz, Omar Poler, Brittney Edmonds, Michael Peterson, Laurie Beth Clark, Emi Freirichs, Sue Zaeske, Nicole Nelson, Jenell Johnson, Sainath Suryanarayanan, Noah Weeth Feinstein, Nan Enstad, and Jenna Loyd. Kelly Ward, Jess Waggoner, Nadia Chana, and Jen Rose Smith: many thanks for holding space in our virtual writing group during the final push. Huge thanks to Stepha Velednitsky for stellar and wise editorial assistance, and to Cora Segal for assistance with the bibliography. Many thanks to wonderful people that I have had the privilege to work with as grad students, including Jimmy Camacho, Jalessa Bryant, Ozhaawashko Blue Sky, Jenny Fierro Padilla, c nelson, Lou Groshek, Sam Miller, and Amy Pearce. I am grateful to my students in the Science and Politics of Reproductive Health, Childbirth in the US, Race Gender, Colonization, and Gender, Women, Bodies, and Health.

At Vassar College, gratitude to colleagues in Political Science and beyond, including Katie Hite, Samson Opondo, Luke Harris, Himadeep Mupiddi, Andy Davison, Mary Shanley, Zachariah Mampilly, Taneisha Means, Diane Harriford, Hiram Perez, Elías Krell, Shona Tucker, Molly McGlennen, and Quincy Mills. Orion Morrison-Worrell provided terrific research support as an undergraduate at Vassar. It's been wonderful to reconnect with alum Alejandro McGhee.

At the University of California Press, profound gratitude to Rickie Solinger, editor of the Reproductive Justice series, for sustained support of the project and over this long haul. Enormous gratitude to reproductive justice movement cofounder, theorist, and leader Loretta Ross's vision and work, which has been so crucial to making the very concept of the series possible. Deep thanks to Khiara Bridges, as former editor of the series, for encouraging words about the project early on.

Many thanks to editor Naomi Schneider for consistent support. Editorial assistant Aline Doline shepherded the final steps of the process with skill and care. Amy Smith Bell's copyedits offered crucial clarity.

Parts of this book benefited greatly from invited presentations at Beloit College, Marquette University, Brown University, the University of British Columbia at Okanogan, the UW-Madison Department of Geography's Yi-Fu Tuan Lecture, UW's Holtz Center for Science and Technology Studies, and the Utah College of Midwives. Pieces of the book were presented at the annual meetings of the Western Political Science Association, the American Political Science Association, and the National Women's Studies Association.

I have learned so much about reproductive justice from and with my WMF Abortion Fund comrades as well as the National Network of Abortion Funds, before and after *Dobbs*. This circle overlaps with beloved comradeships and friendships that have grown through organizing and cherished community here in Teejop/Madison and beyond. Thank you for making political home with me. Huge love and gratitude to Lucy Marshall, Ali Muldrow, Katrina Morrison, Gail Konop, Silvia Martinez, Lexy Ware, Barbara Alvarez, Wendy Hathaway, Isabella Horning, Lizzie Bruno, Sarah Hinkley, Laura McNeil, Angela Marchant, Erica Shroyer, Dawn Matlak, Lorrie Hurkes, Caitlin Yunis, and Josh Jenkins. Abortion access now! Free Palestine! A just and livable world for our children and all children everywhere!

I simply am because of the accompaniment of my beloved friends, loves, and lodestars of my life. Some of whom I have thanked above. Zeina El-Azzi, divine lioness and brightest star, thank you for the beauty and lifelong soul-accompaniment. Antonio Garza, from my core to yours, for your breathtaking and beautiful signature dance with the world, for your YAYYYYYYYY! Heather Rule Day, my companion through the soul-grater of grad school, the glory of flowers, parenting, all of it. For your generous leadership and your magnificent care for the world, thank you, dear Shadee Malaklou.

Shannon Tyman, for exquisite deliciousness, generous hosting, and getting ever more real together. Kristin Forde, my sister in this world, thank you for being the one I want to call. For the walks and heart to heart connection, thank you, Cynthia Lin. Kelly Ward, for being so wildly fantastic in every way—wise friend, badass parent, cosmic adventurer. For moving in the world with magnificent freedom, fearlessness, and dazzle, and for being the most incredible queer auntie to Phoebe, thank you, Sami Schalk. For heart connection, integrity, and humor from our first Divine serendipity, Jess Waggoner. For lifelines of serious thought and glorious delight, Lester Spence. For your wise and constant friendship, Caroline Faria. For life as poetry, Jihad Touma. For always making a home for me, Andrew Whitver and Kevin Brannaman. Thank you for the kinship, the self that I feel in the illumination of your being, for the worlds that you make possible and are.

I am so grateful to and for my family. I simply couldn't have done this without my mother, Liisa Peterson. Thank you for being my amazing mom and the most wonderful grandma possible to Phoebe, my miraculous bright star. To and for Phoebe, I love you infinity! I am so grateful for your strong, bold, and shining self as my life's compass point, its divine and snuggly and stubborn center. Thank you to my truth-seeking brother, Galen, for your companionship and understanding. Thank you so much, my dad, Chris Menzel, for your ongoing support and pride in me. In loving memory of my stepfather, Garret Ihler. Alex Dressler, my trusted co-parent and truly the best dad in the multiverse. My beloved aunt, hero and icon Beth Gilson. Gratitude and love for the Peterson clan, the Menzel clan, and the Ihler clan. In loving memory of my grandparents, Clare Menzel and Bob Menzel, and Ellen Peterson and Bob Peterson, my great-grandmother Gladys, and my uncle Jon Peterson.

· · ·

An earlier version of chapter 2 was published as "'Awful Gladness': The Dual Political Rhetorics of Du Bois' 'Of the Passing of the First-Born,'" *Political Theory* 47, no. 1 (2019): 32–56. An earlier version of chapter 4 was published as "The Midwife's Bag, or, the Objects of Black Infant Mortality Prevention," *Signs: Journal of Women in Culture and Society* 46, no. 2 (Winter 2021): 283–309. Thanks to *Signs* and *Political Theory* for permission to print this material in revised form.

Introduction

Fatal Deflections

In May 1896, Frederick Hoffman, German-born white statistician for the Prudential Insurance Company, published his influential treatise, *Race Traits and Tendencies of the American Negro*. Hoffman's 330-page tract begins by declaring its dedication to the most comprehensive and disinterested scientific investigation: "Only by means of a thorough analysis of all the data that make up the history of the colored race in this country," the introduction reads, "can the true nature of the so-called 'Negro problem' be understood."[1] *Race Traits* presents an unprecedented synthesis of new criminal, demographic, epidemiological, and vital statistics with older anthropometrical studies and anecdotal evidence. Hoffman argues that his statistical methods place his findings beyond dispute: "it is a fact which can and will be demonstrated by indisputable evidence, that of all races for which statistics are obtainable . . . the negro shows the least power of resistance in the struggle for life."[2] Conversely, Hoffman argued, these numbers proved the enduring vitality of the Anglo-Saxon race. As Khalil Gibran Muhammad observes, Hoffman's treatise was pivotal in establishing statistics as objective "proof" justifying the white supremacist racial order, offering unprecedented—and apparently unshakeable—validity to long-standing myths of Black inferiority and deviance, "shaping racial statistics into a powerful, full-blown narrative of Black self-destruction, racial decay, and the futility of reform."[3]

Hoffman's comparative infant mortality statistics, and his interpretations of them, were a key component of these findings.[4] Employing mortality tables from New York City, Brooklyn (two years before the other four boroughs annexed it), Boston, Philadelphia, Baltimore, Washington, DC, New Orleans, Charleston, and Richmond, Hoffman observes that the difference in mortality "for the earliest period . . . is enormous."[5] Black infant survival, he concludes, is compromised throughout the nation: "Nowhere else do we meet with such a frightful infant mortality as we find prevailing among the colored population of the large cities, both North and South."[6] It is clear that compared with their white counterparts, Black infants are faring extremely poorly. Hoffman proclaimed that these much higher rates of Black infant mortality, rather than reflecting the perilous conditions for Black families in these cities—relegation to poor, expensive, and often extortionate housing, withholding of sanitation services, exploitative and dangerous working conditions, uncertain access to good food and clean water, criminalization, medical apartheid, and increasing racial terror—heralded a dying race. As Muhammad writes, this "disappearance hypothesis" came to prevail among white analysts of the so-called "Negro Problem" during the racial nadir of the 1890s.[7]

For Hoffman, this hypothesis relied on the rationale that under enslavement, Anglo "masters" had benignly protected Blacks as a race from the rigors of the "struggle for life." Translating into the idiom of statistical science the comforting myths of slavery apologists like John C. Calhoun, he attempts to erase not only the current death-dealing conditions of Jim Crow city life, but the still-recent horrors of the lash, forced labor, routine sexual violence, and family separation. Black infant mortality rates in the 1890s, for Hoffman, allegedly show that race survival was impossible without that tender "protection."

He thus places great emphasis on the comparison of the newest generation with their elders. He presents age-differentiated mortality tables showing that Black and white mortality rates diverge less among older adults, whereas the gap widens dramatically for infants and children: "the greatest excess of mortality amongst the colored falls on the early age groups."[8]

Hoffman also adduces evidence diachronically, using Charleston's data to compare the "excess mortality" of Black people in 1890 compared with 1848, noting little change in the oldest category age-differentiated vital statistics but significantly increased mortality rates among the young.[9] Although this is only one city for which he presents such data, Hoffman asserts that "we have an abundance of testimony . . . that previous to emancipation the negro enjoyed equal health if not superior to that of the white race"—although no evidence he cites supports such robust health.[10] Since emancipation, in contrast, this "superior" health has only declined, to the point that now "the young generation is the one least fit for race survival."[11] He notes that other analysts have long observed the "excessive mortality of the colored race."[12] However, his inclusion and interpretation of African American infant mortality statistics constitutes new support for this alleged trend of race extinction. Allegedly reflecting both the inherent "traits" of physiological and moral weakness and their correlate "tendencies" of parental deficiency, Hoffman argued that Black infants' mortality rates heralded the fate of the race as a whole.

By the 1920s the disappearance hypothesis no longer held sway in white experts' discussions of Black infant mortality. These explanations no longer propounded inherent biological "race traits" and even brought certain environmental factors into view. They nevertheless remained wedded to a notion of "race tendencies," ultimately blaming the neglect and allegedly harmful behaviors of Black families, especially mothers, and community members—especially midwives. Their explanations thus, like Hoffman's, ultimately deflected attention from the root causes of Black infants' increased vulnerability to death. For example, in a paper given at the 1920 American Public Health Association meeting, published in the *American Journal of Public Health* that year, Dr. Stewart B. Thompson, director of Vital Statistics for the Florida State Board of Health, offered his analysis of "factors that influence infant mortality" in his state, which was not yet included in the country's vital statistics registration area. He noted that Florida's numbers compared favorably with those aggregate numbers, taken largely from the Northeast and the Midwest, noting that the registration area's annual white infant mortality rate was 91 per thousand births, and Florida's was 72, while the numbers for "colored" babies were 149 and 126, respectively.[13]

As was usual in such reports at the time, the striking disproportion between Black and white rates in both areas passed without comment. Yet Thompson did take an unusually fine-grained approach to the question of seasonal causes among Florida infants, graphing mortality in both groups by month for 1917 and 1919. This revealed a significant spike in Black infant deaths in the months of April and May, while white infant deaths remained relatively steady. Thompson had a theory about the cause of this spike: "In many parts of the state," he wrote, "colored women are employed to dig the enormous potato crop which is harvested during the spring of the year. The diggers travel long distances in auto trucks and many camp nearby until the end of the season. All children who are able to work follow their mothers, and of course the little babies are very much neglected; not only improperly fed, but irregularly and often underfed."[14] The everyday violence of postpartum mothers forced to stoop for weeks from dawn to dusk, the brutal normalization of Black child labor, gasoline fumes on the road between sites, and the flimsiest of shelters during the night goes unremarked.[15] The ascriptions of neglect and improper feeding, moreover, shifts the lion's share of the blame from these deplorable conditions onto mothers themselves.

Yet the violence and deprivation that would "of course" prohibit mothers from feeding and caring for their newborns are nevertheless discernible here.[16] In short, Thompson offers an account—albeit unaccompanied with even the barest response to its horror—of the social and economic etiology of Black infant mortality within a racialized labor hierarchy monstrously predatory on Black women's labors and capacities. Apart from this disclosure, however, Thompson's report closely hews to the common explanatory logics of the day, including the era's de rigueur diatribe against "ignorant," unsanitary, and "superstitious" Black midwives, whom he implicitly blames for the "53% of the infant deaths last year . . . reported as occurring from tetanus, convulsions, [and] diseases of early infancy."[17] In one of the grand deflections of the first half of the twentieth century, white health officials throughout the South blamed not poverty or medical neglect—let alone racist terrorization—for high Black infant mortality rates but the alleged ignorance and unhygienic practices of Black midwives, instituting programs of midwife surveillance and control that largely fostered official indifference to the deleterious conditions of Black infant life and death.[18]

Thompson's concluding summary of the causes of infant death makes no mention of the racialized labor regime as a causal factor. Rather, he names malaria and other disease factors common in Florida at the time and emphasizes the Black "midwives with their superstition, lack of education and training" and parental deficits—this time without reference to context or working conditions: "ignorance and lack of care . . . insanitary conditions of the home."[19] He concludes by remarking on Florida's salutary climate: "The mild climate is a factor in reducing the infant mortality rate as it is possible to keep the baby out in the fresh air most of the time."[20] This "fresh air," evoking the domesticated outdoors of screen porches and shaded yards, neatly eclipses the forced exposure of infants in the potato rows and trucks. Thompson thus briefly brings into view a damning account of the fatal impacts of Black infants' social and political milieu, a racialized labor hierarchy in which Black women and children were bound to the very bottom rung, with its life-depleting demands and toxic exposures. Yet the final analysis reverses course completely, repeating the familiar tropes of dangerously ignorant Black midwives and careless parents.[21]

These two foundational explanations for Black infant mortality are distinct—one positing an inherent pathology within the bodies of Black infants themselves, the other focused on malignant maternal behaviors and community birth practices. Yet they each serve as a declaration of innocence on the part of the white commentators. They each allege that the harm that causes Black infant death is located within Black life itself, whether in the particular organism or in the communal lifeways within which it is embedded. Nowhere do the investments, interests, or life-insulating factors that characterize the white ownership class to which these commentators belong appear as part of the story. They do not appear in relation to the white infant mortality rates that, within the comparative frame, appear as the neutral norm, let alone in their relation to the sanctimoniously lamented numbers, the deviant data points, by which they count Black infant deaths. But for a scientific community and citizenry invested in a white national future, these rationalizations conveniently effaced both the conditions that threatened Black infant life and the lived experiences of loss for Black mothers, fathers, kin, and communities.

Throughout this book I argue that these dual ascriptions—inherent pathologies and dangerous practices—comprise the *fatal deflections* on which the biopolitics of Black infant mortality in the United States was founded. These ascriptions prevailed among white physicians and experts in explicit and unapologetic terms during at least the first three decades of the twentieth century. Yet in more subtle ways they have persisted long past this time, and, as I argue, are still discernible in early twenty-first-century approaches. For one brief example, in 2007, the Office of Minority Health initiated a targeted national intervention in response to high infant mortality rates among Black communities, titled "A Healthy Baby Begins with You."[22] As the name suggests, the campaign laid personal responsibility for infant outcomes on Black mothers themselves. Of the "nine risk factors that contribute to infant mortality," seven focused on maternal behaviors or individual characteristics: "Late Prenatal Care, Smoking, Substance Abuse, Poor Nutrition, Obesity, High Stress."

As I detail in chapter 5, this emphasis on *stress* reflected emerging understandings of how racism in the United States can impact Black people across the life course. Yet the intervention prescribed by the campaign nonetheless held individual mothers responsible for their stress levels.[23] Not only did the campaign brochure direct mothers to exercise and eat healthy—obscuring the racial and class geographies of grocery stores, sidewalks and parks, and labor conditions that shape access to these "choices"—and to avoid alcohol and drugs but to "keep stress under control, do pleasant things that will keep you in good spirits." In other words, this national-level public health campaign forwarded a notion of risk apparently isolable to maternal traits and behaviors, decoupled from any mention of systemic racism or economic deprivation. In just the fifteen years since that campaign, the discourse has shifted significantly. Research is establishing ever-clearer causation to the harms of systemic and medical racism in their complex intersections with class hierarchies, sexism, ableism, and other systems of oppression. Yet if not explicitly confronted, the habitual ascriptions of inherent traits and pathological behaviors can still shape frameworks of intervention and protocols of care.

The biopolitics of racial innocence is what I term this long-standing pattern of deflection that characterizes dominant physician and health authorities' explanations of and interventions into Black infant mortality. In her work on the US carceral regime, political scientist Naomi Murakawa defines racial innocence as "practiced blamelessness for the death-dealing realities of racial capitalism . . . maintained through willful ignorance, blame displacement, and liberal reforms."[24] Murakawa's formulation builds on James Baldwin's analysis of US whites' disavowal of the genocidal racism that has constituted them as a people, in a kind of Möbius strip of deadly violence and willful denial: "they have destroyed and are destroying hundreds of thousands of lives and do not know it and do not want to know it. . . . [I]t is not permissible that the authors of devastation should also be innocent. It is the innocence which constitutes the crime."[25] Throughout this book I use the biopolitics of racial innocence to describe the institutionalized mechanisms, habits, and techniques of practiced blamelessness that have at once enabled, obscured, and perpetuated racial capitalism's fatal impacts on Black maternity, gestation, birth, and infancy. As Ruth Wilson Gilmore writes, "the forms and patterns that coalesce into premature death, reveal human sacrifice as an organizing principle."[26]

These fatal deflections set the dominant terms under which the political thinkers and actors whose work is at the center of this book lived, mourned, organized, and worked to transform the conditions that imperiled their children. In different ways they all refused this biopolitics of racial innocence. Importantly, in many ways this expressed a collective refusal. Hoffman blamed Black parents for their own infants' demises just when race leaders W.E.B. Du Bois and Mary Church Terrell themselves became bereaved parents in the 1890s. Du Bois and fellow scholar Kelly Miller challenged this hypothesis at the time in critical reviews of Hoffman's text.[27] Among other strategies, Du Bois situated US Blacks' numbers within international mortality statistics, showing that death rates were equally high for urban poor in several European cities, to argue that Hoffman's conclusions about race decline were erroneous.[28] Moreover, Du Bois's careful studies of Black living conditions in *The Philadelphia Negro*, as well as other studies undertaken under the auspices of

Atlanta University, demonstrated that these numbers were anything but natural.[29]

Along with other Black clubwomen, Terrell addressed the urban conditions that made Black mothers and infants vulnerable, establishing daycare centers, kindergartens, and homes for single women new to the cities.[30] Du Bois and Terrell also contested the biopolitics of racial innocence rhetorically, along with its keystone figurations of Black parental damage, infant moribundity, and white beneficence—emphasizing instead the death-dealing environments and murderous bad faith of whites that menaced their infants' life chances. Rural Southern Black midwives, situated very differently than Du Bois and Terrell in terms of geography, education, and class location, likewise carried out their praxes of care for infants and mothers under the shadow of accusation of being agents of death. Thompson's indictment of midwives in 1920, though present in texts from decades earlier, had become paradigmatic by that date and would be at the heart of the Southern interventions ushered in by the Sheppard-Towner Act the following year. Midwives refused the biopolitics of racial innocence primarily through their practices of community care: what Gertrude Fraser calls their "philosophy of praxis"—though some of their own narrations of this history, reflecting decades after the implementation of midwife control programs, also entail powerful discursive contestations.[31] In the present day, calls for birth justice, which explicitly frame the United States as a hostile environment for Black maternal, infant, and community life, carry this lineage forward in the realms of rhetoric and practice alike.[32]

As with Baldwin's formulation of innocence, these words and deeds reveal the structural nature of these fatal deflections. That is, racial innocence is both produced by and essential to the violence of racial capitalism, which, among its many harms and horrors, underwrites Black infants' unjust vulnerability to preventable death. Together, these accounts make clear that the biopolitics of racial innocence is a key component of *white settler reproductive futurity*—the organization of space, social, political, and economic structures, institutions, laws, and norms to preserve US whites' entitlements to stolen property, intact family, relative health, and wealth from generation to generation, at apocalyptic cost to Black and Indigenous peoples in the United States, and to communities, workers, and life worldwide under those entitlements' monstrous extractive footprint. Though at unjustly vast variance in timescales and intensities of violence, white settler reproductive futurity imperils all human and other-than-human beings and relations on earth—even, eventually, its "innocent" beneficiaries. Yet both in terms of US white citizenly memory and self-regard, and as a defining feature of the white baby as avatar and material locus of intergenerational entitlement, racial innocence preserves, sustains, and serves as alibi for the mass murderous, planet-killing trajectories of commodification, extraction, hoarding, and ongoing theft of lands, peoples, and labor.[33]

Innocence and Reproductive Racial Capitalism

The text from which Baldwin's formulation of innocence is taken, "My Dungeon Shook: Letter to My Nephew on the One Hundredth Anniversary of the Emancipation," in fact thematizes the predatory conditions that both expose Black infants to death and conveniently obscure, for the white public and its governing bodies, any responsibility for those conditions. While the essay's most well-known lines, quoted above, blast the culpability of whites' innocence in the massive destruction of life, Baldwin stages the birth of his beloved nephew—also named James—fifteen years before as a particular and telling scene of innocence's crimes. The lines immediately following those quoted above read: "Now, my dear namesake, these innocent and well-meaning people, your countrymen, have caused you to be born under conditions not very far removed from those described for us by Charles

Dickens in the London of more than a hundred years ago. (I hear the chorus of innocents screaming, 'No! This is not true! . . . '").[34]

Later in the letter, Baldwin puts an even finer point on that causal factor, the disavowed agency of these "innocents" in creating the perilous conditions of birth: "This innocent country set you down in a ghetto in which, in fact, it intended that you should perish. . . . You were born into a society which spelled out with brutal clarity and in as many ways as possible, that you were a worthless human being."[35] These lessons are communicated to the teenage James in "details and symbols," "what white people say about [him]"; but they have also been at spelled out from the start in the *intentionally created* material conditions of his birth, which, also by design, most whites never encounter.[36] As Baldwin, also born and raised in this ghettoized space, writes: "I *know* the conditions under which you were born, for I was there. Your countrymen were *not* there, and haven't made it yet."[37] Their white fellow citizens have created a political, legal, moral, economic, and physical geography that protects them from encountering and comprehending, let alone redressing, the destruction from which their own symbolic and material advantages derive.

As Kirstine Taylor argues, Baldwin's formulation of innocence is not simply about whites' self-serving epistemological or moral refusals of acknowledgment; it is a founding and enduring structural feature of US racial capitalism.[38] In positing Baldwin's notion of innocence as structural, Taylor draws on Cedric Robinson's theorization of racial capitalism: "The development, organization, and expansion of capitalist society pursued essentially racial directions, so too did racial ideology. As a material force, then, it could be expected that racialism would inevitably permeate the social structures emergent from capitalism. I have used the term 'racial capitalism' to refer to this development and to the subsequent structure as historical agency."[39] Jodi Melamed glosses Robinson's concept: "Capital . . . accumulation require[s] loss, disposability, and the unequal differentiation of human value, and racism enshrines the inequalities that capitalism requires . . . by displacing the uneven life chances that are inescapably part of capitalist social relations onto fictions of differing human capacities, historically race."[40]

For Baldwin, innocence is just such a fiction, or more precisely a fictionalizing function. This function has not only been enshrined in law, in white moral sense, and within the hierarchies at the heart of American enterprise, but has taken material form in and as the differential geographies and embodiments that comprise the polity itself, directly shaping life chances and trajectories in the present. Taylor points to Baldwin's emphases, as in this passage, on spatially segregated built environments as key sites of this structural innocence, such that whites tend to be physically distanced and insulated from encountering the bodies and lives, the death and destruction, that undergirds the country's accumulated wealth. Baldwin's repeated use of "conditions" in the passage above, along with his depiction of the ghetto as a deliberate creation, underscores this point. Extending Lawrie Balfour's depiction of Baldwin as a "profoundly spatial thinker," Taylor links his vivid accounts of the built environment with his attention to policing and carceral containment and racialized labor hierarchies. All three of these features of the US polity systematize the violent containment of and extraction of value from Black communities, and white insulation from those scenes of routine predation on which their own entitlements depend.

Taylor argues that, for Baldwin, this is not only a feature of his own mid-twentieth-century moment, but foundational to the country's racial-capitalist origins and enduring structure. The same innocence that consigned his nephew to the category of "worthless human being" inhered in the human rankings that enabled the US polity's founding. For Baldwin, innocence—the deliberate unknowing of what is known too well—has been a central feature of racial capitalism's historical agency from country's origins to the present.

Baldwin's account of structural innocence positions Native genocide and slavery as the "two racial histories of conquest from which racial innocence was created."[41] Upon reaching "these shores," Baldwin writes in "The White Problem," "we did several things in order to conquer the country . . . we promptly eliminated [the Indigenous people]; we killed them." This, for Baldwin, simultaneously instantiated the innocence-preserving myth of the heroic settler and justly vanquished enemy Native; "all those cowboy-Indian stories are designed to reassure us that no crime was committed. We've made a legend out of a massacre."[42] In that same essay, Baldwin makes clear that innocence qua disavowal likewise characterizes the dominant white relation to the enslavement regime that, along with genocide, literally constituted the country, its conquest and its wealth alike: "We enslaved [Africans] because, in order to conquer the country, we had to have cheap labor . . . creating that capital of which we are now so proud, and to which we claim Negroes have never contributed anything." He expands on this process of disavowal in his "Talk to Teachers" that "black men were brought here as a source of cheap labor . . . the white republic had to brainwash itself into believing that they were, indeed, animals and deserved to be treated like animals . . . it was a deliberate policy hammered into place in order to make money from black flesh."[43] Both this brainwashing and the brutal extraction of value that necessitated it, Baldwin argues to his audience, were "indispensable" components of the United States, and they still profoundly shape its material conditions.[44]

In these passages Baldwin figures Black men as the subjects of this essential and disavowed labor.[45] Yet the commodification, dehumanization, and theft of Black women's reproductive bodies, reproductive *and* productive labors, and care are no less foundational to US racial capitalism. Political theorist Joy James's figure of the "captive maternal"—which can be "biological females or those feminized into caretaking and consumption"—foregrounds this predation on the labors that make life possible, and on which the US colonial slave state and its machinery of extraction depend. The "captive maternal" encompasses those "most vulnerable to violence, war, poverty, police, and captivity; those whose very existence enables the possessive empire that claims and dispossesses them."[46] Moreover, these founding and ongoing dynamics of reproductive violence and value extraction have entailed specific forms of racial innocence.[47] In her account of how enslavers asserted claims to captive women's reproductive capacities in the earliest decades of the transatlantic slave trade, Jennifer Morgan identifies a number of interlinked fantasies at work. On the one hand, there is evidence, even in that era, of the still-tenacious mythologies of the fertile and fecund enslaved woman and the lack of African maternal and family ties and feelings, such that enslaved procreation could be justifiably commodified. Alongside these fantasies about African women, however, Morgan discerns a self-regarding fantasy about Europeans themselves: "notions of slave ownership without entanglement or culpability, of endless returns on investments, of the gentle and Christian slave owner."[48]

Such dreams of guiltless mastery—racial innocence, congealing as the categories of chattel slavery hardened—continued to structure slaveowners' responses to high rates of infant death as a feature of the enslavement regime. The figure of the "griefless" African mother soothed slaveowners' qualms about separating and selling commoditized children. Similarly, Morgan writes that "the image of the malevolent and depraved enslaved mother circulated as a salve to exonerate slave owners from their responsibility for the low fertility and high mortality rates among the people they had enslaved, who were suffering the consequences of brutal extractive labor, inadequate food, and unhygienic living conditions . . . the accusation that enslaved mothers and midwives were responsible for the deaths of infants served an important purpose for proslavery writers."[49] Reproductive slavery thus produced both Black infants' acute vulnerability to preventable death and the fictions that deflected responsibility from that deadly machinery.

Morgan writes that "slave owners needed to reroute their attention from the depravity of the slave market to the depravity of Black life."[50] As Hoffman's and Thompson's texts exemplify, this justificatory specter of the depraved and uncaring Black mother persisted well after Emancipation. In fact, the figure of the malevolent Black mother, herself posing the greatest danger to her offspring, still animates policies and institutional protocols that claim to protect Black infants and children. As Dorothy Roberts shows, such policies and protocols, including those of the so-called child welfare system—which Roberts designates the "family policing system"—do not only discursively pathologize Black mothers (especially poor and disabled Black mothers) but criminalize them, terrorizing and traumatizing the very children that these systems purport to protect.[51] This criminalization carries out a key innocence function, as it "blames the most marginalized parents for the impact of race, class, and gender inequalities on their children, obscuring those unequal structures and the need to dismantle them." It is perhaps no surprise, then, that the three core mechanisms that Murakawa identifies in the "practiced blamelessness" of the carceral system more broadly are likewise at work in infant mortality's biopolitics of racial innocence.

These mechanisms—willful ignorance, displacement of blame, and liberal reformism—are perceptible across the entire span of time examined in this book. As in Thompson's assessment of Florida's infant mortality rates, contradictions between description and prescription often mark sites of willful ignorance, as white physicians and public health experts bring relevant conditions into view and/or acknowledge Black communities' unjust exposures to harmful conditions, only to default to racist conventions and stereotypes in their ultimate diagnoses. More subtly, even as new understandings of racism and harmful stress emerge in the present day, recent interventions have nevertheless defaulted to Black mothers' individual responsibility. This willful ignorance thus ensures the persistence of these deadly conditions over time. The *displacement of blame* from economically exploitative and white supremacist structures, as well as medical and other forms of institutional racism, onto Black women, families, and communities themselves is a central feature—perhaps *the* central feature—of the biopolitics of racial innocence. As obstetrician and reproductive justice scholar and organizer Karen Scott and her coauthors observe, "structural racism . . . [is] embedded in 'mother blame' narratives" that often dominate maternity care/neglect for Black women.[52]

Finally, *liberal reformism* manifests through discourses of white official concern—a kind of performance of racial progress—disconnected from structural transformations. Reflecting on white attachment to political dominance in the United States, Juliet Hooker writes that "liberal unwillingness to enact the egalitarian values they profess is a form of white refusal that functions to secure enduring advantage, one that also partakes in white innocence in the form of nostalgia for a time when less was asked of them."[53] Such a dynamic of loud lamentation paired with institutional inertia that sustains protections for white infants and harms to Black infants, characterizes the biopolitics of racial innocence. In many cases, this entails major funding for established agencies and programs in the name of addressing Black infant mortality, even as these agencies systematically fail to address the root causes at work. Meanwhile, the most effective grassroots maternal and infant health work in and by Black communities themselves often goes unfunded or vastly underfunded. Doula and community organizer Hakima Tafunzi Payne, founder of Kansas City's Uzazi Village, terms this parasitic dynamic "disparities pimping," a term that maternal health advocate, breastfeeding counselor, and fellow doula Sherri White originated.[54]

Liberal reforms entail approaches that individualize and atomize both patients and providers, such that the broader context recedes from view. With respect to the former, such approaches "responsibi-lize" the Black maternal body and behavior in ways that, again, seamlessly foster blame. With respect to the latter, we might think of the increasingly pervasive emphasis on implicit bias among individ-ual physicians—an emphasis that, as Tiffany Green and coauthors note, can distract from the more demanding collective efforts needed to shift long-standing racist institutional protocols that operate re-gardless of individual physicians' intentions or biases.[55] Also trou-bling, as Jennifer Nash argues, is the trend of promoting Black doulas as solely responsible for solving the maternal health crisis, while hos-pitals and medical schools fail to transform the deadly racist, sexist, classist, and ableist standards of "care" that are actually killing Black infants and Black mothers and birthing people.[56]

The Biopolitics and Necropolitics of Black Infant Mortality

In naming these dynamics the biopolitics of racial innocence, this book invokes Michel Foucault's designation for the techniques and institutions that modern states use for the administration and optimization of their populations' collective life, beginning—on his account—in roughly the mid-eighteenth century.[57] Foucault devel-ops the concept of biopolitics most explicitly in *The History of Sexual-ity*, volume 1, and his 1975-76 lectures at the Collège de France. For Foucault, this development is marked by the emergence of the new concepts of the *population*, the society's aggregate "body . . . serving as the basis of the biological processes . . . [including] births and mortality . . . life expectancy and longevity."[58] And the concept of *statistics*, literally the "science of the state," makes it possible to measure these collective biological processes.[59] The "biopolitics of the population" is concerned with monitoring and intervening in the collective life of the population through new fields such as public health, hygiene, sanitation, birth control, urban planning, and epidemiology.[60]

Biopolitics is a kind of "positive power," designed to optimize the life and futurity of this newly conceived collective entity, the population, and its continuity over time. But, Foucault argues, these life-fostering techniques and institutions inevitably entail what he terms "state racism": the officially sanctioned classification of particular groups within the polity as inferior, degenerate, abnormal, or otherwise threatening to the "legitimate" population's health and continuity over time, and the attendant subjection of these groups to neglect, violence, and death.[61] The biopolitical state thus fractures collective life along hierarchies of value, fostering the flourishing of the forms of life that it deems valuable, and depriving or directly targeting those that it deems inferior or threatening. While Foucault holds up the Nazi Holocaust as the murderous apogee of biopolitical state racism, he specifies that this killing can take more subtle forms: "the fact of exposing someone to death, increasing the risk of death for some people, or, quite simply, political death, expulsion, [or] rejection."[62] Biopolitical states mete out death via state-sanctioned killing, but also by exposure to toxic conditions and negation of a political status whose claims might register at all.[63] Thus, even as biopolitical states aim to optimize and protect certain lives and relations, they designate zones of "lives . . . less valued, more available to neglect, injury, precariousness, abjection, and . . . violence not conventionally counted as such."[64]

Yet Foucault's formulation of biopolitics itself bespeaks a kind of racial innocence. Morgan makes the point that Foucault's theorization completely erases the precise, highly developed, and state-sanctioned systems of accounting that characterized the management of captive human life and death for centuries. Any understanding of nineteenth- and twentieth-century biopolitical states' rationalized violence must take serious account of the originary political arithmetics in the ledger books of chattel slavery.[65] Morgan's work, along with that of Stephanie Smallwood and other historians of slavery, renders manifest the limitations of Foucault's temporal schema and geographical scope, showing these political arithmetics of life and death, reproduction and the selective management of futurity, to be rooted in brutal human accounting practices that emerged both earlier and elsewhere. Morgan and Smallwood highlight the emergence of such calculations at the very origin of the transatlantic slave trade and European conquest—on the west coast of Africa, on slaving ships, and on plantations in the Western Hemisphere.[66]

Other critics have pointed out that Foucault's own figurations of state racism paid little attention to the fatal impacts of structural inequalities, the quotidian forms of violence, hoarding, impoverishment, exploitation, and marginalization normalized by racial, colonial, economic, gender, and ability hierarchies.[67] His state paradigm ignores ways that biopolitical modes of management in European metropoles in fact originated in, or were fundamentally entangled with, racist and colonial logics, classifications, and protocols.[68] As Joy James notes, Foucault's theorizations of biopolitical racism and colonial violence are striking not only in their neglect of the work of his contemporary Frantz Fanon, but in their effacement of precisely the foundational role of colonial genocides, dispossession, and anti-Black dehumanization and violence for European subjectivity, states, and capital that Fanon illuminates. This neglect seems particularly willful in view of the strong echoes of the latter's insights on colonialism in Foucault's framing of biopolitical racism as a Manichaean state of war.[69] As M Murphy sums it up, Foucault's work "refuses to engage with colonial and postcolonial histories [and] the elaboration of the racial state."[70]

Nevertheless, despite Foucault's own silences, Murphy and other scholars likewise attentive to these omissions have extended and supplemented the framework of biopolitics to parse the ways that states simultaneously foster spaces of both optimization of living being and condemnation to death, and the links between these divergent operations. Infant mortality, first emerging as an affectively laden target of measurement and intervention in the second half of the nineteenth century in the United States, is a biopolitical concern par excellence.[71] White infant mortality became a key locus of psychic and material investment for the white-settler polity, concentrating concerns spanning gender, race, and civilization, national futurity and identity, urbanization, immigration, maternal responsibility and medical authority. Infant mortality statistics operate as what Murphy calls "phantasmagrams": "quantitative practices that are enriched with affect, propagate imaginaries [and] lure feeling."[72] The phantasmagram is a particularly apt term for understanding the racialized imagery and investments that infant mortality statistics conjure. For even as the enumeration of dead white "angels" roused a white public to action, Black infant mortality barely registered as a dominant public concern: figuring as losses on a ledger in the antebellum period, largely left uncounted after the Civil War.[73]

Elaborate funerary rituals and accoutrements for dead infants, in a proliferation of poetry, literary representations, and popular songs, evinced an efflorescence of public feeling. This was accompanied, in the following decades, with public outcry about urban white infant mortality statistics and calls for action to end this "slaughter of innocents," giving rise to major Progressive Era initiatives and culminating in a new federal bureau and the first federal welfare legislation, the Sheppard-Towner Act.[74] As Black infant mortality came into view as an object of state concern in the late nineteenth century, it bore the imprint of the plantation biopolitics that Morgan points to and their necessary fictions about the depravity of Black life. Even as evolutionary frameworks came to the fore in characterizations of the physiological entailments of that alleged depravity, the dangerous deviance of Black mothers and midwives persisted in official interpretations of and interventions into Black infant mortality. Part self-serving scientific innovation, part old wine in new bottles, infant mortality as a key feature of the so-called "Negro Problem" deflected attention and responsibility away from the enduring structures of reproductive racial capitalism.

In twenty-first-century US biopolitics, comparative statistics still show persistently stark inequities between Black and white infant mortality, despite more than a century of interventions and official concern.[75] Even in the service of condemning the current system's fatal impacts, however, reiterating these grim statistics is a thoroughly ambivalent move. On the one hand, these numbers can be deployed as evidence of the persistence of the anti-Black racism and reproductive violence that produce Black infants' acute vulnerability to preventable death. On the other hand, the repetition of statistics itself can do a kind of violence. As LaKisha Simmons argues, "they cannot account for the experience of Black maternal mourning."[76] In addition to eclipsing the ways that these unspeakable losses marked the lives of mothers, fathers, kin, and communities, numbers fail to communicate the legacies of survival, protection, and care that have sustained Black infant life against the odds. On the contrary, given the proclivities of racial innocence among white experts to displace blame and unsee their own institutional implications, the repetition of racially inequitable infant mortality statistics, if not embedded in a thoroughgoing indictment of the current system's impacts on health, can as easily bolster as refute the convenient and profitable mythology of Black maternal and community pathology. As Monica Casper writes, these "numbers . . . drain emotion from loss and fail to inspire care and concern."[77] Like Marx's fetish object, infant mortality statistics on their own tell us nothing of the conditions that precipitated them.[78]

Likewise, the biopolitical idiom of *gaps* and *disparities* itself can obscure as much as it reveals.[79] For one thing, disparities talk misleadingly posits an equivalency between whiteness and Blackness as comparative variables.[80] The comparative frame, central to the biopolitics of Black infant mortality from the beginning, erases the fundamental relation between these numbers and the broader environments that produce them both. In Ruha Benjamin's terms, "vampirically, white vitality feeds on black demise."[81] Furthermore, even as whites' relative vitality accrues from a system of theft and hoarding, the language of the Black-white gap erroneously posits white US infants as the standard of health. They are not, even domestically: Asian American infants overall have significantly better survival rates than white babies in the United States, although all broad categorizations miss major internal differences.[82]

Globally, Singapore, Japan, Anguilla, and France are among the forty-three other countries with better survival rates than white US infants.[83] I include these examples ambivalently, knowing that they may conjure phantasmagrammatic effects of their own—from a "model minority" halo around Asian American birth to white victimry in relation to global comparisons. Nevertheless, they call attention to the false notion of US white health supremacy. Moreover, the disparities paradigm fails to capture the breadth of neglectful and deleterious obstetrical care that all too many mothers and birthing people across the board experience in the United States. Undocumented and working-class Latina mothers and their infants have been particular targets of routinized neglect and violence.[84] Additionally, a kind of eugenic common sense tends to render disabled maternity and infancy beyond the pale of reproductive value and life worth caring for.[85] And while it is of utmost importance not to flatten extreme differences in experiences and outcomes, the pervasive abuse of pregnant people of all demographics, the extreme cesarean rate in the United States, the negligible postpartum support, and the lack of paid parental leave make giving birth and the first year afterward preventably perilous and difficult for nearly all birthing parents.

This is not to minimize the fact that Black, Indigenous, Latinx, and Asian American birthing people, as well as people with disabilities, are more likely to be subjected to obstetric violence and that Black and Indigenous birthing people are far more likely to suffer life-threatening sequelae from the latter.[86] It is rather to emphasize that white people also have deep material and political stakes in refusing and transforming current systems toward care worthy of the name.

Nevertheless, disparities talk around US infant mortality extends this false white standard of health into the statistical realm what I call—extending the analyses of Hazel Carby and Robin Bernstein—the "cult of true babyhood": the iconization of a typically-abled white cherub in devoted maternal embrace, at the heart of propertied het-eronuclear domesticity.[87] The "true baby" sits at the apex of health officials' disavowed hierarchy of life worth, the norm in reference to which medical discourse and education and popular media alike cast Black infancy as deviation or damage.[88] In instrumental relation to the so-called true baby, US health authorities have used the figure of Black infancy to punish Black women coming and going, as a "whit-ened" vulnerable/neglected victim threatened by the Black mother's inadequate care *and* a "blackened" figure of future threat, a potential drain on public resources whose well-being is at best a private mat-ter.[89] As I argue in chapter 1, the true baby has marked a core incom-mensurability among human groupings since the mid-nineteenth century: the ultimate avatar of white settler reproductive futurity and the unacknowledged operative standard in the comparative biopoli-tics of infant mortality. Both alibi and embodiment of racial inno-cence, the true baby is the sanctified idealization of a white suprema-cist property regime that is in fact predatory upon Black life, health, and labor, predicated on the genocide and dispossession of Indige-nous lives, relations, and lands, that devalues and invisibilizes femi-nized care work, that seeks to dispose of disabled lives, and wreaks disaster through US militarism and extractive capitalism worldwide.

Illuminating these mechanisms of predation and routinized violence, some key accounts of Black maternal precarity and reproductive harms have deployed Achille Mbembe's notion of *necropolitics* rather than biopolitics. Mbembe offers the complementary formulation of necropolitics to describe spaces where the death function of biopolitics is most active. Drawing a throughline through various sites beginning in early modernity, from the plantation to colonization in Africa to occupied Palestine, Mbembe addresses the spatial and historical limits of Foucault's formulation, describing the manifold ways that sovereign power expresses itself through routinized killing, violence, and injury, through "the capacity to define who matters and who does not, who is disposable and who is not."[90]

Anthropologist Christen Smith draws on Mbembe to conceptualize the impacts of police violence on the kin and communities of its immediate victims in both Brazil and the United States. Smith focuses her attention on Black mothers in particular—both the specific form of necropower to which they are exposed and the ways that they refuse this violence. Smith posits that the impacts on mothers who must fear and witness police brutalization and murder of their children constitute an invisibilized yet pervasive form of gendered state violence that she terms "sequelae," a health sciences term denoting the aftereffects of acute injury or illness. Through sequelae, states deliberately impede these lifegiving functions; they are "necropolitical mechanisms that terrorize Black mothers and inhibit their ability to further care for Black life."[91] Smith argues that Black mothers—a category in which she includes both gestational mothers and all those who "practice social responsibility for collective care"—are not simply collateral victims of this slower form of violence.[92] Rather, they are "enemies of the state" who challenge the anti-Blackness fundamental to the nations of the United States, Brazil, and beyond through their role as generators and protectors of Black life and kinship. Through sequelae, states deliberately impede these life-giving functions.[93] In terms resonant with this analysis, Erica S. Lawson frames violence against US Black children as a foundational to the racial state's necropolitics and Black activist mothering as a strike against its targeted distributions of death.[94]

Likewise engaging with research on the health harms of racism, Naa Oyo Kwate and Shatema Threadcraft use the framework of necropolitics to describe transgenerational dynamics of assault. Routinized state violence targeting Black communities, like "stop-and-frisk" policing, means that "necropolitics is the more significant power formation in Black space [than biopolitics] within the United States."[95] They turn to the work of health researcher Arline Geronimus, who uses the term "weathering" to name accelerated cellular aging and the wear-and-tear of intensified inflammatory, metabolic, immune, and endocrine processes among Black communities and other communities targeted for state violence, which many public health experts see as at least partially explaining the gaping inequities in Black-white life expectancy, maternal and infant outcomes, and overall health. Kwate and Threadcraft frame weathering, especially for the kin and communities of Black youth targeted by stop-and-frisk, as an invisible but significant enactment of necropower. Although pregnancy is not their primary focus, they highlight research linking the stresses of racism with low birthweight, a primary proximate factor in infant mortality, among other ways that this necropower manifests—in this case, even before birth.

While these accounts call attention to often-invisibilized enactments of necropolitical violence, Zakiyyah Iman Jackson offers a sustained engagement with the cellular and molecular processes at work in these harms. Jackson draws on epigenetics—the interactions between experiences, environments, exposures, and gene expression, which may result in heritable changes—to reconfigure the space and time coordinates of Mbembe's account.[96] As she writes, "Mbembe's spatial reading describes a necropower that compartmentalizes life and death into geographic zones 'epitomized by barracks and police stations,' but in what I describe as necropower's 'boundaries' and 'internal frontiers' are not so much spatialized but corporealized . . . traveling with black(ened) subjects even when they are able to transgress geopolitical-spatialized borders."[97] In other words, these cellular and molecular effects are not pinned to particular geographical locations but rather carried inside the subject. They can thus cause persistent harms even at a geographical remove from the scene of injury. Moreover, they can potentially span multiple generations through epigenetic inheritance, potentially repeating patterns of harm.

In chapter 5, I take a closer look at some of the health sciences research that these accounts are building on, which posits racism as a key factor patterning maternal and infant morbidity and mortality. For now, it is important to note that, in conceptualizing racism itself as a harmful environment, these accounts of necropolitics guard against the perils that can attend studies of fetal development and epigenetics in practice as well as its popular understandings. While (perhaps) bemoaning the conditions that have given rise to health inequities, such approaches can nevertheless figure marginalized bodies and communities as the locus of pathology, implicitly figuring white settler bodily and community health as the innocent standard, leaving the relation between these disparate sites of alleged health and damage unmapped and uninterrogated.[98]

In contrast, these extensions of Mbembe's account render visible what we might think of as the *reproductive necropolitical ordinary* of the United States. They illuminate the diffuse, unspectacular, and multiscalar forces that threaten Black maternal and infant life as part of the broad array of anti-Black necropower. In confronting the pervasive and protean forms that this reproductive necropower takes, they make clear the profound changes that shifting these patterns will require in both the US political order and the medical field. As

Kwate and Threadcraft note, this necropolitical ordinary has not precluded the reach of biopolitical accounting and intervention into Black community life: "The two power formations, biopower and necropower, are not mutually exclusive, as both are deployed to varying degrees in Black space. For example, the longstanding concern with Black births, birth control use, abortions, sex, marriage, and drug rates stand as evidence of the operation of biopower in Black space, though to what end is up for debate."[99]

The biopolitics of racial innocence gets at the relation between these two forms of power, between the preservative and the predatory. Official interpretations of and incitements to Black infant life have largely failed to interrupt the reproduction of the broader necropolitical surround. If Baldwin's geographies of innocence under US racial capitalism obscure the brutality and exploitation that enables white affluence and ease, the biopolitics of racial innocence effaces the political, legal, social, economic, and environmental conditions that predicate white infants' protections on Black infants' exposures.

True Babyhood and the Wages of Innocence

In addition to Baldwin's writings, the framing of racial innocence here builds on formulations of innocence across a number of disciplines. Literary scholar Robin Bernstein's notion of racial innocence describes the nineteenth-century racialization of the category of childhood. "At the mid-nineteenth century," she writes, "writers began to polarize black and white childhood," construing white children as the embodiment of innocence and thus excluding of Black children from childhood itself.[100] George Shulman posits a polarity in his account of Baldwin's "innocence" as diagnosing a set of deeply held psychic and libidinal structures turning on a spectral duo of utter abjection and impossible purity. As he writes, "disavowal creates the blackness that enables whiteness as a form of innocence; one is a

specter of what is disclaimed in life and humanity; the other is a purified identity [Baldwin] depicts as idolatry."[101] And, indeed, Bernstein
highlights key sites of both the idolization of white childhood and its
fundamental dependency on a demonized and grotesque Black juve-
nility as its constitutive other. Bernstein locates two features in particular that structured the binary between nineteenth-century white
"true children" and Black youths: sexual innocence (versus Black
children's alleged knowingness) and susceptibility to pain, as "tender angels" contrasted with "insensate pickanninies."[102]

These bifurcations persist today, as white authorities consistently
overestimate the age of and impute sexual precocity to Black children, especially girls.[103] Physicians' systematic refusals to hear, believe, and respond appropriately to Black patients' pain, including
pediatric patients, as well as the widely-cited pervasiveness of medical students' beliefs in racial differences in sensory capacity, also be-
speak the tenacity of these profoundly harmful myths.[104] The normative white child became simultaneously the bearer of racial meaning
(white racial superiority and a monopoly on the category of the human itself), and the shield against its open acknowledgment: a divine "angel" floating above the turmoil of public contestation.[105] This
iconized white child at once justified and concealed the violent racial
and economic hierarchies, the extraction and predation, that underpinned the material existence of white patriarchal settler households. Conversely, as Ebony Thomas writes, juxtaposing Bernstein's
formulation with Christina Sharpe's meditations on Blackness and
white construals of the human, the white universe declares "the
impossibility of Black childhood."[106]

Innocence as this dual formation, simultaneously an ontological
project—producing hierarchies of human kinds—and an ever-
flowing font for the absolution of racial capitalism's reproductive violence, shaped an emerging US public health establishment and pat-
terned its interventions into infant mortality. The innocence of

"babyhood" per se is also a special case, partially sharing in Bernstein's analysis of the racialization of childhood, yet with distinct features specific to the precarious first year of life. With high rates of infant mortality across all groups in the nineteenth century, even as affluent whites were relatively insulated, white infants' association with angels was particularly strong. Through the crystallization of the angelic white infant taken too soon, sensationalized depictions of poor white babies born to US citizen parents and "whitenable" European immigrants languishing in urban tenements became the object at once of collective mourning and the target of outcry and calls for reform. Initially excluding Black infants from the horizon of reform, by the Progressive Era white experts instrumentalized Black infant mortality rates as evidence of the natural supremacy of whites. Yet this instrumentalization worked in two contradictory directions. Insofar as these experts recognized Black infants' vulnerability at all, they did so in its intimate proximity to their figurations of deviant and blameworthy Black maternity. As described in detail in chapter 1, Hoffman's account posits them as pitiable victims of their mothers' recklessness, carelessness, and immorality. In relation to white infants, however, experts negated both Black infants' value and in some cases their vulnerability. Ironically, within his overarching account of Black evolutionary demise, Hoffman posited that Black children were less susceptible to diphtheria, the disease that killed Du Bois's nineteen-month-old son.[107]

Dorothy Roberts's account of the "crack baby" media frenzy in the 1980s illustrates the persistence of this dual dynamic. On the one hand these babies were to be pitied as victims of their "monstrous crack-smoking mothers," yet another iteration of the long-standing "iconography of depraved Black maternity," born sick and "hopeless." On the other hand, the media simultaneously characterized these babies themselves as dangerous to the body politic: not only—in terms that reveal an ableism inextricable from the racism at work—as dependent tax burdens, but as themselves monstrous and dangerous, unchildlike in their affective deficiencies: "expressionless zombies or uncontrollable demons."[108] Dána-Ain Davis traces a more generalized exclusion of Black infants from the fragility ascribed to white infants, or what she calls the "hardy Black baby thesis" back to the nineteenth-century.[109] As Davis shows, the hardy Black baby figure has persisted in twenty-first-century public health and NICU care protocols alike.[110] Within the biopolitics of racial innocence, Black infancy has marked a site of useful paradox, wherein both an allegedly inherent weakness and a preternatural hardiness can be variously harnessed in the service of denying, justifying, and naturalizing the very conditions that make Black infants disproportionately vulnerable to preventable death.

While my conception of the biopolitics of racial innocence is not primarily psychoanalytic, the dynamics of true babyhood are in some ways of a piece with Du Bois's notion of the "public and psychological wage" of whiteness, developed in 1935's *Black Reconstruction*.[111] Du Bois forwards this notion with regard to white men in the laboring class, as part of his explanation of how cross-class collusion on the part of white workers, who allied themselves with owning-class whites, foreclosed the prospects of an abolition democracy. He writes: "The white group of laborers, while they received a low wage, were compensated in part by a sort of public and psychological wage. They were given public deference and titles of courtesy because they were white. They were admitted freely . . . to public functions, public parks, and the best schools."[112] My account here signals the implication of this dynamic not only within the public realm but also within the unwaged domestic realm of white maternal labors—a kind of private feminine wage.

As Jennifer Morgan has shown, the very constitution of the private realm beginning in early modernity, the homeplace as a site where affective and familial relations were sheltered from both state interference and market exchange, demarcated a space of white reproductive futurity, predicated on the reproductive enslavement of Black women and their exclusion from such protections.[113] It was also constituted through the colonial state and its white settlers' theft of land and genocides of Indigenous peoples. Settler private life only became possible through the destruction and erasure, the literal building-over, of the lifeways cultivated since time immemorial between this continent's peoples and their lands. The colonial regime also legally imposed the political exclusion of white womanhood onto Indigenous women, but without any of its nominal consolations. Namely, these consolations included protection against state invasion of the bodily and home spaces and kinship ties—coded as private and inviolable for white mothers—and the internal and socially validated value vested in normative white maternity. As Heidi Kiiwetinepinesiik Stark writes, "the continued domestication of Indigenous women's political authority was carried out with focus given to the private sphere, constructing Indigenous women as deviant, immoral beings who needed to learn proper forms of domesticity."[114] In truth, the state would never hold the sanctity of Indigenous mothering or kinship as inviolable, even as it held out a distant prospect of contingent privacy conditional on conformity with heteropatriarchal norms.

By the nineteenth century, for typically-abled and married working-class white mothers, this dual benefit of a measure of actual private protection and their legally and socially validated value as bearers of the apex form of humanity might be thought of as a counterpart to the "public and psychological wage" of their men.[115] As Stephanie Jones-Rogers documents, white women slaveowners avidly participated in targeting the reproductive bodies and maternal capacities of Black women as well, through forced wet-nursing and other means.[116] Situating white settler reproductive futurity within this schema renders the political significance of white women's cross-class collusions for these private wages of feminine whiteness both before and after formal emancipation visible as well. It is significant that Du Bois names schools as key materializations of this public wage, for, while funded with public moneys, the care and education of children, as well as the fact of (underpaid) white women as its majority work-force, link it with the white feminine private in key ways that span for-mal emancipation and Reconstruction into the present moment. White women—especially but not only mothers—were the core organ-izers of massive resistance against school desegregation.[117]

The accrual of relatively better health for white working families and their babies, via the destruction and sacrifice of Black and Indig-enous life, while inferior to wealthier white counterparts, also consti-tutes a kind of *physiological* wage, linked to both less actual labors of nursing sick children and some measure of insulation against the in-calculable violence of preventable infant and child loss. As this phys-iological wage congealed into the comparative statistics that—as chapter 1 details—became key to white supremacist public health sci-ence, it helped to establish the white baby as the innocent standard of health, a legacy that lingers in the present day: the infantine ver-sion of what Stephanie Bray and Monica McLemore call "the myth of the default human that is killing Black mothers."[118]

This biopolitical configuration of true babyhood both ideologi-cally hides and materially relies upon concentric violences of the white supremacist settler state. Pressurized, isolating, and over-worked parenting even for typically-abled and economically privi-leged white cisgender mothers is underpinned by the disposability of disabled life, violation and negation of Black, Indigenous, and working-class immigrant-of-color mothering and kinship, imperiled life for transgender parents and transgender children, especially when compounded with racism, violent disregard for poor mothers and children across the board, and the vampiric extraction and caustic flow of capital as the lifeblood of this configuration's perpetuity. As Lisa Beard writes of Baldwin's concept, "white people's 'unutterably exhausting' innocence is widely dangerous—it is dangerous to their own souls, to Black people, to America as a country, and to the entire world."[119]

Innocence and Colonial Futurity

The biopolitics of racial innocence also draws on accounts of innocence that center white colonial and imperial fantasies of benign supremacy.[120] Anthropologist Miriam Ticktin calls attention to the ways that, on the global scale, racial and imperial logics likewise cathect certain child bodies as endangered and vulnerable, while others remain affectively and politically invisible both as children and as deaths.[121] Moreover, within prevailing humanitarian rationalities, these children's aura of innocence "appears outside history and as such, it allows those who work as saviors to ignore the political and historical circumstances that created those victims." Ticktin analogizes this dynamic to Gayatri Spivak's formulation of "white men saving brown women from brown men" such that the white men are absolved of all implication in the violence that they purport to oppose.[122] In the case of infant mortality interventions, this framing could be transposed to "experts saving Black babies from Black mothers (and other caregivers, kin, and communities)." This book's discernment of racial innocence within an ongoing history of biopolitical documentation, analysis, interventions, and policy approaches to Black infant mortality also takes inspiration from Gloria Wekker's analysis of white innocence, anti-Blackness, and colonial disavowal in the Netherlands: the "taken-for-granted, hidden discursive and organizational principles . . . the toxic substructures upholding the worlds of policy making and academic knowledge production."[123]

In critical Indigenous studies and settler colonial studies, innocence describes a history-erasing and violence-enabling form of colonial disavowal.[124] Kevin Bruyneel and Alissa Macoun each call attention to the centrality of innocence in white settler affects, memory, and political practices. For Bruyneel, innocence animates settlers' nostalgia for an illusory past emptied of colonial violence.[125] Macoun enumerates ways that left/progressive white settler researchers in particular disavow their complicity with ongoing colonial projects, which she terms "colonising white innocence."[126] This line of thinking resonates with my attempt, in chapter 5, to think through mainstream health organizations and institutions' recent avowals of structural racism. The concept of settler innocence is influentially formulated—as "settler moves to innocence"—by Eve Tuck and K. Wayne Yang as "those strategies or positionings that attempt to relieve the settler of feelings of guilt or responsibility without giving up land or power or privilege."[127] One such move to innocence is particularly relevant here: "At risk-ing / Asterisk-ing Indigenous peoples," figuring them as on the brink of extinction and/or as mere statistical outliers.[128]

This book homes in on the specific work of innocence in official approaches to Black infant mortality; the interconnections and disjunctures between the US biopolitics of baby-saving efforts and reproductive violence among Indigenous nations and Black communities, respectively, bear much further study. Yet a unifying thread in many late-nineteenth-century studies of both Black and Indigenous infant mortality was precisely a social evolutionary discourse of extinction—the high infant mortality among each group allegedly heralded the moribundity of their respective "race"—neatly eliding alike genocidal settler colonial violence, dispossession, and forced removals of Indigenous nations, and white supremacist terror, criminalization, and super-exploitation of Black communities. Hoffman, in *Race Traits*, also declared extinction nearly inevitable for Indigenous nations due to sexual immorality and race mixing—despite a regretful admiration for their chiefs' "iron will" and "brave and persistent struggle."[129] Moreover, this horizon of extinction gave way to Progressive Era public health interventions that blamed both Black and Indigenous mothers for improper care and feeding, "at-risking" both Black and Indigenous infants in ways that painted white settler society as blameless and beneficent.[130]

These interventions—like Thompson's 1920 report of the American Public Health Association—have construed existing kinship and care relations in these communities as themselves as harmful. Especially targeted were supposedly "uncivilized" maternal practices—including many now vindicated as far more salutary than the protocols being prescribed by US- and US-aligned experts—from on-demand breastfeeding by Native mothers to affectionate Filipina mothering.[131] This has allowed a studied unseeing of the overwhelming violence of the US settler colonial racial state and its political economic imperatives—what Manu Karuka, Juliana Hu Pegues, and Alyosha Goldstein call "colonial unknowing."[132] It has also, in a brutal paradox, figured the often-violent *disruption* of care as "care" itself.[133] As Roberts documents in her work on so-called child welfare, this figuration—counterposed to a self-ascribed "white benevolence"—still underpins the state's protocols of routine child removal among Black and Indigenous families.[134] While enforcing white supremacist norms, in the current day these experts may or may not identify as white. Tanya Katerí Hernández has recently made clear that anti-Black racial innocence is broadly enacted within the broader structure of US white supremacy, including in Latinx communities.[135] Yet as with regard to disparities talk, the dominant paradigm nevertheless retains the innocent white "true baby," ensconced within a propertied and typically-abled nuclear family, as its normative core.

In view of these multifarious ways that innocence serves to warp and obstruct human interconnections, as living beings who share a single planet, is there any room for innocence at all? I argue in chapter 2 that Du Bois discerns a positive form of innocence in his son Burghardt—one that, rather than foreclosing that interconnectedness, in fact entails its full inhabitation. This innocence is literally opposed to the pernicious forms of white innocence that deny and attempt to sever our relatedness, attacking collective life at the root. According to the *Online Etymology Dictionary*, "innocence"—meaning "doing no evil; free from sin or guilt" and "childlike simplicity"—emerged in the mid-fourteenth century; these meanings in turn derive from the Latin negation of *nocere*, "to harm." The root of *nocere* is the Indo-European *nek-*, "death." Before its inflection with Christian judgment and duality of good and evil, *innocent* expresses a principle of nonharm; further back, it is linked with life itself, and it is this sense that might be said to best correspond with the expansive force that Du Bois attributes to his son, both in life and after his passing. As to whether this is a formulation worth taking up despite the perils of the term, I leave readers to decide.

Reading these formulations of racial innocence together brings into focus key modes of practiced blamelessness in the face of racial capitalism's fatal impacts on Black infancy. The biopolitics of racial innocence effaces the polity's structural predation on Black maternal and infant life, erases historical and ongoing institutionalized reproductive violence, and exiles Black infants themselves from the realm of babies as unique, precious, and deserving of protection and care. In their different ways, through rhetoric and via praxis, Du Bois and Terrell, Jim Crow–era Black midwives and contemporary birth justice advocates, have contested these deadly dynamics.

Overview of Chapters

Fatal Denial posits that the biopolitics of racial innocence perpetuates and obscures the causal conditions of Black infant death, and it tracks crucial expressions of Black political thought and praxis against that innocence and toward transformed conditions of life and horizons of care. In chapter 1, I sketch the nineteenth-century emergence of an important figure animating the emerging white public awareness of infant death as a political problem. Extending Hazel Carby's revision of white feminist critiques of the antebellum "cult of true womanhood," I draw on historical accounts of nineteenth-century cultures of mourning and funereal practices in both white bourgeois households and on Southern plantations to argue that the new category of "true babyhood" in antebellum decades was figured as white—utterly unique, fragile, and precious. Because "true babyhood" was crucial in galvanizing public concern for infant mortality after the Civil War, the first decades of governmental interventions to improve infant survival largely excluded Black babies. This exclusionary ontology of "true babyhood" shaped the evolutionary logics and statistical interpretations that characterized Progressive Era reproductive necropolitics of Black infant mortality. The exemplary text here is Hoffman's influential 1896 treatise, *Race Traits and Tendencies of the American Negro*, an elaborate attack on Black maternity and infancy in particular. Khalil Gibran Muhammad demonstrates the text's importance in cementing a new white consensus about Black criminality. I show the additional centrality of its representations of Black mothers as culpable for high infant mortality rates, in both their embodied "traits" and deviant "tendencies."

Chapter 2 closely engages with "Of the Passing of the First-Born," Du Bois's elegy for his beloved son in *The Souls of Black Folk*, written under the shadow of both Hoffman's statistical assaults and the terrors of lynch law. In addition to a portrait of parental adoration and agonized bereavement, the elegy is a striking account of innocence. More precisely, Du Bois stages an interplay between three forms of innocence: Burghardt's infantine innocence as an expansive orientation to joy, interconnection, and belonging, doomed by the forced imposition of the color line; the racial innocence of the whites who appear briefly but consequentially on Burghardt's funeral day; and Nina Gomer Du Bois's feminine and maternal innocence, which shades into troubling tropes of respectability. At the same time, the elegy contains elements that militate against this masculinist Victorian propriety. In the interplay between Du Bois's own "crushed" boyhood innocence and the preservation of Burghardt's innocence through his early death, Du Bois articulates an anguished ambivalence that situates him in a tradition in Black political thinking and rhetoric, largely authored and focalized through Black mothers, of political ambivalence regarding the death of children.

Chapter 3 turns to leading Black organizer and clubwoman Mary Church Terrell's narration of maternal bereavement and infant loss in her 1940 autobiography, *A Colored Woman in a White World*, as well as in key speeches from the racial nadir of the 1890s and early 1900s. Contemporary and sometime collaborator with Du Bois, Terrell suffered three infant deaths in the first five years of marriage. Terrell's first decade of political struggles on behalf of Black Americans during these years were thus marked by profound grief and loss. Her text highlights the affective impacts of the Jim Crow environment, tracking the material effects of those feelings themselves. Terrell's narrations of infant death and maternal bereavement are part of a broader rejoinder to and a reworking of conceptions of heredity and environment that prevailed from the 1890s until at least the 1920s. Within prevailing white supremacist understandings of human development and racial hierarchy at the turn of the century, higher levels of what was termed "impressibility" corresponded with higher civilizational status, with normative white women cast as the most delicately sensitive, as the most evolved forms of feminine being.[136] Terrell not only invokes this notion of impressibility—sometimes reinscribing its hierarchical terms—but also reconfigures it in key ways. In linking the somatic and intergenerational with the infrastructural, her account demonstrates the resonances between long-standing theories of maternal impressibility and today's emerging understandings—both better and worse—of racism and epigenetics.

Chapter 4 turns to Black midwifery in the Jim Crow South. Under the 1921 Sheppard-Towner Act's maternal and infant health programs, Southern public health officials concentrated funds on controlling Black community midwives as scapegoats for high infant mortality rates. The standardized medical bags that Southern Black midwives were required to carry are highly visible in the archive: in public health manuals and reports, photographs from midwife trainings, in midwives' own oral histories, and even in a widely circulated training film from the 1950s. The chapter centers this fetishized object in the Southern conscription of Black midwives into a racist surveillance regime that trafficked under the name of "care." Midwives were disciplined through frequent bag inspections; moreover, the bag was a fetish object for white public health officials, standing in for more substantial health interventions. While midwives used bags as tactics of contestation and care—for example, smuggling forbidden remedies and tools to births—the bag's trajectories as both surveillance technology and fetish allowed enforced poverty and racial terror to disappear from the etiology of Black infant mortality, positioning Black women themselves as the inhuman agents of Black infants' demise. At the same time, I draw on Simone Browne's notion of *sousveillance* to describe the midwives' deployment of the bags as life-support objects.[137] I then draw connections between this paradigm and current conditions, in terms of both the persistent pathologization and blaming of Black motherhood and the radical care of present day Black midwives and birth workers working at the grassroots to nurture and sustain Black infant and maternal life.

Finally, chapter 5 turns to the present moment. I examine the ways that the biopolitics of racial innocence may persist in explicitly antiracist official rhetoric and interventions currently emerging that seem to reverse these patterns. Increasingly since the early twenty-first century, and with almost explosive acceleration since the presidential election of 2016 and the summer 2020 uprisings against police murders of Black people, there has been a dramatic shift among medical and public health experts toward *avowing and indicting* structural and institutional racism as the root cause of persistently high rates of Black infant and maternal mortality. This acknowledgment is not by any means new. As sociologist Alondra Nelson notes, there is a long "tradition of black health advocacy in which pragmatic matters of disease and healing . . . were coextensive with broader political matters (e.g., challenges to racism)."[138] This longstanding analysis, however, is now everywhere in health policy, scholarship, and advocacy. Unlike even a decade ago, structural and systemic racism as primary causes of health inequities are now front and center in the leading medical and public health organizations and publications.[139] Particularly in the wake of the summer of 2020 and in the intensified attention to the atrocious racial geographies of COVID-19 vulnerability and treatment, institutional avowals, mea culpas, and commitments to racial justice abound, released by nearly every medical or health organization.

What does this turn mean? What will it mean for practices on the ground? Chapter 5 analyzes the way that, even as recently as the 2007 Office of Minority Health campaign, "A Healthy Baby Begins with You," federal health authorities primarily blamed Black mothers themselves for their infants' deaths. In contrast, the 2022 White House Blueprint for Addressing the Maternal Health Crisis exemplifies the growing consensus that, as Dr. Joia Crear-Petty and her coauthors sum it up, "racism, not race, [is] a root cause or driver of health inequities."[140] The leadership of Black doulas, midwives, obstetricians, nurses, and other health care workers across the United States who have long been spearheading crucial and transformative work has come into prominent public view. The birth justice movement is gaining ground, and its influence is even felt in the White House's

Blueprint. Yet institutional change is slow—and given their long history and continued political economic utility, it is worth considering how the long-standing habits of racial innocence, including Black mother-blame and individual responsibility, as well as other long-standing fatal deflections, might persist in new forms.

1 *The Cult of True Babyhood*

Innocence and Infant Mortality

In 1909 the newly formed Association for the Study and Prevention of Infant Mortality (AASPIM) held its first meeting. A culmination of decades of efforts to combat scandalously high levels of infant mortality, particularly in Northern cities, the association gathered leading white physicians, nurses, social workers, health statisticians, and sanitary reformers. Over the next several years, this group would spearhead a bold agenda to improve infant survival, sharing data at annual conferences and coordinating local efforts in the urban North. Yet even as Black infant death rates were generally included in the mortality data gathered by members, they spurred little comment or action. Particularly telling was a paper at the inaugural conference titled "The Influence of Race on Infant Mortality," focused on the situation in Boston. While the city's Black population figures and disproportionately high Black infant mortality rate are included in the data tables, they are glaringly absent from the document's analysis and commentary. The paper itself compares only native-born whites with "alien races," especially Irish, Italian, and Jewish immigrants.[1] This is certainly not because data were lacking. Black infant mortality had garnered intense attention by this time. As this chapter highlights, these statistics were central to scientific justifications for Jim Crow like those of Frederick Hoffman, as well as to the political work of Black social science in the service of uplift, like that of W.E.B. Du Bois.

AASPIM's preoccupations with race as a factor in infant mortality was explicitly rooted in eugenics.[2] From its founding, the organization included a eugenics section and counted among its members and contributors some of the most influential eugenicists of the day, including Charles Davenport, founder of the Eugenics Record Office, and Harry Laughlin, leading proponent of eugenic sterilization. These prominent men of science, however, were simply the most public names within an organization robustly committed to controlling heredity and improving racial quality. Spurred by the specter of "race suicide," eugenicists worried that allegedly genetically inferior groups—including immigrant groups enumerated in the Boston report, as well as those deemed "feebleminded," mentally and morally deficient, and dependent—would outpace the Anglo-Saxon bloodlines of what they termed, in a signature settler colonial erasure of Indigenous presence, the "native" citizenry of the United States. As a resolution of the eugenics section at the 1911 meeting stated, given that the "ultimate ideal" of infant conservation work was "to aid in the effort to produce the highest type of physical, social and intellectual man," the members "earnestly advocate[d], by means of individual efforts for creating public sentiment, by public instruction . . . moral suasion . . . by effective segregation and . . . by legislation authorizing even surgical procedure, the prohibition of procreation to the racially unfit." Conversely, they prescribed a positive eugenic program for the "encouragement . . . to greater productivity among the best elements of our stock."[3] As Richard Meckel notes, there were tensions and debates among eugenicists about the proportion between the influences of heredity and environment, the kind and degree of intervention required.[4] Yet the AASPIM's proceedings also reveal an implicit consensus that Black infant mortality was outside the purview of negative and positive interventions alike.[5]

As Rana Hogarth makes clear, it is important to situate Progressive Era eugenic interventions within a longer history of anti-Black scientific racism, including antebellum justifications for slavery.[6] I propose that the wholesale exclusion of Black infants from this thrust of preventative concern rested on an older ideological figure of "true babyhood." This figure marked a polarity between white public sentiments and conceptions of white infants and Black infants—even as there was complexity within and around the category of whiteness that became encoded within evolutionary mythologies of Anglo-Saxon purity and deficiencies of "inferior" European immigrant groups. Extending Hazel Carby's critical engagement with the "cult of true womanhood," I posit that a parallel "cult of true babyhood" emerged during the decades of the nineteenth century before the Civil War.[7] This defined white infants as adored and uniquely precious but highly vulnerable future citizens, whose lives required special protections and whose deaths occasioned profound grief. "True babyhood" was a key figuration as the biopolitics of racial innocence took shape in the late nineteenth century, entailing a new and thoroughly racialized public understanding of infant life and death. It profoundly shaped the way that infant mortality as a political problem came into white public view, first through white baby-saving campaigns and subsequently through Progressive Era statistical and social scientific accounts. Within this latter approach, true babyhood took on key evolutionary meanings as well as shoring up a new sense of white innocence, making possible the fatal deflections of statistical comparison that shadow the biopolitics of Black infant mortality to this day.

This exclusion was precipitated by a new understanding of and emotional investment in white infancy, and corresponding disinvestment in Black infancy, which emerged with enduring force among the white public during the decades preceding the Civil War. In her classic analysis of enslavement and gender in the nineteenth century in *Reconstructing Womanhood: The Emergence of the Afro-American Novelist*, Hazel Carby demonstrates the power of the antebellum "Cult of True Womanhood" as racial and sexual ideology. White feminist historians had characterized it as a project of patriarchal control, primarily relevant to white women's experiences; in fact, Carby argues, the signature virtues of "true" women took form and meaning only in opposition to characteristics ascribed to enslaved Black women: "a nexus of figurations which can be explained only in relation to each other."[8] Moreover, while foregoing accounts had by and large taken true womanhood to task as a false representation of white women's actual lives, Carby homes in on its ideological functions, in the work it did to resolve the contradictions inherent in the chattel slavery system.[9] She then shows how Black women writers themselves confronted the binds of true womanhood.

I draw on and extend elements of Carby's analysis to argue that a companion ideology of "true babyhood" emerged alongside, and in inextricable relation to, true womanhood: an adored and uniquely precious but highly vulnerable individual, whose life required special protections and whose deaths occasioned profound grief. I flesh out the analogies and interplay between these two interlinked figurations of endangered innocence, their Black counterpoints, and their respective political functions.

Carby's "Slave and Mistress": True Babyhood as Ideology

In "Slave and Mistress: Ideologies of Womanhood Under Slavery," the second chapter of *Reconstructing Womanhood*, Carby sets out to examine the "mythical aspect of the requisites of womanhood . . . in the context of the cultural and political power of sexual ideologies under slavery."[10] For "in order to perceive the cultural effectivity of ideologies of black female sexuality, it is necessary to consider the determining force of ideologies of white female sexuality."[11] Two opposed but co-constitutive codes of sexuality, motherhood, and womanhood emerge and congeal in the "figures of the slave and the mistress."[12] These are key factors within which Black women's own narrations must be understood, as the matrix within which Black women writers "addressed, used, transformed, and, on occasion, subverted the dominant ideological codes." From the start, Carby clearly states that her emphasis will be on the ideological function of stereotypes. Unlike accounts (of which many examples follow) that seek to measure the "accuracy" of literary stereotypes as reflections of reality, Carby argues that her analysis presumes that "stereotypes . . . function as a disguise or mystification of objective social relations" arising from "particular viewpoints under specific historical conditions."[13] She stresses the importance of identifying the distinct sets of constraints in operation for a man writing a slave narrative, a woman writing a slave narrative, and a white Southern woman writing a diary. In particular, Black women "embody the tension between the author's desire to privilege her experience and being able to speak only within a discourse of conventionally held beliefs about the nature of black womanhood."[14]

Carby opens her discussion by recapping what had by then become a classic figure of white feminist historiographical critique, namely the "cult of true womanhood." Carby cites white feminist historian Barbara Welter's 1969 essay on true womanhood, which enumerates its "four cardinal virtues" as "piety, purity, submissiveness, and domesticity," reinforced through the dominant literary works of the day.[15] Carby's complex notion of ideology comes clear in her parsing of two aspects of the cult of true womanhood. The first is its dominance and pervasiveness as a governing convention. The second, however, describes an ontological valence: it "describe[ed] the parameters within which women were measured and declared to be, or not to be, women."[16] Carby thus interweaves a cultural studies approach to ideology as the everyday common sense, structures of meaning and feeling within material systems of domination with a Black feminist theorization of the "Western" or white supremacist category of woman qua human that was emerging in the 1980s and early 1990s.

In her 1982 essay "Interstices," Hortense Spillers writes that "slavery did not transform the black female into an embodiment of carnality, as the myth of the black woman would tend to convince us, nor, alone the primary receptacle of a highly profitable generative act. She became instead the principle point of passage between the human and the non-human world."[17] Later in the essay, Carby likewise makes this connection explicit in her reading of Mary Prince's narrative.[18] Carby argues, however, that these "virtues" were constituted through their opposition to characteristics ascribed to enslaved Black women: "In order to perceive the cultural effectivity of ideologies of black female sexuality, it is necessary to consider the determining force of ideologies of white female sexuality: stereotypes only appear to exist in isolation while actually depending on a nexus of figurations which can be explained only in relation to each other."[19]

Through the schematic account that follows, I argue that it is likewise necessary to consider the ideological function of white *infancy*, in order to understand the ideology underpinning the seemingly paradoxical exclusion of Black infants by 1909 from the mainstream of white public concern. The ideology of true babyhood christened the white typically-abled baby as the tender bearer of the great national and racial destiny. It also ratified the heteronuclear white settler family as the only milieu where this destiny could be cultivated. The cult of true babyhood thus figured this family structure as utterly benign, the very home of innocence, at once obscuring the violent conditions that produce and sustain it and casting other kinship formations as corrupt.

This is, of course, not only about figuration. Carby's account is concerned with the function of this ideology in structuring the material relations of labor and kinship, captivity and domination under the enslavement regime—the literal spaces and flesh and blood bodies enmeshed in these relations. Black women's coerced and devalued labors made the cult of true babyhood possible both symbolically and materially. Tending to the actual white human infants in whom so much social and political value was vested entailed the violent extraction of their time and capacity to care for their own children and communities, and even their own capacities for pregnancy and day-to-day reproduction of their own selves in a state of health. Harriet Jacobs's account of her Aunt Nancy's multiple miscarriages, stillbirths, and infant losses under the tyrannical demands of tending her mistress's children names its violence clearly: upon her aunt's death, Jacobs writes that "she had been slowly murdered."[20] Jacobs's nineteenth-century narration reflects a pattern entrenched over centuries.

As Jennifer Morgan makes clear, the so-called private realm for white women's economically devalued—but increasingly ideologically vital—labors of white mothering began to crystallize, in early transatlantic modernity, as simultaneously a place of forced labor and terrorization for enslaved African women, predicated on the disruption and negation of their own kinship ties. As Morgan writes: "Enslaved women had no relationship to the private and the domestic, to the realm outside the market; such a relationship was fundamentally impossible . . . the family lives of enslaved people always served to demarcate the boundaries of the emergent terrain of bourgeois affective private relations through their exclusion from this terrain."[21] By the mid-nineteenth century the sacred inviolability of the bond between the middle-class, typically-abled, married white mother and her baby was subtended by the legal and social violability and negation of Black maternity; the literal, embodied lives of these white mothers and their babies simultaneously relied upon and disavowed the theft of Black women's labors and life force. Dorothy

Roberts's distinction between "spiritual and menial housework" also captures this distinction, as well as the ways that it persists into the present. "The racial division that tracked the dichotomy between spiritual and menial housework," Roberts writes, "resolved the ideological contradiction between the purified ideal of virtuous womanhood and the reality of dirty household tasks."[22]

As both Morgan and Roberts make clear, this also meant that reproductive embodiment and labor were deeply politicized terrains for Black women both under slavery and in its aftermath. Black women's bids for the protection and sanctity of their own children, kinship on their own terms, and bodily autonomy—through both overt and more quotidian and subtle forms of refusal—militated against this routinized reproductive violence. However, as Morgan notes, the historical record largely obscures the details of Black women's modes of insurgency.[23] Angela Davis's foundational "The Black Woman's Role in the Community of Slaves" posits that the structural position of enslaved Black women as both the forced reproducers of enslaved human commodities and keepers of community life meant that their work to sustain the latter was inherently militant, a strike for life and the possibility of freedom against death in captivity.

As Alys Weinbaum argues, this theorization grounded a line of Black feminist analysis and praxis—including Roberts's work—that centers bodily autonomy and kinship on Black women's own terms as core tenets of liberation. Roberts cites Davis's text as she elaborates a lineage of refusal of the racist dichotomy of spiritual white "homemaking" versus menial "housework" on the part of "menial" workers from enslavement to the present day: not only did "slave women's devotion to their own households def[y] the expectation of total service to whites," but more recent domestic workers "transformed the personal meaning of their work" as a bid for their own daughters' education and freedom from this form of externally degraded work, and ultimately "shattered the divide between spiritual and menial housework."[24] Chapters 2 and 3 highlight the respective political responses of elite Black leaders W.E.B. Du Bois and Mary Church Terrell, as they each grieved their own infants in the shadow of white supremacist attacks on Black maternity, family, and feeling. In chapters 4 and 5, I examine important insurgent continuities within the realms of Black midwifery and birthwork. In what follows, I limn a key structure of reproductive extraction, violence, and racialized hierarchy of infant life and loss that set the stage for this insurgency.

White Infant Death and the Cult of Domesticity

Infant death was a central part of all family and community life throughout the nineteenth century, just as it had been throughout the previous centuries. But Nancy Schrom Dye and Daniel Blake Smith demonstrate in their analysis of white women's diaries and letters in the US North that even as mortality remained nearly constant, the conventional understanding of infant life and death shifted significantly over the nineteenth century, corresponding to the profound economic and ideological transformations of the white middle- and upper-class household. They write that "despite the continuous reality of infant death, mothers' responses to sickness and death in their families changed significantly over time as cultural explanations for infant death and definitions of maternal roles changed."[25]

For white families of at least moderate means, the decades of transition between the pastoral power of the eighteenth century and the biopolitical regime of the later nineteenth century saw "extensive mothering" give way to the more constricted nuclear family form, reflecting significant changes in the political and libidinal economy of the household. As paid work moved outside the home, white antebellum women were incited to live up to the ideal of true womanhood—guardians of the newly hived-off domestic sphere, embodiments and protectors of private morality against the encroachments of a profane public world.[26] But also in this milieu, the true baby emerged: the adored, precious, and vulnerable white future citizen. Like true womanhood, true babyhood reflected the new notion of the household as a private space of sentiment and noninstrumental relationships, walled off from the competitive amorality of commerce and public life. Viviana Zelizer writes that as "the increasing differentiation between economic production and the home transformed the basis of family cohesion . . . the sentimentalization of childhood was intimately tied to . . . the increasing domestication of middle-class women in the nineteenth century."[27] Carl Degler writes of these transformations within the family: "Exalting the child went hand in hand with exalting the domestic role of woman; each reinforced the other while they raised domesticity within the family to a new and higher level of respectability."[28]

By the mid-nineteenth century white women's diaries and letters reflect this decisive shift in the conceptualization of even newborn infants, figuring them as *adored* members of the family unit, objects of the most profound emotional investment. This adoration, a vastly intensified relation between white parents and infants, was a key element of the new figuration of true babyhood. The nineteenth-century journals showcase a dramatically heightened focus on the personalities, appearance, and daily activities of their babies from birth on.[29] The circulation of birth announcements, including the sex, birth date, and name of the baby, signifying the recognition of newborns' definite place within family relations and broader social networks, also came into vogue during this period.[30] Whereas eighteenth-century parents often expressed their provisional detachment from infants in denominations like "little stranger," these later writings reflect a culture of intense attachment.[31] This included nicknames ("birdies," "chicks," "pets"), celebration of baby talk and adoption of infantine pronunciations, and maternal thrills at developmental milestones.[32] In short, conventions not unlike those that define the prevailing sense of parenting today. Mother Fanny Longfellow, wife of Henry Wadsworth Longfellow and daughter of a prominent Boston family, notes in February 1848 that "Little Fan has a tooth and climbs by chairs upon her feet"; in March, "Baby looked at me and smiling said 'Mama' then put her finger in my mouth."[33] Calista Hall's "Little Frances grows more interesting every day. She will try to say everything you tell her too [sic]. Ask her whose baby she is and she will say Pa and Ma."[34]

This new adoration of infant life, however, brought with it unprecedented dread at the prospect of infant death. Mid-nineteenth-century mothers evinced deep attachments to much younger infants. From her postpartum bedchamber, Longfellow wrote of the newborn Fanny that that "she is as charming as these fresh spring days," with "a sweet little face just beginning to show there is a soul behind it."[35] Elizabeth Child posited a reciprocal attachment from the very first time that she and her newborn gazed at one another: "while I looked you opened your eyes . . . and as they met mine I thought they mutely recognized the new tie."[36] This immediate attachment was matched by profound apprehension about the loss of new babies, even "frightened," as Dye and Smith write, "of the intensity of their feelings for infants whose lives seemed so fragile."[37] Caroline White wrote of her fears about the fragility of her own newborn son in 1856: "He is so tender—and I do not feel ready to part with him—short time as our relation to each other has existed."[38]

While diaries reflect private joys, fears, and tragedies, the attention and attachment to infant life and the "magnification of mourning" that attended infant death were what Ann Cvetkovich and others have called "public feelings."[39] This referred to shared or common emotional states that arise among particular subjects within and in relation to political economic, political, cultural, and social conditions.[40] The explosion in what Ann Douglas calls "consolation literature" during the mid-nineteenth century testifies to the affective investment in true babyhood as a large-scale phenomenon. Consolation literature includes "actual mourners' manuals ... prayer manuals, poetry, hymns, fiction and biographies whose purpose is clearly consolatory."[41] Douglas's opening example is a widely circulated 1836 poem by Lydia Sigourney, "Twas But a Babe," which dramatizes the scene of the devoted mother at her infant's death.[42] Douglas also highlights the new funerary conventions for infants and children in particular that came into vogue during these years, highlighted in the consolation literature. These included elaborate new metal caskets, cushioned satin linings, and gentler lock-and-key closures rather than hard wooden coffins with their "remorseless screws and screwdrivers."[43] The new rural cemeteries, beginning with Mount Auburn in Cambridge (where, as it happens, Longfellow's infant was buried), were also "rapturously described" in the consolation literature. Unsullied, like an extension of the idealized domestic realm, by the calculating hustle and bustle of urban life, they emblematized "the idea that the living, and the dead, still 'cared'" for the precious individual soul after it had departed for God's own green pastures.[44]

Preciousness

The cult of domesticity "went hand in hand with the new conception of children as precious."[45] Crucially, as Zelizer demonstrates, this is a conception of value that is beyond price: what she calls the "economically worthless [but] emotionally 'priceless' child."[46] Previously seen as future contributors to the household economy or as future supports for elderly parents, infants and children were gradually expelled "from the cash nexus" in the latter half of the nineteenth century and first decades of the twentieth. "In an increasingly commercialized world," Zelizer writes, "children were reserved a separate noncommercial place. The economic and sentimental value of children were thereby declared to be radically incompatible."[47] From birth on, children came to be seen as emotionally and morally valuable in themselves, irreplaceable individuals whose proper nurture "precluded instrumental or fiscal considerations"—a process that Zelizer terms "the sacralization of childhood."[48] Although her study focuses on the years 1870–1930, she acknowledges that among the same cultural vanguard for whom the cult of domesticity could be materially realized, this process was realized earlier: "By the mid-19th century, the construction of the economically worthless child had been largely accomplished among the urban middle class."[49] The hard division that developed between the realm of exchange and the newly sacralized realm of infancy and childhood decisively expelled enslaved infants from this aspect of true babyhood. True babyhood was beyond price; in white public feelings, enslaved infants were fungible.

One hallmark of this pricelessness was a new stress on the unique individuality of each infant. This sentimental valorization was signaled, among other things, by the disappearance of the custom, still prevalent in the eighteenth century, of naming infants for siblings who had previously died; no longer was it the case that "another child replaced the lost one."[50] Seen a century before as only provisionally present in the world, at least until they had survived the perilous first few years, now at birth they were already "full-fledged, albeit physically fragile, individuals."[51] Among other things, the convention of the birth announcement, the presentation of a particular new life inscribed with the date of birth as well as name and patronymic, not only affirmed the genealogical belonging of white infants of a certain class but marked the entry of the infant into a publicly recognized realm of biographical personhood. The priceless individuality of true babyhood, entailed the immediate ascription to newborns of an eventful chronology, signaling their membership in the human and social world.

Nineteenth-century journals strikingly illustrate this new biographical personhood of infants and very young children. Elizabeth Sedgwick, writing in the 1820s, kept, as she wrote, "a journal of my child's life extending even to the minutest action and the slightest unfolding of her character."[52] She makes clear the link between her daughter's status as a biographical subject and her pricelessness, the latter entailing the former: "The smallest events of her life have had their peculiar interest for us, who have been watching her as parents always watch their heart's treasure."[53] In Fanny Longfellow's journal, from the 1850s, the denomination of "biography" is literal. After a hiatus from previously extensive personal journaling as a single and then childless woman, she titles her new diary, upon return to writing after the birth of her youngest, "Chronicle of the Children of Craigie Castle"; the volume is entirely "given over to the unfolding of her children's personalities and to notes on their activities and behavior."[54]

The biographical personhood of infants is also signaled by a strong sense of their earthly futurity, piously absent in earlier accounts: an anticipation of adult characteristics and even their potential contributions to society. Reflecting the prevailing structures of citizenship and the sexual dimorphism that Kyla Schuller calls attention to as the supposed hallmark of civilization, these projections are distinctly sexed. Longfellow describes her infant daughter mostly in terms of her physical characteristics: "Little Fan . . . is only a round merry plaything with dark blue eyes, a cunning little mouth and a very intelligent eager air."[55] Similarly, Calista Hall evokes the white feminine attribute of charm.[56] She describes her own baby Frances as "a little rogue."[57] In contrast, Longfellow discerns in her young sons' behaviors distinct ideals of manhood: the elder is a "man of action" who promises to have a rich and noble nature," while the sensitive and affectionate younger toddler inclines toward the contemplative; a friend calls him "the little philosopher," and his mother judges that he "promises to be the poet."[58] Welter writes that "America depended on her mothers to raise Christian statesmen."[59] The projections recorded in these diaries not only illustrate the new white maternal role as nurturer of future citizens, but the imagined future value of white infants' individual citizenly attributes.[60]

The newly biographical infant adds an additional explanatory dimension to the "magnification of mourning" sketched above. As Zelizer notes, French historian of childhood and society Philippe Ariès "refers to a nineteenth-century 'revolution in feeling' by which 'the death of the other,' particularly the death of a close family member, was defined as an overwhelming tragedy: 'The death which is feared is no longer so much the death of the self as the death of another.' The death of a young child was the worst loss of all."[61] As entirely unique individuals, infants were now fully-fledged "others" whose loss left an irreparable rent in the fabric of the world. Longfellow's lament "every room, every object recalls her, and the house is desolation" foreshadows the deep depression to which the grieving mother would succumb for the entire year following her infant daughter's death.[62] "Almost all of Longfellow's diary notations for the next year dwelt on little Fanny's death and the fear that her remaining children would die. She could not look at them, she wrote, without imagining them in their own small graves. . . . Her daughter's death remained the central event in . . . Longfellow's life."[63] What else but endless mourning could commemorate the death of a priceless and irreplaceable infant? While not all parents suffered such permanent devastation, Longfellow's response emblematizes the experience of infant death that shadowed true babyhood: no longer a merciful escape from inevitable mortal suffering but rather the traumatic loss of a unique human futurity.

Vulnerability Requiring Action

If true babyhood was adored and precious, it was also a figure of vulnerability, not only deserving of love from its caregivers but in need of special protections. Considered in itself, nineteenth-century infant vulnerability to sickness and death was in itself more a matter of continuity than of change. David Stannard observes that typical Puritan parents in the seventeenth and eighteenth centuries could expect one-quarter to one-third of their offspring to die in early childhood.[64] Even as nineteenth-century parents underwent Ariès's "revolution in feeling," their infants continued to die at rates comparable to those of their more taciturn forebears.[65] Yet we have seen that an intensified fear of infant death—as well as magnified grief if the worst should happen—accompanied parents' intensified affective investment in infancy.[66] Accompanying this intensified fear was a more sweeping transformation of the very notion of infantile vulnerability: a new conviction that infant death could potentially be prevented, given the proper precautions. The figure of true babyhood entailed a new understanding of infant death, not as natural or divinely ordained but shaped in large part by human—and especially maternal—agency. Enslaved Black infants, in contrast, remained sutured to the logic of the commodity, by which, as suggested above, a considerable quantum of death was simply one unavoidable pecuniary factor among others.

We have linked the adoration and pricelessness of true babyhood to the political and libidinal economic changes in the middle-class white household; this new attribute of *vulnerability requiring action* was a product of two interlocking factors, both related to the cultural shifts already described. The first was the rise of medical science, entailing a secularization of attitudes toward corporeal health. The relationship of this development to gendered changes in the household economy is complex. On the one hand, new forms of medical-scientific expertise, available only to men, entailed the discrediting, or at least subordination, of women's vernacular health-care knowledge and practices, and the related casting of women as suited only to auxiliary and basic quotidian aspects of health care. There is in this sense a division that arises between "public"/masculine medical authority and "private"/feminine subservience.[67] Tracking similar developments in France during this period, Jacques Donzelot writes of the emerging "privileged alliance between doctor and mother," citing physician and hygienist Fonssagrives's "ambition to make women into accomplished nurses . . . the doctor prescribes, the mother executes."[68]

On the other hand, as Judith Leavitt stresses, childbirth and infancy were objectively dangerous times of life, and women with the means to do so actively sought new medical techniques that promised to reduce danger and suffering for themselves and their loved ones (even as the positive consequences of these techniques remain questionable from some contemporary perspectives).[69] The second development, more obviously connected to the cult of domesticity, was a new sense of maternal responsibility for child well-being broadly construed, including not only their offspring's moral but also their corporeal health, which would help to ensure the future of the nation. This responsibility was signaled by, among other things, the new proliferation of child-raising manuals, demanding the addition of certain forms of "domesticated" scientific knowledge to the repertoire of virtuous motherhood. The paramount importance of breastfeeding was particularly emphasized. As an 1844 infant care manual admonished, "The first and most important truth . . . to be impressed upon mothers, is, that the constitution of their offspring depends on natural consequences, many of which are under their own control."[70] Both of these developments, as Dye and Smith observe, entail a "growing belief that human agency could shape and control the natural order."[71]

In 1848, Fanny Longfellow, whose record of profound grief is introduced earlier in this chapter, had called in a doctor to try to save her dying infant; this doctor had attempted a variety of "heroic medical measures, including large doses of mercury."[72] Longfellow herself spent several sleepless nights at the baby's bedside. Afterward, significantly, she wrote that she was "haunted by thoughts of what might have been avoided, the most pitiless of all."[73] Not God but the right combination of maternal and medical interventions might have served to save her infant daughter. As one of the many home medical guides designed for nineteenth-century mothers put it: "No one can for a moment believe that the excessive and increasing infant mortality among us, is part of the established order of nature, or of the systematic arrangements of Divine Providence."[74] The figure of true babyhood entailed a new conception of infant death as a largely *unnecessary* evil, an avoidable injury, a sign of vulnerability improperly attended to.

Infant Death and Enslavement

An abundant archive of nineteenth-century parental writings thus testifies to the fact that white infants—true babies—were precious and, if they died, irreplaceable; the preponderance of records of Black infant deaths reveal little of the suffering that attended them. In *Laboring Women*, Jennifer Morgan cautions that we cannot know the meanings of motherhood or infant loss for early modern enslaved African women.[75] Sasha Turner elaborates: "Absent from the archives are enslaved women's feelings about childbearing, and how the specter of death that hovered over the womb shaped maternal desires and practices," as many enslaved women could expect to lose half of their newborns.[76] Turner delves into Caribbean plantation records and slaveowners' letters, and observations of funerary practices for the traces of maternal experience potentially legible against the grain, "engag[ing] with archival fragments using a rhetorical strategy to tell a story of mothers' fear, grief, and apprehension while calling attention to the challenges of such narration."[77] Given the pervasiveness of infant death for all demographic groups in the seventeenth and eighteenth centuries, records suggest that elite white parents practiced a self-protective detachment from their newborns. Turner calls attention to the vastly more complex and brutal reality confronting enslaved mothers, whose infants were not only more likely to die given hostile conditions, but as legal chattel were also always potentially lost to them as kin.[78]

The complexity of Black maternal experiences under the death-dealing conditions of enslavement is a key theme in Black women's writings. In her 1861 *Incidents in the Life of a Slave Girl*, Harriet Jacobs employs the prevailing sentimental idiom to express a bitter ambivalence as the protagonist watches over her infant son: "I could never forget that he was a slave. Sometimes I wished that he might die in infancy. God tried me. My darling became very ill. . . . I had prayed for his death, but never so earnestly as I now prayed for his life. . . . Alas, what mockery it is for a slave mother to try to pray back her dying child to life! Death is better than slavery."[79]

This closing conviction is expressed perhaps most dramatically in accounts of Margaret Garner, the enslaved mother who killed her baby rather than allow its recapture.[80] At the same time, Turner warns that "all too often, narratives for motherhood among enslaved women are frozen in a 'heroic pose', and the quest to capture the s/hero's 'unbending defiance' sidelines the complexities and vulnerabilities of enslaved subjects."[81] Attuned to these complexities, vulnerabilities, and experiences, historian LaKisha Simmons examines Works Progress Administration interviews with former enslaved people to listen to experiences of loss from mothers and kin, witnessing the horror of enslavers' casual murders of infants as well as the murderous conditions of enslaved infant life, and how these experiences shaped parents, siblings, and kin who lived to tell. Simmons situates these historical accounts within the continued atrocity of vast and preventable inequities in mortality and survival. In so doing, her account joins a lineage of Black organizers, scholars, and practitioners who have pointed to Black infant death as a form of everyday anti-Black violence spanning the eras of enslavement and formal emancipation. White terror, gender-based racial violence, and economic coercion persisted as core features of a political landscape fundamentally hostile to Black life, kinship, and reproductive health.

The antebellum period saw true babyhood becoming a unifying affective formation that manifested in new mothering practices for living infants as well as in elaborate funerary rituals for dead infants. This laid the groundwork for white infant mortality as a significant site of what Kyla Schuller terms "sentimental biopolitics" for the white polity in the latter half of the nineteenth century, as infant mortality among poor urban whites and European immigrants became the target of outcry and a locus of increasing public and private resources.[82] Meanwhile, Black infant mortality garnered little white public attention. In the South, as historian Wangui Muigai writes, "disputes over the underlying causes and the losses incurred illuminated the ways slaveowners regarded enslaved infants as assets of little worth but whose economic value was expected to appreciate over time."[83] These disputes often entailed ascriptions of Black maternal negligence—a pattern of blame still discernible in official approaches to Black infant mortality today.[84] Yet while excluded from broader biopolitical concern, and subject to slaveowners' brutal calculations, enslaved people maintained their own ways of honoring infant death, including both African burial rites and Christian funerary practices.[85]

In the eye of enslavers, as Saidiya Hartman writes, "the concept of 'injury' did not encompass the loss of children"; "the reproduction and conveyance of property decided the balance between the limited recommendation of slave humanity and the owners' rights of property in favor of the latter."[86] If, as Zelizer argues, "the economic and sentimental value of children were . . . declared to be radically incompatible," then enslaved infants could not properly be considered children.[87] They could not be included in the ontological category of (true) babyhood. Within this political ontology and structure of feeling, the status of enslaved infant life was diametrically opposed to that of white infants: not precious and irreplaceable but a fungible, essentially substitutable good. Births of enslaved infants were recorded in the plantation ledger along with other gains in property—not, of course, occasioning formal or informal social announcement. The noneventfulness of enslaved infant birth points to the broader exclusion of Black infants—in the white public imagination and slaveholding practices—from the biographical individuality of true babyhood. Frederick Douglass opens his *Narrative* with a reflection on slaveowners' active exclusion of enslaved people from the linear temporality of human biography through depriving them of the knowledge of their own birth dates: "I was born in Tuckahoe . . . Maryland. I have no accurate knowledge of my age, never having seen any authentic record containing it. By far the larger part of the slaves know as little of their age as horses know of theirs, and it is the wish of most masters within my knowledge to keep their slaves thus ignorant."[88]

Even in abolitionist literature, "excessive attention to heart wrenching scenes of family separation through sale obscures the suffering mothers also felt when their children 'not named, dead' were forgotten well before the ink that inscribed the loss in the plantation ledger died."[89] Chris Dixon writes of the centrality of the violated maternity of enslaved women to abolitionist discourse; along with the brutal treatment of pregnant women, the horror of such forced separation played a central role in these representations. Female abolitionists in particular employed such images both to elicit empathy in their audiences, and in representing their own empathetic responses as mothers themselves, drawing "connections between the suffering of women within their own coterie, and the horrors inflicted on slave mothers."[90] Harriet Beecher Stowe connected her own sorrow at the death of her child with the death of enslaved children in *Uncle Tom's Cabin*. Abolitionist Mary Grew wrote to Helen Garrison soon after the death of the latter's own young child in 1848, describing the comparison that she (Grew) had made, in a speech at an antislavery meeting, between her friend's profound "affliction and sorrow" and the situation of enslaved mothers, the latter "torn from their dear ones, not by the gentle hand of the death-angel, but by the merciless grasp of the traffickers in human souls; and it seemed almost a contrast, rather than a comparison, for the one became almost joy and blessedness beside the deeper bitterer woe of the other. And I told the audience that it seemed to me that in our sorrow, better than in our joy, we can sympathize with our enslaved brothers and sisters."[91]

Dixon argues that Grew, even while pointing to the incommensurability of the respective situations, "was certain that suffering on the part of abolitionists would enable them to better empathize with slaves."[92] Is it not the case that this empathy, the attempt by analogy to inhabit the full feeling of this worse-than-death dislocation, is predicated on the attribution of the characteristics of true babyhood to enslaved infants? Certainly this was the sincere intention of Grew and her abolitionist sisters-in-arms. Hartman, however, warns of the "difficulty and slipperiness of empathy" on the part of those whose humanity is unquestioned for the enslaved subject. Empathy is "a projection of oneself into another in order to better understand the other." However, given "the vulnerability of the captive body as a vessel for the uses, thoughts, and feelings of others the humanity extended to the slave inadvertently confirms the expectations and desires definitive of the relations of chattel slavery . . . [and] the fungibility of the captive body." The danger of an "obliteration of otherness" attends such empathetic exercises, such that "the white witness of the spectacle of suffering affirm[s] the materiality of black sentience only by feeling for himself" or herself, and "by virtue of this substitution the object of identification threatens to disappear."[93] The suffering of the enslaved mother and infant becomes a sentimental resource for Grew; given the depth of its horror as a point of contrast, it transmogrifies the bereavement of free white mothers upon the deaths of their children—which, as we have seen, was devastatingly profound—into "almost joy and blessedness."

Grew's characterization of sympathy as requiring sorrow connects to the related question of "why the site of suffering so readily lends itself to identification. Why is pain the conduit of identification?"[94] Hartman concedes that on the one hand, given the constitutiveness of violence to the maintenance of the system of slavery, this makes sense. Yet on the other hand, the invocation of the acutely suffering body as the point of identification also "risk[s] . . . fixing and naturalizing this condition of pained embodiment."[95] Hence, contrary to the intentions of the empathizer, this reinforces the distance between the enslaved body in pain and the protected body of the white subject. Representations of the mother and infant violently separated, analogously, may have helped to fix and naturalize the Black maternal-infant dyad as always already disrupted, always already pathological—especially given the maternal deficiency so widely attributed to Black women. Moreover, given that these scenes of suffering are designed to elicit the maximum affective response, "the violence of slavery or the pained existence of the enslaved, if discernible, is only so in the most heinous and grotesque examples and not in the quotidian routines of slavery."[96]

With regard to enslaved infant life and death, the vast majority of enslaved infant mortality and suffering was in fact due not to the "merciless grasp of traffickers in human souls," but to the unspectacular wearing-away of a vitality born compromised, to the everyday violence of those quotidian routines. These representations, while certainly portraying Black infants as subject to violence, may also have inadvertently reinforced the nonrecognition of Black infants' vulnerability to the same ordinary harms as white babies. While they may indeed have stirred indignation, inspired sorrow, and generated sympathy, these same feelings themselves may have further affirmed the distance between true babyhood and the enslaved Black infant.

Sentiment and Statistics: The Biopolitics of True Babyhood

The cult of true babyhood under the chattel slavery regime entailed one particular emergence of the (infant) human; it also laid the groundwork for, and was folded into, the emergence of a new, statistically defined human and its others after emancipation. White scholars, physicians, and other specialists used mortality statistics to enshrine the object status of Black infants after the legal emancipation. Far from moderating these harms, white medical men and scientists were often at the forefront of their perpetration and justification. For when Black infant mortality belatedly entered the white public view, it did so as part of a broader "condemnation of Blackness"—to use Khalil Gibran Muhammad's phrasing—as white health statisticians like Frederick Hoffman proclaimed that the much higher rates of Black infant mortality, far from cause for alarm or intervention, heralded a dying race: what Muhammad terms the "disappearance hypothesis."[97] Statistical methods during the nineteenth century had already offered new rationales for the existing system of slavery as "protecting" Black people in the evolutionary struggle of "races." After leading the Union to victory as soldiers and workers, the US government denied freedpeople food, shelter, clothing, and even quarantine protocols. The resulting magnitude of freedpeople's suffering and death lent unprecedented weight to this notion.[98] Though challenged at the time by Black leaders, these rationalizations effaced both the conditions that threatened Black infant life and the lived experiences of Black maternal, parental, and community grief.

Many whites already believed before the Civil War that the system of enslavement "sheltered" Blacks from the consequences of their alleged evolutionary inferiority, and that emancipation would inevitably lead to the extinction of the race.[99] But the magnitude and visibility of African American suffering and death in the postwar period lent unprecedented weight to this notion: "Thousands of emancipated slaves [were] dying from smallpox, starvation, exposure, among other ailments. . . . [J]ournalists, scientists, doctors, politicians, and ordinary white Americans . . . could then point to the problems that emancipation engendered."[100] Needless to say, whites "did not consider structural poverty, medical neglect, and lack of basic necessities as the cause of illness and death among the ex-slave population."[101] This hypothesis became a self-fulfilling prophecy, as many white physicians used it to justify actions undermining Black survival and good health.[102] The decades following the Civil War also witnessed a proliferation of medical studies of the apparently fatal effects of emancipation.[103] As Evelynn Hammonds and Susan Reverby write, "Throughout the late 19th century and into the 20th century poor health and lack of access to health care, coupled with theories of innate weakness, followed African Americans out of the rural South and into the cities. The housing segregation, crowding, and heavy manual labor faced by Black men and women took their toll as infectious diseases spread."[104]

Saving Babies as White Settler Reproductive Futurity

Just as imminent African American extinction pervaded American medical, anthropological, and social scientific thought, there was an enormous groundswell of public outrage over the high rates of native white and European immigrant infant mortality, through the 1870s, 1880s, and 1890s. By the late 1850s, Northern US cities were regularly characterized in the press as killing fields for babies, "infant abattoirs."[105] It is striking that this was often framed as the "slaughter of innocents"—even though this disproportionate mortality occurred not just among the poor, but especially among the foreign-born poor. For instance, one of the first studies, carried out in Boston in 1855, showed that 641 of the 971 infant deaths that year were offspring of impoverished immigrant families.[106] Reflecting public anxieties among US-born whites about the fitness of European immigrant groups for inclusion in the national body, the discourse accompanying these studies apportioned a great deal of blame to the allegedly filthy habits of the Irish and other "unacclimated foreigners" only much later putting a stronger accent on poverty than on culture. Racialized notions of parental apathy were also common among reformers. For instance, an 1864 health official in Boston dismissed the possibility of education as a solution for improving the endemic "disregard of the laws of health" among immigrant populations, as "such attempts will result as similar attempts have always resulted, in perfect indifference and apathy."[107]

Prefiguring Cybelle Fox's account of the trifurcated structure of pre–New Deal relief programs for European immigrants, African Americans, and Mexican Americans, however, public measures for the improvement of the conditions of urban immigrants was never a question.[108] For instance, even as the reformer quoted above deplored the ineducability of immigrant parents, his solution was "rigid oversight and control of the erection of dwellings."[109] However different these immigrant families may have been in habits and customs, their citizen children were not to suffer for the sins of the fathers. As a sanitary reform movement in the name of lowering infant mortality gathered steam through the 1880s and 1890s, culminating in the formation of the American Association for Study and

Prevention of Infant Mortality (AASPIM), the focus remained largely on improving the conditions of the European-born immigrant poor in Northern cities.[110]

The white public excluded Black infants' deaths from the increasingly public sense of tragic loss that shadowed white infancy, even as enslaved Black infants in the antebellum and postwar periods died at rates far exceeding those of white infants.[111] Public health officials, sanitary reformers, medical personnel, and other experts attributed white deaths to environmental or remediable cultural causes, and municipal and state efforts to prevent them proliferated. At the same time, Black mortality statistics from Southern cities were seen as confirmation of the disappearance hypothesis, and efforts to reverse the trend as a waste of resources better invested in the futurity of the white citizenry.[112] Thus public health experts took up Black infant death not in terms of human suffering but as part of a larger scholastic question of *when* and *how* the ultimate extinction of African Americans would take place. A "proprietary expertise in all matters relating to black morbidity and mortality" in white Southern experts reflected the lingering effects of Blacks' commodity status under slavery.[113] While the high rates of death among the infants of European immigrants in the North in themselves spurred intervention, "discussion of black infant mortality centered on the disparity between white and black infant death rates" and debates over the precise mechanisms of inherited racial traits.[114] In Omar Ricks's phrasing, Black infant deaths were "counted without counting."[115] It should be noted that, even as it was Southern experts who most actively propounded the disappearance hypothesis, the leading national medical and public health journals gave them prominent place.[116] The study of racial disparities in these journals—though contested by Du Bois, Kelly Miller, and many others—originated in debates entirely uninterested in preventing Black infant death and the suffering of Black families and communities that this entailed.

These racist evolutionary notions corresponded with sciences of racial measurement, including pelvimetry, according to which Black women's allegedly "primitive" pelvises, unlike those of "civilized" white women, were supposedly conducive to easy births—further justifying medical disinvestment in Black reproductive health.[117] Laura Briggs's account of nineteenth-century gynecology's opposition between "overcivilized" white women and "savage" nonwhite women—particularly Black women—illuminates the ways that this category was a key biopolitical one as well, in its connections to patriarchy, medical power/knowledge, and political economy.[118] While diagnoses of reproductive "diseases of overcivilization" such as hysteria and neurasthenia justified white women's exclusion from higher education and their consignment to the domestic sphere, the complementary construction of nonwhite women as reproductively hardy and insensate construed them as ideal subjects for both medical experimentation and hard labor.[119] It also justified the obstetrical neglect of nonwhite women, who—despite this ascribed hardiness—suffered disproportionate maternal morbidity and mortality, when intervention would actually have been warranted.[120]

As Muigai documents, countervailing projects of care existed at the municipal level, such as the Bureau of Child Guardians, founded in 1892 in Washington, DC. These intersected with deep networks of communal childcare by which Black communities supported maternal and infant well-being, especially among women recently arrived in cities from the rural South. Many Black physicians worked concertedly to support Black infant life.[121] In addition, as Hammonds and Reverby note, "African Americans made demands on the local and federal governments, built up mutual aid societies, and formed separate medical and nursing schools when denied access to those controlled by Whites."[122] Yet Black infant mortality nevertheless remained high—a result of concerted medical neglect, legally enshrined economic exploitation and deprivation, and continued white violence.

True Babyhood by the Numbers: Hoffman's
Race Traits and Tendencies

Prudential Insurance Company statistician Frederick Hoffman's influential 1896 treatise, *Race Traits and Tendencies of the American Negro*, was a quintessential expression and promulgation of the turn-of-the-century ideology of true babyhood. Whereas true babyhood figured white infants as adored, inherently precious, and vulnerable future citizens, Hoffman figured Black infants as neglected, devalued, carriers not of a racial future but as doomed specimens of a moribund race. His 330-page tract begins by declaring its dedication to the most thorough and disinterested scientific investigation: "Only by means of a thorough analysis of all the data that make up the history of the colored race in this country," its introduction reads, "can the true nature of the so-called 'Negro problem' be understood."[123] *Race Traits* employs new statistical methods as evidence of Blacks' peculiar double role as both exception and threat to the (white) nation's evolutionary progress. Khalil Gibran Muhammad has demonstrated that *Race Traits* was pivotal for the tethering of Blackness to criminality in the 1890s, a legacy that has profoundly shaped present racial and carceral geographies, policies, and conventional wisdom.[124] I argue that Hoffman's readings of Black mortality statistics, and infant mortality in particular, harness these statistical findings to three distinct though interconnected necropolitical rationalities that exclude Black infants from true babyhood: physiological, affective, and actuarial.

Race Traits and Tendencies of the American Negro appeared in the pages of the prestigious *Publications of the American Economic Association* in May 1896, the same month and year as the *Plessy v. Ferguson* decision. In his introduction to the work, Hoffman cites his German birth and education as a guarantee of freedom from the racial bias that may taint demographic studies of Blacks by white Americans.[125]

Muhammad locates this framing "in the tradition of an Alexis de Tocqueville," noting that Hoffman "marketed himself as a clear-eyed, plainspoken, unbiased foreign observer of American race relations and demographic trends."[126] Thus he sought empirical unassailability for his conclusion that "in vital capacity, the most important of physical characteristics, the tendency of the race has been downward. This tendency if unchecked must in the end, lead to a still greater mortality, a lesser degree of economic and social efficiency, a lower standard of nurture and a diminishing excess of births over deaths. A combination of these traits and tendencies must in the end cause the extinction of the race."[127]

Race Traits presents an unprecedented synthesis of new criminal, demographic, epidemiological, and vital statistics with older anthropometrical studies and anecdotal evidence. As Muhammad notes, it was "the first time" statistics would secure a place in American race-relations discourse, one that would prove "permanent."[128] Hoffman argues that his statistical methods place the extinction hypothesis beyond dispute: "it is a fact which can and will be demonstrated by indisputable evidence, that of all races for which statistics are obtainable . . . the negro shows the least power of resistance in the struggle for life."[129] As Muhammad documents, contemporary white readers viewed the evidence Hoffman presented as unassailable.[130] Hoffman's synthesis and interpretation of infant mortality statistics were a key component of these findings.

Medical historian Nancy Stepan reminds us that "the scientists who gave scientific racism its credibility and respectability were often first-rate scientists struggling to understand what appeared to them to be deeply puzzling problems of biology and human society."[131] There is no reason to doubt that Hoffman earnestly believed in his own personal impartiality, or in the urgency of his findings for the good of humanity—in his narrowly circumscribed conception of the term. At the same time, *Race Traits* was not a professionally disinterested project. New state laws in the late 1880s had barred the racially differentiated life insurance rates and benefits that insurance companies had instituted a decade earlier, and Prudential Life Insurance Company was in the process of denying life insurance to all African Americans on the grounds of their "excessive mortality."[132] Hoffman had compiled a range of African American vital statistics in 1892 and rendered conclusions firmly in support of the disappearance hypothesis. Attributing to African Americans a "gross immorality, early and excessive intercourse of the sexes, premature maternity, and general intemperance in eating and drinking," the treatise argued that "the whole body politic of the colored race is undermined and finally doomed."[133] "What else but final extinction," he asked, "can be the future of the negro, thus presenting all the evidences of a dying race?"[134]

Prudential hired Hoffman two years later, expecting him to demonstrate the inherent moribundity—and hence noninsurability—of Black life.[135] *Race Traits* thus helped to translate the disappearance hypothesis into the terms of unmanageable actuarial risk, to the financial benefit of Prudential. Beyond pecuniary considerations, however, Hoffman's influential text abetted his firm's policies in positioning Blacks outside what François Ewald calls the "insurantial imaginary."[136] In the United States at the end of the nineteenth century, this imaginary cast the new technologies of mutuality and risk-sharing through insurance companies as necessary components of citizenship.[137] The elaboration in *Race Traits* of an actuarial rationality of exclusion, which dovetailed with more familiar physiological, moral, and affective rationalities, helped to crystallize the postemancipation reconfiguration of Blacks as outcasts from both the nation and the human.

A lexical note: by "rationality," I mean, borrowing Ewald's succinct definition, "a way of breaking down, rearranging, ordering certain elements of reality."[138] A rationality always presupposes an ontology: the always-partial selection of elements that qualify as the reality that is to be ordered. In human affairs a rationality presupposes a *political* ontology, given that both this selection and its ordering reflect the valuation of certain forms of life above others. They also retroactively justify it. If this ordering has any purchase in the world, it is achieved through the exercise of power. Hoffman's rationalities each explain and reinforce the biopolitical order of racial Darwinist white supremacy by figuring Black infants as lacking a key feature of the true baby.[139]

Exclusion from Futurity: Hybridity as Moribundity

The true baby embodied the future of the nation and the race; while vulnerable as newborns, this vulnerability signaled the imperative to cultivate each baby's infantine life force so that, as adults, they could carry that destiny forward. In contrast, *Race Traits* figures Black infant mortality as a sign of a moribund race. "The vitality of the negro," Hoffman writes, "may well be considered the most important phase of the so-called race problem; for it is a fact which can and will be demonstrated by indisputable evidence, that of all races for which statistics are obtainable . . . the negro shows the least power of resistance in the struggle for life."[140] He notes that other analysts have long observed the "excessive mortality of the colored race."[141] But his inclusion and interpretation of African American infant and child mortality statistics constitutes new support for the alleged trend of race extinction. This is achieved through a synthesis of mortality statistics from Northern and Southern cities broken down both by race and age categories, allowing not only for accurate interracial comparison but intraracial comparison between different stages of life.[142]

Employing mortality tables from New York City, Brooklyn (two years before the other four boroughs annexed it), Boston, Philadelphia, Baltimore, New Orleans, Charleston, Richmond, and Washington, DC, Hoffman observes that the difference in mortality "for the earliest period . . . is enormous."[143] Black infant and child survival, Hoffman concludes, is compromised throughout the nation.[144] He writes: "Nowhere else do we meet with such a frightful infant mortality as we find prevailing among the colored population of the large cities, both North and South."[145] Compared with their white counterparts, Black infants are faring extremely poorly.

Hoffman's larger point resides, however, in the comparison of the new generation with their elders. In all of the age-differentiated mortality tables, differences between Black and white mortality diminish sharply among older age groups, whereas "the greatest excess of mortality amongst the colored falls on the early age groups."[146] Why is this so significant, in Hoffman's view? Because substantial proportions of Black people over the age of forty-five, who are more like whites in terms of their death rates, were born and raised in slavery. He presents Charleston's age-differentiated vital statistics, showing a significantly increased "excess mortality" of younger Blacks in 1890 compared with 1848, but little change in the oldest category.[147] Hoffman thus asserts that "we have an abundance of testimony . . . that previous to emancipation the negro enjoyed equal health if not superior to that of the white race."[148] He reiterates the point multiple times: "the excess [mortality] is greatest for the first generation, and least for the third. . . . It would seem therefore, that the young generation is the one least fit for race survival."[149] Then, a page later, he writes: "mortality is most excessive . . . among those who largely represent the present generation, born or raised during the period of freedom . . . [among] those who were under the influence of the conditions of servitude. . . . [W]e find a greater power of resistance to disease and death than among the generation following emancipation and the participation of the negro in the active struggle for life."[150] Saidiya Hartman argues that, along with what she calls the fungibility of the enslaved Black body, a primary form of the negation of

Black subjectivity under slavery was the total appropriation of the *spatial extent* of the enslaved body: "the extensive capacities of property—that is, the augmentation of the master subject through his embodiment in external objects and persons."[151] We might say that Hoffman's post-emancipation negation of Black existence operates rather through the denial of African Americans' collective *temporal duration*, figuring the Black body's vital persistence as being eaten ineluctably away. Hoffman attributes the post-emancipation decline primarily to sexual licentiousness; Black people, and Black women in particular, have mistaken sexual license for liberty, resulting in constitutionally compromised mixed-race offspring. He devotes significant space to ruling out environmental factors, such as altitude, population density, or unsanitary conditions as major causes of infant mortality.[152] Deaths from prematurity and stillbirth among African Americans in his representative cities of Washington, DC, and Baltimore, double to triple the white rate, like the similarly disproportionate "deaths from inanition, debility, and atrophy," are "largely the result of inferior organisms, which . . . is one of the most pronounced race characteristics of the American Negro."[153] At the root of this organismal debility is the racial impurity of North American Blacks, a factor Hoffman claims has increased sharply since emancipation. The race is "hopelessly mixed"; in this sense, "true" Blacks are in fact already practically extinct: "the infusion of white blood, through white males, has been widespread, and the original type of the African has almost completely disappeared."[154] This mixing is not, for Hoffman, the result of the widespread sexual violence over centuries of slavery but rather the high levels of prostitution among African American women. Hoffman claims that prostitution is the most prevalent form of Black female sexual activity.[155]

In the opening discussion of population trends in *Race Traits*, Hoffman uses the maps attached to the "Hull House Papers" to show that Blacks tend to live in neighborhoods with the highest density of "houses of ill repute."[156] Apparently ignorant of restrictive housing policy, he claims that Blacks "choose" to live in the shadow of these brothels and willingly constitute their primary occupants. In Hoffman's depiction marriage simply has no place at all within the sexual lives of Black people, which are at best carried on casually, but most often as prostitution: "an immense amount of concubinage and prostitution prevails among the colored women of the United States . . . a fact fully admitted by the negroes themselves. . . . Of the two evils, prostitution for gain prevails the more widely."[157] Black sexual relations are essentially immoral and aberrant. Hoffman devotes significant space to endorsing Southern writers' accounts of the bestiality of Black male rapists, for instance.[158] However, these allegedly frequent attacks apparently do not yield any issue.[159] It is principally Black female prostitution with "white males of a lower type" that produce the moribund hybrid offspring that signal the decline of the race: "In the irregular sexual relations of the present day prostitution for gain is the prevailing rule, and one of the determining causes of the inordinate mortality."[160]

Hoffman argues: "It is largely to the frequency of illicit intercourse between white males and colored females that we must attribute the wide prevalence of syphilis and scrofula among the mixed population, as well as the excessive mortality, the lower fecundity, the increasing tendency to consumption and other tubercular diseases, the smaller chest expansion and vital capacity. All are the consequences of a union of two races in violation of a natural law."[161] Hoffman's multiple repetitions of the allegation of miscegenational prostitution testify to Jared Sexton's observation that "a certain superintensity of attention, an exorbitant single-mindedness concerning the centrality of interracial sexuality to all things" "characterizes the discourse of white supremacy and anti-Blackness."[162] But even in relations between Black men and women, Hoffman paints casual illicit encounters as the rule, not least because most are degenerate hybrids themselves.[163] Both in its flouting of matrimony and its transgression of the "law of similarity," which Hoffman claims leads unlike races to have a natural mutual aversion, Black sexual relations are "outside of the pale of the moral law."[164] Consequently, it has "very seriously affected the physical and moral characteristics of the colored race. *These consequences fall most heavily on the offspring.* The children of colored women and white men, of whatever shade of color, are morally and physically the inferiors of the pure black. It has been stated by [Josiah] Nott and proved by subsequent experience, that the mulatto is in every way the inferior of the black, and of all races the one possessed of the least vital force."[165]

This passage is typical in that Hoffman entangles physiological and moral factors in his diagnoses of the cause of decline. Nevertheless, he offers a litany of medical testimony focused purely on the degenerate physique of biracial persons. For example, he quotes a doctor at the New York Reformatory who claims "color exercises an influence in disease resistance. Thus, other things being equal, the white opposes the greatest resistance; next comes the full blooded negro . . . while the mulatto is most susceptible, as if the inferior elements of two colors combined in him produced a strain ill-calculated to resist disease."[166] Pairing this data with Civil War–era studies claiming biracial recruits have a smaller lung capacity, Hoffman asserts that "the inferior vitality of the mixed race is . . . sufficiently proven."[167] Those of mixed race are "inferior even to the pure black," he writes.[168] This "inferior vitality" manifests most acutely in the "wide prevalence of syphilis and scrofula among the mixed population, as well as the excessive mortality, the lower fecundity, the increasing tendency to consumption and other tubercular diseases, smaller chest expansion and vital capacity."[169] In support of these claims, Hoffman lists a number of "excerpts from the report of the Provost-Marshal General," featuring the notes of Civil War army doctors from across the Union:

There are few if any pure Africans [in Vermont], but a mixed race only. They probably lose in vitality what they gain in symmetry of form by admixture; they die early of scrofula or tuberculosis . . . as a general rule, any considerable admixture of white blood deteriorates the physique and impairs the powers of endurance, and almost always introduces a scrofulous taint . . . a genuine black is far superior in physical endurance to the mulatto or yellow negro; the last named are with few exceptions, scrofulous or consumptive. . . . The colored men, as far as my observation goes, make excellent soldiers. . . . The mulatto, however, is comparatively worthless, subject to scrofula and tuberculosis.[170]

In line with the dominant theories of his day, Hoffman acknowledges the notion that white blood improves the Negro mind, citing brain weight studies.[171] But "whatever the race may have gained in an intellectual way," he writes, "which is a matter of speculation, it has been losing its greatest resources in the struggle for life, a sound physical organism and power of rapid reproduction."[172] These "physiological consequences alone," Hoffman warns, "demand race purity and a stern reprobation of any infusion of white blood." He returns to this theme in the work's conclusion, writing that "the mixture of the African with the white race has been shown to have seriously affected the longevity of the former and left as a heritage to future generations the poison of scrofula, tuberculosis and most of all of, syphilis."[173] This "hopelessly mixed" race cannot hope to compete for survival against pure African stock (if any can be found), let alone against the vastly superior Anglo-Saxons.

The pride of pathological place given to miscegenation and syphilis, however, clearly signal that these physiological aberrations from Anglo-Saxon biological norms cannot be considered in isolation from their moral counterparts. In fact, Hoffman is explicit about this: "All the facts obtainable which depict truthfully the present physical and moral condition of the colored race," he writes, "prove that the underlying cause of the excessive mortality and diminishing rate of increase in population is a low state of sexual morality."[174] If inferior organisms are the proximate cause of race decline, immorality might be said to be the ultimate cause.

Regarding the pathological causes of disproportionate Black infant mortality rates, Hoffman not only dismisses environmental factors but introduces a racially bifurcated reading of disease more broadly. He approvingly quotes the assessment of the registrar-general of Antigua: among Blacks, the latter writes, the so-called causes of infant mortality "are not diseases at all but merely names, all of which have nearly the same meaning . . . parents, who in the majority of these cases are broken down by disease consequent on vice, immorality, and debauchery . . . impart such enfeebled constitutions to their offspring that they cannot live a few months even under the most favorable circumstances."[175] The disease of Black infants cannot even be read or classified according to the same etiological processes that define disease among whites. Disease, as commonly understood to apply to the human organism, here loses purchase even as a proximate cause. Quoting the Antiguan physician, Hoffman implies that the erroneous assimilation of Black disease to the individualized disease process in non-Blacks misrecognizes the real pathology, which is phylogenetic in nature: namely, the literally corrosive "vice, immorality, and debauchery" of the race as a whole.

A racially bifurcated epistemology of disease does not of course originate with Hoffman. Jim Downs identifies a similar dynamic in his comparison of the lax governmental and medical responses to smallpox epidemics among freedpeople during and after the Civil War with the disciplined response to the disease among poor, mostly immigrant communities in Northern cities.[176] The larger backdrop to this bifurcation is the nineteenth-century medical commonplace that the allegedly profound anatomical and physiological differences between Blacks and whites testified to the former's evolutionary inferiority, or even an innate inability to evolve at all.[177] (Scientists nonetheless performed experiments on African Americans for the benefit of white patients.)[178] Hoffman's innovation here is to tie this organismal difference to a phylogenetic moral depravity through the statistical links that he establishes between vice (prostitution in particular), illegitimacy, and infant death. He attributes "excessive infant mortality" to "an immense amount of immorality, which is a race trait, and of which scrofula, syphilis, and even consumption are the inevitable consequences." Hoffman writes:

> So long as more than one fourth . . . of the births for the colored population of Washington are illegitimate . . . [compared to] only 2.6 per cent. of births among the whites . . . it is plain why we should meet with a mortality from scrofula and syphilis so largely in excess of that of the whites. And it is also plain now, that we have reached the underlying causes of . . . enormous waste of child life. It is not in the conditions of life, but in the race traits and tendencies that we find the causes of the excessive mortality. So long as these tendencies are persisted in, so long as immorality and vice are a habit of life of the vast majority of the colored population, the effect will be to increase the mortality by hereditary transmission of weak constitutions, and to lower still further the rate of natural increase, until the births fall below the deaths, and gradual extinction results.[179]

Hoffman's statistics suggest three-quarters of African American births occur within the bounds of matrimony, but he claims this is an artifact of self-reporting. "The actual number if known would of course, give a much higher rate," he concludes.[180] Hoffman here extends the insights borrowed from Antigua, figuring tubercular and venereal diseases not as infectious agents but as virtually arising from within rather than contracted from without—inevitable consequences of Blacks' inherently vicious sexual practices.

Beyond serving to explain the causes of race decline, however, Hoffman's depiction of this sexual immorality also draws a hard line between the norms governing Anglo-Saxon existence and the aberrant contours of African American bodies and lives. Hazel Carby's analysis of the "cult of true womanhood" sheds light on the exclusionary gender work done by Hoffman's depictions of vicious Black womanhood in particular.[181] Critically extending Barbara Welter's analysis of "true womanhood," which centered without avowing the whiteness of that womanhood, Carby examines the bifurcation between the standards of "true womanhood" to which planter-class white women were held and the non-womanhood (in addition to non-personhood) to which enslaved Black women were consigned. Responding critically to feminist historians' inattention to the fundamental whiteness of the figure of true womanhood, Carby describes this figure as not merely an impossible ideal but "as a dominating image, describing the parameters within which women were measured and declared to be, or not to be, women."[182] White women were tasked with producing citizens and ensuring the channels of property inheritance, while enslaved Black women were forced to reproduce property itself.[183] If the former were bound to reproduce a patriarchal *fixity*—of the family form, of property relations—the latter were forced to be both embodiments of and vessels for what Hartman calls the essential *fungibility* of Black life as a form of capital.[184]

In the literary sources that Carby cites, depictions of contrasting physical attributes signal this ontological distinction: golden-haired lightness versus shadowy darkness, fragility versus a mannish strength. But the most obsessive emphasis was placed on "purity," without which, Welter writes, a female was "no woman at all, but a member of some lower order."[185] One of Carby's principal interventions is to show that this "member" was the Black female herself, whose "overt sexuality . . . excluded [her] . . . from the parameters of virtuous possibilities."[186] Carby shows that this exclusion was essential, the constitutive limit of that virtue: "Existing outside the definition of true womanhood, black female sexuality was nevertheless used to define what those boundaries were."[187] Hoffman's diametrically opposed characterizations of Black and white womanhood reflect the persistence of this antebellum structure of femininity. Black women in his account are, through the moral and constitutional effects of this fundamental immorality, responsible for the fall of their race; the evolutionary superiority of Anglo-Saxons hinges on "chastity in woman," the feminine counterpart to "self reliance in man."[188] Hoffman thus conjoins "true womanhood" to his racial Darwinist narrative, joining it to his evidence of physiological African American decline. But he adds an emotional dimension to this diagnosis.

The Affective Rationality of Exclusion

More precisely, Hoffman imputes a *lack* of emotional connection, tenderness, or love to African Americans' intimate relationships, citing this affective deficit as a third causal factor behind high Black infant and child mortality. He conscripts the alleged prevalence of prostitution into a narrative of increasing Black affective deficiency as an aspect of race decline. "All the data at my command," he writes, "show that physically the race [under slavery] was superior to the present generation, and no physical health is possible without a fair degree of sexual morality . . . *in which affection played at least a small if not an important part.* In the irregular sexual relations of the present day prostitution for gain is the prevailing rule, and one of the determining causes of . . . inordinate mortality."[189] Hoffman has already provided abundant evidence of the fatal consequences of prostitution in terms of disease (*qua* heritable compromised constitution). Here he posits a lack of finer feelings that, among civilized subjects, underpin not only the bonds of matrimony but the vital investment in the life of the next generation. Quoting sociologist Herbert Spencer, Hoffman makes this point explicit:

> In societies characterized by inferior forms of marriage . . . there cannot develop to any great extent that powerful combination of feelings . . . affection, admiration, sympathy . . . which in so marvelous a manner has grown out of the sexual instinct. And in the absence of this complex passion, which manifestly pre-supposes a relation between one man and one woman, the supreme interest in life (the raising up of members of a new generation) disappears. . . . a prevalent unchastity severs the higher from the lower components of the sexual relation: the root may produce a few leaves, but no true flower.[190]

Hoffman thus posits that lacking the mutual "affection, admiration, sympathy" that naturally arise within civilized white conjugal relations, Black parents have no affective resources to bestow upon their progeny.

He makes explicit the link between this alleged affective deficit and "the excessive mortality of colored children" by quoting at length a series of annual reports by a Savannah, Georgia, health officer to his superior: "[1890] The neglect of children by negro parents is so often apparent to your health officer that he must call your attention again to this matter. In many instances they will not call in a physician when the city provides them free medical attendance . . . . [1891] Fifty per cent. of the children who die never receive medical attention . . . the parents will not call in a physician, claiming the children died before they could go for a physician."[191] The officer's report reaches a more desperate pitch in 1893: "For years the city of Savannah has furnished gratuitous medical advice and medicine, and the negroes persistently refuse to accept them, at least for their children.

Can the city do more? Is there any other move to make save that of appeal to the law to force parents to care for their offspring?"[192] By 1894 the health officer paints this failure to care as not only immoral but criminal: "We must have stringent laws covering the criminal neglect of negro parents who allow their children to sicken and die."[193] Hoffman makes a small qualification: "The indifference as to medical attendance in cases of illness of their children is due to ignorance rather than to criminal neglect."[194] However, he nevertheless attributes fatal power to this parental neglect: "in our Southern cities" just as in "British Guiana . . . Antigua, [and] Trinidad . . . the excessive infant mortality among the colored population is largely the result of individual neglect, as well as in part due to inherited organic weakness."[195] Not only sexual immorality, not only the degenerate hybridity that is its fruit, but also Black parental apathy toward their casually conceived offspring, lead to the fatally "diminished power of vital resistance among the young."[196]

In elaborating out the essential whiteness of "true womanhood," Carby calls attention to the intertwined material and affective dimensions of what was perhaps the fundamental denial of relationality during the epoch of slavery: "the simultaneous existence of two definitions of motherhood: the glorified and the breeder."[197] Pushing to a deeper level feminist historian Ann Berg's argument that "love of home, children and domestic duties are the only passions ['true women'] feel," Carby shows that in addition to their figuration as fundamentally impure, Black women's exile from consideration as subjects of such homely passions served to reinforce their exclusion from womanhood.[198] Moreover, Carby shows that this negation extended to the very possibility of Black feeling more broadly. She demonstrates that revulsion at the cruelties of slavery tended to coexist with the contempt for Black personhood in antebellum white women's writings. She thus argues that white womanly sentimentality— even as it decried the spectacle of Black subjection to violence—

tended to affirm, rather than bridge, the ontological distance between whites and African Americans.

"The terrain of sensibilities was highly contradictory," Carby writes. "A sensitivity that was heightened into an awareness of slavery as a brutal social system often existed simultaneously with a rejection of the humanity of slaves as brute creatures. A display of finer feelings worked to affirm the superiority of white sensibilities, and of white people as a group, over and above the slaves who were constructed as being incapable of harboring feelings or of generating grief."[199] Hartman identifies a similar dynamic at work in antislavery writers' depictions of brutal scenes of punishment in bondage, in the professed service of inciting horror and empathetic outrage among a white readership. Even among committed abolitionists, she argues, the fixation on scenes of spectacular Black suffering tended to confirm the "humanity" of the white spectator, affirming the unbridgeable distance between the white spectator and his or her addressees (as empathetic-ethical subjects) and the Black slave (as suffering abstraction, as fungible embodiment of pain).[200]

Likewise, in Hoffman's account, the affective lack that defines both the sexual and the parental relation among Blacks stands in sharp contrast not only to white conjugal and family relations, but to Hoffman's own self-stylization as an emotionally affected witness. Like Carby's exemplary sensitive white mistress, who narrated her own recoiling at the spectacles of slavery's most brutal aspects, Hoffman peppers his account with attestations of pity and distress.[201] High rates of Black infant mortality in are "frightful."[202] They are an "enormous waste of child life."[203] Hoffman's most vivid emotional response, however, dwells not on mortality as a statistical abstraction but on a quasi-sociological description of Blacks' death rites.

Pauper funerals . . . are extremely frequent among the colored population and nowhere else does absence of thrift so clearly manifest itself. . . . Whoever has witnessed the pauper funeral of a negro, the bare pine box and the common cart, the absence of all that makes less sorrowful the last rites over the dead, has seen a phase of negro life and manners more disheartening perhaps than anything else in the whole range of human misery. Perhaps only the dreary aspect of the negroes' "potter's field," the low sand hills, row after row . . . unrelieved by a single mark of human kindness, without a flower and without a cross . . . may be more sad and gruesome than the display of almost inhuman apathy at the funeral. By this I do not wish to be misunderstood as saying that the negro is entirely indifferent, for he is not, and mourns the loss of a near one as sincerely as the member of any other race, but his indifference is to a condition imposed on him not on account of his poverty, but on account of his lack of thrift.[204]

Like Carby's tenderhearted white mistress, recording her own sudden physical illness in response to the sight of a slave on the auction block, it is Hoffman, not the Black mourners, who is, to repurpose Lauren Berlant's formulation, "the subject of true feeling."[205] However, while even the mistress's sentiments, in Carby's account, constituted at least a superficial critique of the system of chattel enslavement—albeit a critique ultimately annulled by its predication on Black subhumanity—it is clear that the "gruesome" spectacle Hoffman narrates is not a scene of white violence but of the alleged inhumanity of Black life, and death, itself. It is no Jim Crow equivalent of the auction block but the depravity of Blacks themselves, their failure to mourn properly, their neglect to mark the deaths of their near ones with even the barest "mark of human kindness," a rude cross or humble nosegay. Hoffman's allegations of the lack of appropriate conjugal and parental feeling during life here finds a vivid counterpart in the desolate scene of "almost inhuman apathy at the funeral," the unadorned pine box and cart and the unbroken expanse of anonymous mounds. Just as Hoffman's contrast between Black prostitution and Anglo-Saxon chastity carried the antebellum racial bifurcation of sexual morality into the Jim Crow era, the affective deficit that he imputes to Blacks, literally from cradle to grave, inscribes the legal arelationality of the enslaved into the fatal behavioral aberrations of emancipated Black subject.

A similar affective configuration would also be a political signature in slightly later infant mortality prevention efforts among Native Nations and in contexts of US imperialism. Expressions of distress at high infant mortality signified the deep and innocent benevolence of US authority and hence, as high numbers "startle us," in the words of Cato Sells in his 1916 pamphlet *Indian Babies: How to Keep Them Well* such that "our" affect testifies to the nonimplication of the United States in the root conditions of this death.[206]

Not Precious but Devalued

But there is more: the mentions of thrift that bookend the passage, the strange contradictory acknowledgment of African American mourning juxtaposed to the allegations of apathy and indifference. Through these rather puzzling formulations, Hoffman fashions a crucial link between his ascription of affective deficiency and the faculty of providence or thrift, which Blacks proverbially lack. "Thrift" is a key term in Hoffman's text, which he holds up, like "self-reliance" and "chastity," as "the essential virtue of Indo-Germanic races."[207] "Thrift," Hoffman writes, "is the result of self help . . . self-denial and self-sacrifice, developed . . . only after a struggle against adverse conditions which would have reduced a race less sturdy [than Euro-Americans] to barbarism and savagery."[208] Black people, he implies, have been so reduced, for not thrift but pauperism, "the natural and inevitable result of crime and immorality" that characterizes Black existence.[209] He describes the pauper funeral with such melancholy fascination, marked at the outset by two parallel absences: the absence of thrift and "the absence of all that makes less sorrowful the last rites over the dead." This "all" appears to signify in part the gravestones and flowers of the proper funerary proceedings. But in view of the emphasis on thrift, it also seems to comprise the more intangible element of providence. What could make death "less sorrowful" for the civilized man than the prospect of posthumous provision, for dependents and one's own interment alike?

Like Herbert Spencer's assessment of Black parental disinvestment in "the supreme interest in life (the raising up of members of a new generation)," pauperism signifies not only the absence of forward-looking self-sacrifice but an impoverishment of feeling: a lack of shame, a lack of pride, a lack of concern. It is thus not only the pitiful plainness of the pine box and cart but the visible fact that public funds provide them, a sign of shameless dependency even in death. More broadly, Hoffman has been suggesting throughout, proper shame in the face of immoral behavior—or, if the deceased is a child, had the parents exercised more care—might have prevented the death itself. The "inhuman apathy" of the funeral is not, as Hoffman himself acknowledges, an absence of bereavement for the deceased, but rather a gruesome display of indifference to the improvidence that precipitated both the death and the penury. Hoffman thus dramatizes an inextricable link between failures of sentiment and their failures of providence.

In one sense, Hoffman is doing nothing new here; Blacks' alleged lack of providence and foresight was an old pro-slavery chestnut.[210] But having bound Black peoples' alleged affective deficiency to their moral and physiological decline, Hoffman's link between thrift and sentiment allows him to fold this proverbial improvidence into the logics of the extinction narrative. Facing a bleak physiological outlook due to undeveloped moral faculties, Blacks are allegedly incapable of the sentiments that would properly attach them to the future, or goad them to reverse their fate. Hoffman the actuary is thus able to provide a tightly woven case for categorically disqualifying Black people as insurance risks.[211] Because African Americans were indeed yoked to death-dealing life and work conditions, this may have worked to the financial benefit of Prudential and, in terms of professional advancement, Hoffman himself.

Beyond its immediate actuarial implications, however, Hoffman's disqualification of Blacks from the insurantial imaginary arguably wrought additional harms. Ewald writes that the "insurantial imaginary" can also be a "political imaginary."[212] This is in part because it establishes a form of collective human control over the vicissitudes of fortune. Most of all, however, it is because the institution of insurance calls the collective itself into being: "The work of the insurer is, precisely, *to constitute [a] population* by selecting and dividing risks . . . mak[ing] each person a part of the whole . . . . the constitution of mutualities."[213] If the quintessential object of biopolitics is the population, then insurance, from the late nineteenth century on, is a biopolitical technology of white settler reproductive futurity, projecting the security of the included forms of life (and the vulnerability of the excluded) into successive generations. Hoffman's characterization of Black people as incapable of providence excludes them from this mutuality—an exclusion that still resonates today in the stratifications of health-care coverage and the racialized dichotomization of Medicare as legitimate benefit and Medicaid as stigmatized marker of dependency.[214]

While officially only pertaining to the privately constituted "population" of Prudential subscribers, *Race Traits* was one of the most influential treatments of the race question for the next few decades.[215] Justifying racial and economic domination and medical neglect in a climate of increasingly rampant white terror, Hoffman's actuarial analysis helped to establish a long-standing pattern of policy obstructions to African American families' intergenerational economic security.[216] Moreover, the treatise prefigured the broad exclusions and differential policy treatment of African Americans as the welfare state expanded over the first six decades of the twentieth century.[217]

W.E.B. Du Bois and Frederick Hoffman: Science Wars

Hammonds and Reverby posit a defining opposition between Hoffman's work and Du Bois's *The Philadelphia Negro*, arguing that the contention between the logic of inherent "race traits" and the latter's emphasis on social environment "would continue to frame explanations by public health experts."[218] Additionally, Du Bois responded directly to Hoffman. Seven months after its publication, Du Bois reviewed *Race Traits* in the *Annals of the American Academy of Political and Social Science*. The review's tone is measured; it opens with the generous statement that given the increased interest in social scientific treatments of the "Negro Question," *Race Traits* will be "welcomed as one of the first fruits of this interest."[219] Nevertheless, the review ultimately judges the text "of doubtful value," a product of poor scientific work and multifariously misleading.[220] Hoffman's data is flawed, argues Du Bois. He writes that "most persons will at the outset be disposed to criticize the air of perfect conviction that pervades Mr. Hoffman's conclusions and . . . would feel surer of the author's fairness and judgment if he candidly admitted the contingent character of his broader conclusions."[221] There are methodological problems as well; Du Bois cites apparently well-known doubts about the accuracy of the Eleventh Census, and the fact that urban statistics do not reflect the vital conditions of the still-rural majority of Blacks—these data constituted two of Hoffman's principal sources.[222] "Much light and emphasis have undoubtedly been thrown on many points by his numerous and well-arranged tables," Du Bois writes, but "Mr. Hoffman has by no means avoided the many fallacies of the statistical method."[223] More archly, Du Bois continues, "this method is after all nothing but the application of logic to counting, and no amount of counting will justify a departure from the severe rules of correct reasoning."[224]

Du Bois uses international comparisons to cast doubt on Hoffman's conclusions that African Americans are moving inexorably toward extinction. "Throughout this discussion," he writes, "Mr. Hoffman continually forgets that he is comparing two special classes, the one usually vigorous and intelligent the other with unusual disadvantages [urban Black people]." And yet Hoffman bases his claims on a comparison of each population's relative increase, failing to note that, in fact, "compared with most modern nations the decennial increase of American Negroes has been large . . . higher than the decennial increase of England and Wales."[225] Moreover, even conceding the "immense infant death-rate" and overall "dangerous excess" mortality of urban Blacks that Hoffman's statistics demonstrate, "one cannot . . . agree with the author that this excessive death-rate threatens the extinction of the race. Compared with death-rates elsewhere it is not remarkable."[226] Making pointed reference to the European extraction that Hoffman cites as proof of his own objectivity, Du Bois continues:

> Mr. Hoffman knows that the large cities of his own German fatherland showed an average death rate of 27.50 in 1880–85, and some cities like Munich, a rate as high as 32.80 in 1878–80. Indeed Montreal, Naples, Belfast, Buda-Pesth, Breslau and Madrid, all have shown within a few years, death-rates which equal and often surpass that of American Negroes in cities. Moreover it may be doubted if the sanitary conditions of the Negro portions of Southern cities are, on the whole, as good as the conditions in the above-mentioned municipalities.[227]

Returning to the point about Hoffman's focus on the urban population, Du Bois criticizes Hoffman's extrapolations; he insists that "no careful student would think of judging the death-rate of Germany from that of Munich. . . . Yet Mr. Hoffman commits very similar mistakes; he bases his arguments as to the threatened extinction of the Negro almost solely on city death-rates, and argues that an increase in these death-rates means an increase in the general Negro death-rate. Such logic would be erroneous, even if Mr. Hoffman proved that, following the recent rush of Negroes into cities, their death-rate there had increased. Even this point, however, the author assumes on insufficient proof."[228] Du Bois similarly dismisses Hoffman's emphasis on out-of-wedlock births, noting that "Rome, Munich, Vienna, Stockholm, Paris, and Brussels have all shown more startling percentages of illegitimacy than the Negroes of Washington" and that Washington is not necessarily representative.[229]

As for the allegedly increased criminality and improvidence of Black people, Du Bois foregrounds evidence that conduces to alternate readings of Hoffman's own data. First, Du Bois points out, Blacks are not a monolithic mass: these are "not facts pertaining to 'the race' but to its various classes, which development since emancipation has differentiated."[230] Moreover, crime is no "race tendency" but the fruit of a systematic thwarting of legitimate attempts at advancement: as "a dogged Anglo-Saxon prejudice had shut nearly every avenue of advancement in their faces, the energies of many undoubtedly found an avenue in crime." Beyond these considerations, "the criminal statistics" themselves "raise the whole question as to how far black and white malefactors are subjected to different standards of justice."[231] As to the question of improvidence, Du Bois writes, most Blacks' current state of poverty should be unsurprising, given their situation after the war. In fact, reversing Hoffman's conclusion, Du Bois argues that Blacks' modest accumulation of property, demonstrated by Hoffman's own statistics, in fact testifies to a remarkable degree of thrift and hard work in deeply difficult circumstances. Overall, he concludes, Hoffman's treatise brings together some new and important data, but its conclusions are of little value, as they lack the "careful study and deep insight" that these questions require.[232] And they are based on "the unscientific use of the statistical method."[233] The work, perhaps more than anything, points up the need for better scientific work: Du Bois thus calls for a federal "Department of Negro Statistics in 1900, and . . . careful monographic study of the Negro in limited localities and from particular points of view."[234]

Du Bois assumed the editorship of the *Atlanta University Studies* the year this review was published, overseeing precisely the kind of fine-grained sociological study of African American life he called for.[235] Moreover, he was already in the midst of the intensive study of urban Black life that would become *The Philadelphia Negro*. Using just the comparative data that Hoffman neglects, Du Bois emphatically refutes the disappearance hypothesis: "That the Negro death rate at present is anything that threatens the extinction of the race is either the bugbear of the untrained or the wish of the timid."[236] Missing from both the review and Du Bois's contemporaneous sociology, however, is any comment on Hoffman's depiction of unwed Black mothers' pathogenic immorality. In fact, as Kevin Gaines argues, *The Philadelphia Negro* prominently features "a problematic linkage of poverty and immorality," blaming especially "the absence of the patriarchal black family."[237] Du Bois, like Hoffman, diagnoses a "lack of respect for the marriage bond" that caused "sexual looseness . . . adultery and prostitution" in poor urban Blacks.[238] While vehemently contesting Hoffman's conclusions, Du Bois largely echoed his characterization of unwed lower-class Black women as dangers to the social body.

As Khalil Gibran Muhammad makes clear, however, Du Bois was no lone voice in contesting the self-satisfied racial innocence of Hoffman and his ilk. He was part of a cohort of educated middle-class and elite young Black women and men who, within the shadow of the racial nadir, "used their pedigrees and talents as personal testimonies to the race's infinite capacity for citizenship and excellence."[239] Among the Black women who contested such harmful racist, sexist, and classist interpretations of data at the time were Mary Church

Terrell, to whose writings we turn in chapter 3, and her cofounders of the National Association of Colored Women (NACW). Treva Lindsey situates Terrell and her NACW colleagues' interventions within a polyvocal movement toward New Negro Womanhood, which comprised a wide range of strategies, praxes, and rhetorics, and combined calls for greater gender and sexual autonomy with refutations of racist and misogynist stereotypes: "Within a New Negro women's ethos, freedom from ideas about the inherent hypersexuality of black women as well as freedom from sexual norms and conventions intertwined."[240] NACW cofounder Ida B. Wells drew on statistical science itself as a political strategy. While not tracking infant mortality, Wells's pathbreaking statistical studies of lynching took powerful aim at the white supremacist gender mythologies on which Hoffman rested his case; her bold analyses markedly diverged from the masculinist elitism of Du Bois's writings of this era as well.

As Joy James writes, "Wells-Barnett critiqued the racial-sexual politics of interracial sex and the duplicity of the legal system and its complicity in lynchings in language few male or female race leaders dared to use."[241] Wells's fiery editorial in the aftermath of the 1892 Memphis lynching of her friends Thomas Moss, Calvin McDowell, and Henry Stewart—and the local journals' deceptive coverage of the atrocity—declared that "nobody in this section of the country believes the old thread-bare lie that Negro men rape white women. If Southern white men are not careful, they will overreach themselves . . . a conclusion will then be reached which will be very damaging to the moral reputation of their women."[242] Forced into exile, her press destroyed, in the wake of this editorial's publication, Wells undertook a massive project of data gathering, synthesis, and analysis that not only substantiated this claim but laid the groundwork for decades of anti-lynching politics. While she was not a trained sociologist, Wells was clearly in dialogue with the emergent social science of the day and its implications within a climate of intensifying anti-Black racial terror. As she writes archly in the preface of her second anti-lynching pamphlet, *A Red Record*: "The student of American sociology will find the year 1894 marked by a pronounced awakening of the public consciousness to a system of anarchy and outlawry which had grown . . . to be so common, that scenes of unusual brutality failed to have any visible effect upon the humane sentiments of the people of our land."

Jacqueline Goldsby argues that "*A Red Record* exploits the credibility of sociological empiricism," pointing up the failings of purportedly neutral reporting of "facts" in terms that inure readers to the human lives, the unspeakable violence and the suffering, behind the numbers. While Wells's accounts drew prestige from the scientific objectivity that her fin de siècle readers ascribed to statistics, her framings and narrations were designed to stir rather than inure. Lynching reportage in the white press was part of the problem; Wells "remodel[ed] its conventions . . . to recuperate news writing's value as an ethically motivated source of public power."[243] Muhammad observes that it would have been nearly impossible for Hoffman not to know of Wells's work, as they were each developing their statistical innovations during these years—including drawing on the same lynching data—albeit toward opposite ends; needless to say, he did not cite her.[244]

Anna Julia Cooper, philosopher, educator, and clubwoman alongside Terrell and Wells-Barnett, attended directly to health and mortality statistics. Cooper called attention to the racism that underpinned allegedly objective scientific work and drew conclusions that supported her agenda of social reform. Situating Cooper within a scientific and political context shaped by Hoffman's "objective" prognostications and Francis Galton's eugenic philosophy, Vivian May writes that at numerous points in *Voice from the South*, "Cooper suggests that both the scientific method and quantitative forms of measurement, especially statistics and assessment testing, often serve as masks for biased preconceptions and bigoted cultural assumptions . . . showing repeatedly that seemingly neutral perception is patently biased."[245] In

Cooper's essay "What Are We Worth?" she situates Washington, DC's Black infant mortality statistics—the same data-set that Hoffman would draw on—within the broader environment of state-sanctioned poverty, segregation, and unsanitary conditions. She thus prefigures Du Bois's own insistence, contrary to Hoffman's contentions, on environmental causes rather than inherent racial traits. She uses these statistics to indict the structural violence of Jim Crow property regime, with white landlords bearing particular culpability, and to ground an urgent call for wealthier Blacks to redistribute wealth toward better living conditions for their impoverished brethren.[246] Cooper not only prescribed this to her readers but joined theory to praxis herself as part of Washington, DC's Alley Sanitation Committee.[247]

James observes that even as Du Bois's own analysis came to depart quite radically from the Victorian paternalism of these earlier writings, his problematic gender politics persisted in new ways. While Du Bois drew on the intellectual work of Wells and Cooper, he largely failed to cite them. As noted at greater length in chapter 2, even as Du Bois came to espouse what James terms a "profeminist politics," both his written work and his organizing tended to erase, rather than uplift, the "achievements of women such as Cooper and Wells-Barnett from the political landscape."[248] Those achievements by Terrell, Cooper, Wells-Barnett, and their political women contemporaries are thus even more stunning, given that they contended with masculinist obstructions from "Race Men" like Du Bois alongside the racist and misogynist harms and deflections encoded in the "cult of true babyhood."

From Science to Rhetoric

In a speech to the American Academy of Political and Social Sciences in November 1897, Du Bois summed up his devotion to scientific investigation: "true lovers of humanity can only hold higher the pure ideals of science, and continue to insist that if we would solve a problem we must study it."[249] Two years later, however, David Levering-Lewis writes that Du Bois experienced a crisis of faith in the power of objective science. Once optimistic about the power of scientific work to dispel irrational prejudices and racial mythologies, Du Bois had begun to feel deflated in the face of a hardening "national white consensus," newly bolstered with scientific authority, that Blacks were less than fully human. As Du Bois recounts in his autobiographical *Dusk of Dawn*, the lynching of Sam Hose in Atlanta in 1899 gave this consensus brutal immediacy:

> At the very time when my studies were most successful, there cut across this plan which I had as a scientist, a red ray which could not be ignored . . . a poor Negro in central Georgia, Sam Hose, had killed his landlord's wife. I wrote out a careful and reasoned statement concerning the evident facts and started down to the Atlanta Constitution office. . . . On the way news met me: Sam Hose had been lynched, and they said that his knuckles were on exhibition at a grocery store farther down on Mitchell Street, along which I was walking. I turned back to the University. Two considerations thereafter broke in upon my work and eventually disrupted it; first, one could not be a calm, cool, and detached scientist while Negroes were lynched, murdered and starved; and secondly, there was no such demand for scientific work of the sort that I was doing.

In the wake of this event, Du Bois felt that he could no longer confine himself to the tower of academe, at a sterile distance from these horrors, generating objective data for an audience whose interest was dubious at best.[250] Two months after Hose's lynching, Burghardt Gomer Du Bois died of diphtheria at the age of two. In the wake of these two deaths, Cornel West writes, Du Bois's "Enlightenment worldview faltered."[251]

Du Bois did not give up on scientific pursuits; however the *Atlanta University Studies* continued. But Levering-Lewis casts *Souls of Black Folk* precisely as the fruit of Du Bois's new commitment to additional tactics. Although Levering-Lewis does not cite it here, Hoffman's text was a prominent and influential synthesis of the "ethos, science, and propaganda of racial dehumanization" he posits Du Bois sought to challenge.[252] Now, Levering-Lewis recounts, Du Bois "resolved to write of the genius, humanity, and enviable destiny of his race with such passion, eloquence, and penetration that the claims of African-American inferiority would be sent reeling, never to recover full legitimacy and vitality."[253] The loss of Burghardt occurred in the midst of Du Bois's turn toward more directly persuasive approaches. His rhetoric of paternal loss in the context of the cult of true babyhood, and its claims to white innocence, is the focus of the next chapter.

2 Three Forms of Innocence in W.E.B. Du Bois's "Of the Passing of the First-Born"

In January 1897, when his review of Frederick Hoffman's *Race Traits and Tendencies of the American Negro* was published, W.E.B. Du Bois was not yet a father; his wife, Nina Gomer Du Bois, was not yet a mother. Living in Philadelphia, that spring would see the beginning of Gomer Du Bois's pregnancy. On October 3, their son, Burghardt, was born at Du Bois's mother's house in Great Barrington, Massachusetts. The following year, Du Bois accepted a position at Atlanta University and the young family moved south to that city. Burghardt turned one in Atlanta and continued to grow and thrive over the southern spring, against a background of stark segregation and racial terror.[1] When Burghardt was eighteen months old, he contracted diphtheria.[2] After his parents faced a devastating denial of medical care, Burghardt died on May 22, 1899. Holding a small funeral for him in Atlanta, his parents took his body back to Massachusetts for burial. "Of the Passing of the First-Born," the eleventh chapter of *The Souls of Black Folk*, is Du Bois's elegy for his beloved son.

The shortest chapter in the book, the elegy is a portrait of parental adoration and agonized bereavement. It is a paean to Burghardt's beauty and being, the divine force of life that his father beheld in him. And it is a bitterly observed comment on the spreading poison of the color line that works to negate beauty, to extinguish life, and to deal death and horror in many forms. Beyond and through the interweave of these elements, the elegy is also a striking account of innocence. More precisely, in the text Du Bois stages an interplay between three forms of innocence. The first, most fully and delicately rendered, is Burghardt's innocence. Described in terms of Burghardt's infantine vision and being, this allows readers a window into the expansive orientation to joy, interconnection, and belonging that is the birthright of every human yet is warped and thwarted by the forced imposition of the color line. While deploying some of the prevailing sentimental tropes of infant and child innocence that, as discussed in chapter 1, underpinned the white "cult of true babyhood," Du Bois's account far exceeds a mere rendering of his baby in terms acceptable to a white readership. Through his account of Burghardt's innocence, Du Bois also invokes the innocence of his own childhood and its destruction by racism as a lifelong assault on the soul.

Du Bois juxtaposes this true innocence with the racial innocence of the whites who appear briefly but consequentially on Burghardt's funeral day. These passers-by look upon the beflowered funeral procession, at the sorrow of the bereaved parents, and render it ugly with a word—refusing to comprehend the shared pain and death that would both connect them to human life and loss across the color line and demand accountability for a violent system. This scene replays in key ways Du Bois's own early initiation into the cruelties of the color line. In both cases, whites' casual, almost reflexive reinforcement of the color line and refusal to countenance the damage that they inflict accords with Baldwin's indictment of white innocence, as the foundational disavowal that both denies and perpetuates the massive destruction of Black life. Also in both cases, the white feminine plays a key role.

If these two forms of innocence might be said to stand in clear opposition to one another, the third form of innocence in the elegy is more politically paradoxical. This is Nina Gomer Du Bois's feminine and maternal innocence. Rendered a perfect angel of the hearth, strikingly concordant with the standards of "true womanhood," "girl-wife" Gomer Du Bois speaks only one line in the elegy, just after Burghardt's death. This more troubling form of innocence hearkens to the childlike associations of the word. Du Bois writes in his autobiography that his wife was devastated by the loss, but in the elegy her pain remains unarticulated and backgrounded.[3] Gomer Du Bois's "true womanly" innocence potentially invited elite white readers to see their own experiences mirrored in that of the Du Bois family, thus attuning them to both the devastation of this loss and the injustice of its circumstances. Yet Du Bois's expansive account of infantine innocence as compassing the interrelatedness of being here takes on a more constrained character that both shades into respectability and resonates with his professional patterns of feminine silencing.

Yet the elegy also contains elements that militate against this masculinist Victorian propriety. In the interplay between Du Bois's own "crushed" boyhood innocence and the preservation of Burghardt's innocence through his early death, Du Bois articulates an anguished ambivalence. Contrasting sharply with prevailing white paternal conventions of bereavement, this equivocal grief situates him in a tradition in Black political thinking and rhetoric, largely authored and focalized through Black mothers, of political ambivalence regarding the death of children. As Wangui Muigai shows, this tradition posits these deaths as at once an unspeakable loss and a release from the conditions of war on Black life under US white supremacy and racial capitalism.[4] I consider the ways that his particular expressions of ambivalence both align with and depart from this lineage. In this chapter I offer a brief summary of the elegy. I explore each of the three valences of innocence and then turn to Du Bois's ambivalence and to the elegy's relation to this Black maternal lineage of diagnosis and response to the necropolitical conditions into which Black infants in the United States are born.

Burghardt's Elegy

Du Bois's account of paternal loss opens with a dual reference to the maternal. Nearly every chapter of *The Souls of Black Folk* pairs a European poem with a Sorrow Song from the Black American tradition. "Of the Passing" pairs "Itylus" by Charles Swinburne—from a Greek myth, in the voice of a bereaved mother who, mourning a slain child, has been turned into a nightingale—with the spiritual, "I hope my mother will be there in that beautiful world on high." Both of these citations invoke the actual or prospective death of a child, and the chapter's narrative itself begins with a biblical allusion to a birth that is already bound to sacrifice. As David Levering-Lewis and Shamoon Zamir both point out, the chapter's opening lines cast Burghardt's birth in eschatological terms: "Unto you a child is born."[5]

Du Bois's response is vertiginous. He writes: "the fear of fatherhood mingled wildly with the joy of creation." Yet he also styles himself the secular public man, "unconsciously wandering" at a distance from the "sanctuary" of the birth chamber. Nina Gomer Du Bois, unnamed in the chapter, is the pious, chaste, and all-giving heart of the home; the new father, speeding home, thinks "in awe" of her womanly sacrifice, of she "who at my bidding had offered itself to win a life, and won." On his arrival, her "wan" face testifying to the depth of this ordeal, Du Bois finds her reclining on the "altar" on which this offering had been made, his Madonna and child.[6] A stranger to the mysteries of the nursery, he wonders, "perplexed," at "this tiny formless thing . . . all head and voice," and deems it at first "a ludicrous thing to love." Emphatically not so, however, his "girl-mother": "her I loved . . . she whom I now saw unfolding like the glory of the morning—the transfigured woman."[7] This glory lights the way to his own transfiguration: it is "through her [that] I came to love the wee thing, as it grew and waxed strong; as its little soul unfolded itself . . . and as its eyes caught the gleam and flash of life. How beautiful he was, with his olive-tinted flesh and dark gold ringlets, his eyes of mingled blue and brown, his perfect little limbs, and the soft voluptuous roll which the blood of Africa had moulded into his features." The first movement of the elegy is in some ways a conversion story, a story of falling in a sacred love, becoming alive to his son's own unique and particular being. Du Bois writes that "we were not far from worshipping this revelation of the divine, my wife and I."[8]

The chapter is a play of shadow and light, and a gloomier passage narrates the family's sojourn in the South. After this celebratory description of Burghardt's beauty, Du Bois's register shifts from adoration to ambivalence: "Why was his hair tinted with gold? An evil omen was golden hair in my life. Why had the brown of his eyes not crushed out the blue? For brown were his father's eyes, and his father's father's. And thus in the Land of the Color-Line I saw, as it fell across my baby, the shadow of the Veil."[9] This shadow, which has shaped Du Bois's own parental perceptions, augurs only crushing cruelty and constraint under a racial rule that grants neither true personhood nor liberty to its Black citizens: "Within the Veil was he born, said I; and there within shall he live,—a Negro and a Negro's son. Holding in that little head—ah, bitterly!—he unbowed pride of a hunted race, clinging with that tiny dimpled hand—ah, wearily!—to a hope not hopeless but unhopeful, and seeing with those bright wondering eyes that peer into my soul a land whose freedom is to us a mockery and whose liberty a lie."

Yet the family nevertheless creates a space of soft and protective nurturance. Du Bois, quelling for the moment "the unvoiced terror of [his] life," shows Burghardt the twinkling stars. Gomer Du Bois dedicates herself to maternal duties: "Her own life builded and moulded itself upon the child; he tinged her every dream and idealized her every effort. No hands but hers must touch and garnish those little limbs . . . no voice but hers could coax him off to Dreamland."[10] Moreover, the bright revelations of Burghardt's being extend beyond the domestic space into his encounters with his broader milieu. Burghardt is "sturdy and masterful . . . filled with bubbling life." He moves in reciprocal fascination and wonder with his expanding world, and "the world" itself "loved him" too.[11] All who encounter him are enchanted— women, men, and children alike—and he adores them in return, his joyful embrace yet unencumbered by the color line's divisions.

This sunny time comes to a devastating end. While not mentioned in the elegy itself, a white mob tortured and lynched Black Atlanta resident Sam Hose in April 1899, mere months after the Du Bois family arrived in the city.[12] Less than a month later, Burghardt contracted the illness that would end his own short life. Death comes most literally in the form of diphtheria, which Hoffman, ironically, had characterized as a "civilized" "white" ailment. The elegy does not mention this ailment but narrates the anguished weeks as Burghardt sickens and begins to waste away. The anxious parents do all that they can, and Du Bois himself, as Burghardt reaches a crisis, seeks in vain for medical care in that segregated city. The ministrations of the "gray physician" are futile, and Burghardt breathes his last on the morning of May 22, 1899.[13]

The parents are struck down by this loss. Gomer Du Bois, "the world's most piteous thing—a childless mother," "writhe[s]" in the "chamber of death." Du Bois at first rails against death's invasion of his "one little coign of happiness," his one refuge within the cold "dull land that stretches its sneering web about me".[14] He then shifts registers; in one of the most striking passages of the elegy, Du Bois writes of the "awful gladness in [his] heart" that, in leaving earthly life so early, Burghardt escaped the manifold deaths that the white world held in store: "my soul whispers ever to me saying, 'not dead, not dead, but escaped; not bond, but free." No bitter meanness now shall sicken his baby heart till it die a living death, no taunt shall madden his happy boyhood. Fool was I to think or wish that this little soul should grow choked and deformed within the veil.".[15]

After articulating this ambivalence, however, Du Bois reconsiders, musing that "he might have borne the load more lightly than we." Yet when the bereaved parents hold a small funeral, it is marred by just such a corrosive instance of "bitter meanness": "Blithe was the morning of his burial, with bird and song and sweet-smelling flowers. . . . And yet it seemed a ghostly unreal day. . . . We seemed to rumble down an unknown street behind a little white bundle of posies, with the shadow of a song in our ears. The busy city dinned about us; they did not say much, those pale-faced hurrying men and women; they did not say much,—they only glanced and said, 'N———!'"[16] Unwilling to bury their son in this hostile place, where even "the earth is so strangely red," the parents depart for Massachusetts to bury their baby there instead. Du Bois ends the elegy envisioning rejoining with his son after his own death, the two meeting again "above the veil."

Burghardt's Innocence/Du Bois's Innocence

"Innocence" appears only twice in *The Souls of Black Folk*, neither time in chapter 11. Yet the chapter is rife with signifiers of Burghardt's innocence. First, there is the innocence and truth of his perception, which, as yet untainted by the color line, witnesses the truth of human interconnection and innate worthiness of attention and love. This is expressed most consistently through descriptions of Burghardt's visuality, both his way of looking and his eyes themselves. Closely associated with this perceptual innocence is the innocence of his being, his as-yet undisturbed dignity and at-homeness in the world, the "wild pride of being," that racism has done its best to destroy in Du Bois himself.

Burghardt's innocence expresses of the "joy of creation" that pulses through Du Bois—albeit intermixed with fear—at the news of his son's birth. A kind of species-being, it manifests the true and unspoiled interconnectedness between human souls and with their broader environments. Finally, there is the innocence of his physical being. In his depiction of Burghardt's beauty and vitality, Du Bois borrows from, but complicates and redeploys, key features of the cult of true babyhood, including iconic golden hair and blue eyes. In dwelling on the physical features of his son's baby perfection, Du Bois resignifies purity: from the obsessions with blood of Hoffman and his ilk to the promise of transcendent hybridity. The etymology of "innocence" comes to the fore here. *Innocent* derives from the Latin *innocentem* . . . "not guilty, blameless; harmless"; before its medieval Christian association with childhood, at its foundation it is the negation of *nocere*, harm. Furthermore, the Indo-European root of *nocere* is *nek*—death. The elegy's depiction of Burghardt's innocence is thus also a meditation on life against death in its many forms.

Burghardt's Gaze

Burghardt's blue-brown eyes are in a sense the fixed stars around which the chapter turns. Before speeding to the birth chamber at the chapter's opening, Du Bois ponders how his baby would look and feel: "I wondered . . . what were its eyes." They are innocently penetrating: "bright wondering eyes that peer into my soul." Even as a tiny infant, Burghardt's "eyes caught the gleam and flash of life." Others, too, found this infant gaze transfixing: "men looked gravely into his wonderful eyes." And as mother and father stood beside his little deathbed, Burghardt "turned toward us with great eyes" and they knew that death was near. After the death, Du Bois reflects: "I might have known that yonder deep unworldly look that ever and anon floated past his eyes was peering beyond this narrow Now."[17] As the final passage makes clear, Du Bois is elegizing not only Burghardt's physical eyes but his way of looking. While, as discussed below, the Veil has woven itself irreversibly into Du Bois's own optical faculty, Burghardt does not yet see the painful deception of the "land whose freedom is to us a mockery and whose liberty a lie." He simply "watched the world with wondering thoughtfulness," for "he knew no color line . . . the Veil, though it shadowed him, had not yet darkened half his sun. He loved the white matron, the loved his black nurse; and in his little world walked souls alone, uncolored and unclothed."[18]

Burghardt's innocent infantine vision invokes Du Bois's own sunny outlook in babyhood, before the color line cleaved soul from soul. This association is bolstered by the description, near the close of the elegy, of Burghardt's life as "perfect . . . sweet as a summer's day beside the Housatonic." This geographical reference recalls the author's brief description, in the book's first chapter, of his own childhood loss of innocence on the banks of that river: "It is in the early days of rollicking boyhood that the revelation first bursts upon one, all in a day, as it were. I remember well when the shadow swept across me. I was a little thing, away up in the hills of New England, where the dark Housatonic winds . . ." We will return to that particular brutal revelation in its connection to the white passers-by at the funeral. Yet locating the moment not only in time, when Du Bois was young schoolchild few years older than Burghardt, but also in space, on the banks of that river, is significant. In the opening chapter, Du Bois mentions the Housatonic only in association with the falling of the color line's shadow. In the elegy, through the simile between Burghardt's "perfect life" and the sweet "summer's day beside the Housatonic," Du Bois offers the reader a glimpse of his own childhood's joyful perception "before the Veil." Burghardt's eyes thus have a redemptive quality. The realities of the racial state have rendered impossible this innocence of perception in Du Bois himself, alchemizing his original vision into "second-sight." Through his narration of Burghardt's innocent way of seeing, Du Bois accesses, and offers the reader, a glimpse of his own innocence before the cruel incursion of the color line.

The existential truth of Burghardt's vision, which the edifice of the racial state is designed to disavow and destroy, is preserved by death in this innocent before.[19] This points in turn toward the possibility of a future political optic after the Veil: "when men ask of the workman, not 'Is he white?' but 'Can he work?' When men ask artists, not 'Are they black?' but 'Do they know?'" Du Bois's "awful gladness," then, is in part about the preservation of this way of seeing.[20] As we see below, Du Bois dramatizes the ways that the color line has woven itself inextricably into his own vision. Yet he is able to witness the world anew for a time, through Burghardt's "great eyes."

Burghardt's Being

Burghardt's unhindered vision arises from his unconstrained mode of being; just as he has not learned to see himself as "a problem," he has not yet had to inhabit the "strange experience" of being one. This hearkens back, as in the case of his vision, to the very first page of *Souls*, where Du Bois the father writes that "except perhaps in babyhood, and in Europe," his "problem" status has ever stood between himself and the white world. Just as the elegy reclaims the Housatonic landscape in a kind of redemptive circuit, the elegy links the baby Du Bois, undescribed in the pages of *Souls*, with the closely observed and adored baby Burghardt. In witnessing his son's expansive embrace of the world, Du Bois himself is taken back to that original oneness with creation, which the racial order has stolen from him.

This originary interconnectedness is linked in the essay to *love*. Du Bois signals his separation from this oceanic feeling as he initially finds this tiny new being "ludicrous to love." Du Bois enters the postpartum scene at a perplexed emotional distance from the "winking, breathing, and sneezing" newborn.[21] He writes that it is through his husbandly love for his wife that he comes to love Burghardt in body and soul.[22] Du Bois's descriptions of his son track this progression:

from an alien "wee thing" that he designates as "it," to a particular soul unfolding, to the exultant emphasis on the baby as both physically comely and male: "How beautiful *he* was." This gateway to fatherly devotion parallels prevailing civilizational notions of hetero-patriarchal matrimony, reinscribing love as the refined ambit of more developed "races."[23] Yet if it is this respectable love that initially enables his expanding appreciation of Burghardt as a distinct and precious life, the notion of love throughout the rest of the essay expresses something far less contained: an unbroken reciprocity between beings.[24]

Burghardt loved the world, and "the world loved him." Aligning with his vision, his love is not yet tainted with the categories of the color line; its expansive reach remains unhindered. He thus loved indiscriminately: "He loved the white matron, he loved his black nurse; and in his little world walked souls alone, uncolored and unclothed." Among adult humans, Du Bois represents expressions of this love along unsurprising gender conventions, echoing the domestic division between Du Bois and Gomer Du Bois. Yet this interchange was not limited to men and women; children, too, sensed his gifts and "hovered and fluttered about him." Nor is it limited to human connection, but expands out to other beings in his world; he loved also the "great green trees." These in turn seem to observe and mourn his passing; "the great green trees he loved, stood motionless" at the moment of his soul's departure. Though only a year old, Burghardt is drawn to beauty more broadly; after his passing, Gomer Du Bois comforts herself by saying: "He will be happy [in heaven]; he ever loved beautiful things." The love that Burghardt both emanates and invites returns to Du Bois a horizon of possibility that the father's own serial injuries had seemed to foreclose.

If, as argued above, Du Bois's anguished ambivalence is in part about the preservation of his son's precious innocence of vision, it is also about preserving that originary state of love in and with the world. Unlike Du Bois, Burghardt's innocence as interconnectedness is preserved; he will never have to experience white society's cruel shredding of this birthright of belonging. Du Bois writes: "In the poise of his curl-crowned head did there not sit all the wild pride of being which his father had hardly crushed in his own heart? . . . Well sped, my boy, before the world had dubbed your ambition insolence, had held your ideals unattainable, and taught you to cringe and bow. Better far this nameless void that stops my life than a sea of sorrow for you."[25]

Du Bois quickly pivots to recant these words, saying that Burghardt "might have borne his burden more bravely than we,—aye, and found it lighter too, some day; for surely, surely this is not the end." Even in the face of this terrible loss, Burghardt has left a mark on his father with his innocence of being, his expansive interconnectedness, his love: "I—yea, all men—are larger and purer by the infinite breadth of that one little life."

Burghardt's Body

Burghardt's beauty is not only metaphysical. It is also expressed in his bodily being, in his "gleam and flash of life," which the elegy again and again renders in its everyday divinity. Against prevailing white supremacist civilizational and evolutionary notions of racial purity, Du Bois deliberately thematizes Burghardt's beauty and strength as expressing the promise of his hybrid lineage. Like his way of seeing, Burghardt's physicality itself has a redemptive quality; the sexual violence that his admixture of African and European features bespeaks is nevertheless washed clean in Burghardt's innocent being—echoing the messianic language of the opening. Hybridity was politically charged when Du Bois wrote *Souls*. For Hoffman and other race scientists, racial mixing was allegedly responsible for African American moribundity. The law of the land confirmed this consensus: in 1883's *Pace v. Alabama*, the Supreme Court unanimously upheld state anti-miscegenation laws, holding that "amalgamation of the two races, produc[es] a mongrel population and a degraded civilization."[26] As Juliet Hooker writes: "All strands of scientific racism" at the time "coincided that miscegenation led to degeneration and that crossing between so-called superior and inferior races should be avoided at all costs."[27]

Against this consensus, Du Bois depicts Burghardt as a vital embodiment of racial mixture. Golden curls and blue eyes were the trademarks of juvenile innocence and purity in the day's sentimental literature.[28] Du Bois appropriates these features to glowingly depict his son: "his olive-tinted flesh and dark gold ringlets, his eyes of mingled blue and brown, his perfect little limbs, and the soft voluptuous roll which the blood of Africa had moulded into his features."[29] This description emphasizes hybridity with increasing intensity: "dark gold" moves slightly away from convention, and the mingled colors are suggestive, but the "blood of Africa" is unequivocal. Burghardt radiantly embodies the dual heritage that the white world would simultaneously deny and condemn to death. In direct contrast to Hoffman's claims that "the mulatto is . . . of all races the one possessed of the least vital force," Burghardt is magnificently vital.[30] He is "sturdy and masterful . . . filled with bubbling life." This depiction contrasts the more somber play of color in the "gray physician" who fails to save Burghardt's life. While also neither Black nor white, the gray represents a kind of deathly blurring, in contrast to Burghardt's golden radiance.

This depiction of Burghardt replicates in prose Du Bois's pointed inclusion of light-skinned African American babies and children in his early twentieth-century photographs. Evelynn Hammonds argues that "Du Bois used . . . photography, to make visible the evidence of race mixing that white society denied."[31] Such evidence threw into doubt clearly legible racial categories as well as the degeneration hypothesis.[32] Burghardt's eyes are not only—like the photographs—category-blurring in their coloration, however, but materialize the transcendent and redemptive qualities of his own infant gaze. While sharing in the images' political claims about actually existing hybridity, the elegy also points toward the transformative prospects of hybridity for a more just and truthful polity. This aspiration finds an echo in chapter 14 of *Souls of Black Folk*, which casts racial mixing as the corporeal aspect of a nation that must be affirmed as the collaborative work of Blacks and whites: "Actively we have woven ourselves with the very warp and woof of the nation,—we fought their battles, shared their sorrow, mingled our blood with theirs, and generation after generation have pleaded with a headstrong, careless people to despise not Justice, Mercy, and Truth."[33] Melvin Rogers points out that Du Bois here "projects a vision of the nation (now hybridized) that might be born anew."[34] Burghardt, in his "wild pride of being," embodies the nascent hope of that hybrid nation.

This celebratory description of Burghardt's racial mixture thus prefigures what Hooker calls Du Bois's "mulatto fictions" such as those in 1920's *Darkwater* and the 1928 novel *Dark Princess*, in which "representations of mixture enable Du Bois to imagine (and, he hoped, thereby facilitate the construction of) alternate, better worlds . . . racial utopias that dare to imagine a world not dominated or defined by whiteness."[35] In both his aspect and his innocent perspective, Burghardt embodies the promise of such a world. Claudia Tate connects the elegy for Burghardt and *Dark Princess*; she characterizes the birth of the mixed-race messiah to the Black American protagonist and his royal South Asian mate in the latter as a "grandiose repetition" of Burghardt's birth and the "prophetic aspirations" that accompanied it.[36] In both cases the "figurations of transgressions across the color line were indelibly bound up with questions of futurity."[37] The differences between them chart the shifts in Du Bois's terms of futurity itself, both geographical and political—from survival as part of the national future in "Of the Passing" to global, proto–Third World future in *Dark Princess*.

At the same time, Hooker notes that "the racial utopias depicted in [Du Bois's] mulatto fictions were rife with internal contradictions."[38] And indeed, some of the criticisms applied to these later writings on mixture complicate the elegy's subversive celebration of Burghardt's hybridity. Alys Weinbaum points out the heteronormative logics that underwrite Du Bois's representations of hybridity in the 1920s and the elegy likewise couches the family's mixed genealogies within an unimpeachably proper heterosexual union.[39] Du Bois's portrait of Burghardt also partakes in the colorism many critics have noted, even as it blurs racial categorizations. Tate observes: "Although Du Bois consciously racializes as dark the overdetermined feminine ideal in his creative writings, this intention is invaded by an effect of the white standard of female beauty . . . using as uplift symbols ideal dark women who are, in actuality, golden-hued."[40] As we will see, some of this bleaching is woven into Du Bois's idealized depiction of Nina Gomer Du Bois. Farah Jasmine Griffin likewise highlights the patriarchal colorism that pervades even Du Bois's most overtly feminist writings.[41] His photographic and textual iconographies of mixture in babies and children can be read similarly, largely conforming to white standards of appearance even as they blur the color line. Burghardt, scion of "black fathers," is nevertheless "golden-hued."

This celebration of hybridity is thus at least partially structured by masculinist and colorist hierarchies. Yet in casting Burghardt as a radiant embodiment of racial impurity, Du Bois counters allegations of Black moribundity. Like his vision, which sees the "uncolored" truth of souls, Burghardt's hybridity resignifies purity itself. Purity in this sense has nothing to do with bloodlines preserved from amalgamation; rather, it obviates the illusory boundary between whiteness and Blackness and binds beauty not to color but to life itself. It thus foreshadows Du Bois's later visions of a world where whiteness has lost its power both to divide and to conquer.

White Innocence: The Glance versus True Seeing

Having laid out the glory of what could be—what is manifest, if ephemerally, in Burghardt's boundless being—the elegy reveals passing whites' casually cruel dismissal of the funeral procession in its profound destructiveness. These whites' failure of vision is the vicious converse of Black citizens' "second-sight." These whites are unable to countenance both beauty and loss, life in its divine mystery. Their own story of innocence requires a denial of human interconnection. In the whites' benighted vision, there are no grieving parents, no family, no feeling, no funeral. Among Atlanta Black communities, families lost one of every four babies born in 1900. But for whites, too, funerals were terribly common; about one of every five white babies died before reaching their first year. This brings to mind Olúfẹ́mi O. Táíwò's principle of the violence of racial capitalism: "for every three children of theirs that [racial capitalism/colonial state power] kills, [it] will kill one of yours."[42]

White innocence requires a willful unseeing of this shared vulnerability and a profound disregard for both Black life and Black death that is also a disregard ultimately for all children, white children included, because even the latter's value and nondisposability is contingent on embodying the narrow normative characteristics bound up in the futurity of the racial state. This occluded white vision is marked in the elegy with the term "glance." This blinkered glance is the visual correlate of the "mockery and . . . lie" of the racial present and diametrically opposed to Burghardt's "far-seeing" eyes. The word "glance" appears five times in *Souls of Black Folk*. Two occurrences are neutral or warm.[43] Three uses, however, occur with particular relation to white innocence. Two of these glances come from white people, one in chapter 1 and one in "Of the Passing"; the third, also in "Of the Passing," is the glance of Du Bois himself. I discuss the first two instances in relation to one another, and then turn to the third.

The first occurrence is in the "calling-card incident" of chapter 1, ushering the young schoolboy Du Bois into the shadow of the color line. The second falls across Burghardt's beflowered casket and his grieving parents. Having evoked, through mention of the Housatonic and babyhood, Du Bois's own earliest years, there is likewise a notable resonance between these two forceful manifestations of white cruelty and unseeing.

In the incident in chapter 1:

In a wee wooden schoolhouse, something put it into the boys' and girls' heads to buy gorgeous visiting-cards—ten cents a package—and exchange. The exchange was merry, till one girl, a tall newcomer, refused my card,—refused it peremptorily, with a glance. Then it dawned upon me with a certain suddenness that I was different from the others; or like, mayhap, in heart and life and longing, but shut out from their world by a vast veil.[44]

And in chapter 11:

Blithe was the morning of his burial, with bird and song and sweet-smelling flowers. . . . And yet it seemed a ghostly unreal day,— the wraith of Life. We seemed to rumble down an unknown street behind a little white bundle of posies, with the shadow of a song in our ears. The busy city dinned about us; they did not say much, those pale-faced hurrying men and women; they did not say much,—they only glanced and said, "N____!"[45]

The first passage witnesses the innocent Du Bois among other boys and girls, joined together in the innocent extravagance of decorative cards bearing their names. The "tall newcomer" singles out Du Bois as pariah; his name-card unacceptable, his name obviated, his person unworthy of contact and social exchange. "With a glance" she unsees him as fellow child and schoolmate; "peremptorily," without the need for a second look or consideration. Her own purity, her white feminine innocence, requires the negation of his overture. In the name of this purity, she contaminates the actually innocent extension of the calling-card, rendering it an obscene overture to miscegenation. In so doing, Du Bois in turn learns that, to her eyes, he indeed reduces only to that threatening cypher. Her glancing eyes are the initiation into the "eyes of another," the unseeing glance of the whole imprisoning racial state edifice.

The first passage opens as "merry," the second morning, similarly, "blithe." But unlike his participation, until interrupted, in the merriment on that Massachusetts day, the grown Du Bois and his wife are estranged from the idyllic surroundings: haunted, out of joint with the glorious weather, disoriented in the city streets. It is in this vulnerable moment that the passing whites "glance" at the funeral procession. Failing to see the human loss and grief, the flowers on the tiny casket, just as the "tall newcomer" fails to see the young Du Bois, they dismiss the scene "peremptorily" as irrelevant to their own kind, unworthy of sympathy or being seen. Bringing to mind Baldwin's formulation of innocence—that white supremacist and racial capitalist social order is "destroying hundreds of thousands of lives, and they do not know it and do not want to know it"—their casual insult resounds as both abomination and denial. In both cases this white glance that self-servingly denies the shared realities of life across the color line contrasts sharply with the "all-seeing" vision of Burghardt (and by proxy the young Du Bois).

It is also significant that the hurrying passers-by include both men and women. As detailed below, Du Bois reinforces gender conventions through dualisms of space, sense, and action. Gomer Du

Bois is the keeper of the hearth, at home in the domestic, and communicates through touch and sound. In contrast, Du Bois's relationship with Burghardt revolves around the visual, extending into the prospect of prophetic vision and great acts to carry forward his paternal legacy. Outside the family among loving community, this duality holds as well; men, like Du Bois, look into Burghardt's "great eyes," but women "kissed his curls." The white passers-by at the funeral, however, are equally men and women out in public; like the tall newcomer, they refuse the souls before them in a public act of dismissal and disregard. The agency of white women as well as men is significant. At other moments in *Souls,* Du Bois praises white women, as in the missionary teachers in calico that flock to the post-Emancipation South.[46]

Conversely, it is white men whom Du Bois paints as most directly responsible for violence, as in the wealthy and dissolute father and son in the short fiction "Of the Coming of John," or the cruel clergymen in "Of Alexander Crummel" who thwart the young Crummel's strivings. Through these two *glances* and the resonances between them, however, the "glance" comes clear as a way of looking that preempts true seeing, and whose destructive power both white women and men equally wield. If Burghardt's gaze encompasses the truth of souls' fundamental interconnection, the glance is a technique of division that accords with, justifies, and bolsters the racial capitalist ranking of life: white—regardless of gender—makes right. This meaning coincides, though with a difference, with the third usage, occurring in the elegy. This is Du Bois's own glance as the family arrives in their new Southern home. As noted, after describing Burghardt's hybrid beauty, Du Bois's tone shifts to one of suspicion and estrangement: "I held him, and glanced at the hot red soil of Georgia and the breathless city of a hundred hills, and felt a vague unrest. Why was his hair tinted with gold? An evil omen was golden hair in my life. Why had not the brown of his eyes crushed out and killed the blue?—for brown were his father's eyes, and his father's father's."[47]

In dramatic counterpoint to his earlier appropriation of idealized white childhood's gold and blue, Du Bois now reverses their public significations of innocence. Gold no longer heralds the angelic but augurs "evil." And departing from the previous language of harmonious intermingling, the "blue" that should be "crushed" alludes to the history of white sexual terrorism—though as an antagonism between rival paternities, in terms that erase the maternal line and abstract from the embodied realities of rape and reproductive predation. Burghardt's initial portrayal suggests both blurring and transcendence of the color line; here Du Bois depicts a rigid and embattled boundary. The lines that follow further dramatize Black parental anguish, a painfully educated anticipation of violence that defies assimilability across the color line. Delight in the "unbowed pride" of Burghardt's little head is alloyed with the lived certainty that some future day will see it bowed. Adoration of his "tiny dimpled hand" is made bitter with the knowledge that the white world would seek to crush all that is precious, innocent, and good in Burghardt, just as they had with Du Bois himself.[48] As Thomas Dumm keenly observes, "for Du Bois, the formulation of grief is already written into the life of the child who is mourned."[49]

Unlike in the case of the white glance, however, the object of Du Bois's glance is not a fellow human denied acknowledgment, not a Black boy in his eagerness or Black parents in their loss. Rather, it is toward the perilous ecology in which Du Bois and his family find themselves, the red earth and urban hills of Atlanta. The passage may be an allusion to Sam Hose's lynching, as the "hot red" of the soil evokes words closely associated with blood, and the end of the elegy repeats this figuration: "We could not lay him in the ground there in Georgia, for the earth there is strangely red."[50] The "breathless" city might be the roil of the white mob or the forced breathlessness of

the victim. As he turns his gaze to his son's hair and eyes, he reposi-
tions himself in a kind of momentary antagonism toward these features. In this case, however, it is the signifiers of white purity that are
rejected. If the "tall newcomer" had rendered obscene the child Du
Bois's innocent impulse to friendly exchange, the blue and gold here
themselves signal harm and intimate predation. It might be said that
Du Bois is turning the hostile glance back toward the white world itself. Du Bois quickly shifts, in closing line of the passage, back into
fatherly attention, pointing out the stars and singing to his son. The
momentary recoil at his son's features, however, nevertheless dramatizes the ways that the racial order destroys human connection, is
underpinned by violence, and renders true and lasting innocence
impossible.

Gomer Du Bois's Feminine Innocence

Early on in the chapter, the literal distance of the professional Du
Bois from the scene of the birth dramatizes the gendered separation
of spheres. The figuration of the birth chamber and bed as "sanctuary" and "altar," upon which Nina Gomer Du Bois had offered herself as willing sacrifice, further entrenches this spatial duality and
their respective depictions as pious and profane. In diametrical opposition to the notion of Black women as immoral, as propounded in
Hoffman's account, Gomer Du Bois embodies the very essence of
true womanhood, the pure and innocent "girl-wife" glorified and
transfigured through her motherly destiny. The passage's glancing
description of her physical appearance arguably invokes canonical
literary depictions of white feminine suffering through her postpartum depiction as "wan," signifying pallor.[51] This detail accords with
Shawn Michelle Smith's analysis of the images of light-skinned single women in Du Bois's photographic project, published in 1900,
Types of American Negroes, Georgia, USA. Smith argues:

White supremacists posed the light-skinned woman of color as both the object and the instigator of interracial mixing, as both the sign and cause of racial degeneration. . . . Du Bois reclaims the image of the pale African American woman so highly fetishized in racial hierarchies, re-presenting her as a woman of grace, elegance, and refinement. . . . His photographs celebrate her innocence and purity, to then contain and circumscribe her sexuality by laying out the future roles she is to assume within a patriarchal African American family.[52]

Gomer Du Bois's depiction in the inner sanctum of the birth chamber is thus a kind of postmatrimonial afterimage of these virginal portraits.

While the two parents were united in their devotion, Du Bois likewise bifurcates their rites of worship along gender conventions. Du Bois depicts his wife as consumed by the signature passions of virtuous maternity: "Her own life builded and moulded itself upon the child; he tinged her every dream and idealized her every effort. No hands but hers must touch and garnish those little limbs; no dress or frill must touch them that had not wearied her fingers; no voice but hers could coax him off to Dreamland, and she and he together spoke some soft and unknown tongue and held it in communion."[53] Du Bois depicts himself as a devotee at this same altar, but his own liturgy is distinctively masculine. Nina and Burghardt are literally knit together in prelinguistic unity; if her hands must themselves lose contact with the infant's body, the dresses and frills that she makes serve as soft prostheses. In contrast, musing alone above an already sleeping Burghardt, Du Bois's own arm stretches not toward the babe but toward the future; and it is not homely fibers but the tiny arm of Burghardt himself that extends the father's reach, as Du Bois extends that of his own "black fathers." Where Nina babbles along with Burghardt in a private language, Du Bois hearkens to the "voice of the prophet," bearing some great message for the people within the

Veil, in the "baby voice" of his heir. For Nina, Burghardt constitutes the immersive and immediate present; for Du Bois, he is the future.

These gendered characterizations of feminine stasis and masculine action, immediacy and futurity, private and public frame the account of Burghardt's illness and death as well as his life. His mother nurses him at the bedside; the father goes out to seek the doctor the night of the final crisis. Even after the terrible final breath, the passing from the world that changes nothing and everything, the parents' respective devastations follow this pattern. Nina, "the world's most piteous thing—a childless mother," inarticulately "writhe[s]" in the "chamber of death," while Du Bois rails against his fate, emphasizing his life of active public endeavor in the face of great adversity. In an anguished triple apostrophe to Death, he cries out at the cruelty of its intrusion into the very home itself; willing to risk all in public strivings, Death has instead invaded his "one little coign of happiness," his one refuge—*domus sua cuique est tutissimum refugium*—within the cold "dull land that stretches its sneering web about me."[54]

Gomer Du Bois's feminine innocence is perhaps most on display in the way that the elegy counterposes the two parents' respective pronouncements on their son's afterlife: "She who in simple clearness of vision sees beyond the stars said when he had flown, 'He will be happy There; he ever loved beautiful things.' And I, far more ignorant, and blind by the web of mine own weaving, sit alone winding words and muttering, 'If still he be, and he be There, and there be a There, let him be happy, O Fate!'"[55] This is Gomer Du Bois's only spoken line in the elegy. On the one hand, Gomer Du Bois's "clearness of vision" is of a piece with the optic of innocence ascribed to Burghardt—especially as it is juxtaposed with Du Bois's "ignoran[ce]" and "blind[ness]." This blindness is linked to a cynical lack of faith, in contrast with Gomer Du Bois's certainty that heaven awaited her beloved son. On the other hand, there is discernible here a kind of dissimulation; if mother and son share a clarity of perception, hers is reduced and infantilized as "simple" and childlike, while Burghardt's actual infant gaze bespeaks "infinite breadth." And even in his self-deprecation as ignorant, unseeing, and faithless, Du Bois paints himself as beyond such naïve beliefs.

This accords with the bifurcation of roles in the elegy's closing stanza, in which Du Bois mourns that, unlike the wretched and orphaned of the race, "Love sat beside his cradle, and in his ear Wisdom waited to speak."[56] From the foregoing, it seems as though these two virtues correspond, respectively, to mother and father. It is not necessary to read Gomer Du Bois alone as personifying Love; especially given its breadth, earlier in the essay, as lifegiving interconnection, both parents may be the source. But the foregoing also argues against a similar sharing of Wisdom between the two. This is especially the case in light of Burghardt's description as carrying forward the "dream of [Du Bois's] black fathers" into a prophetic destiny. This rigidly gendered self-stylization aligns with Hazel Carby's argument that in *Souls'* figuration of Black thinkers and leaders, Du Bois's "conceptual framework . . . encompasses only those men who enact narrowly and rigidly determined codes of masculinity."[57] The elegy invites elite white readers' sympathy on the grounds of the Du Bois household's scrupulous conformity with late Victorian bourgeois conventions of morality and affect. Gomer Du Bois's feminine innocence not only counters allegations of Black Americans' moral and affective deficiencies; it also sets the stage for a reversal of this judgment, casting whites themselves as morally deficient and grotesquely unfeeling. It levels this challenge, however, by replicating some of the elitist and gender-oppressive elements of the prevailing biopolitical order.

Melvin Rogers's account of *Souls of Black Folk* as a work of rhetoric helps to clarify this dilemma of persuasion. Rogers writes that "*Souls* attempts to craft a common horizon for author and reader from which shared emotional judgments regarding racial inequality might be reached."[58] With Du Bois's gender conventions in view, it becomes clear that this "common horizon" can entail regressive features alongside the democratic and justice-oriented values that Rogers highlights. Gomer Du Bois's innocence in "Of the Passing" both serves as an instance of the persuasive and affective work that Rogers explicates and draws attention to the oppressive elements that this mode of political speech can smuggle in. In considering *Souls* as a work of rhetoric, Rogers foregrounds its appeal to the feelings of white readers in particular: "the power of *Souls* is bound up with its aspiration to persuade through an appeal to affirmative and negative emotional states, namely, sympathy and shame. Indeed, it is precisely Du Bois's quest to evoke in the reader sympathy for the suffering of black folks and shame in being complicit in their suffering."[59]

The elegy's alignment with prevailing norms of bourgeois masculinity and femininity may have been key to both this sympathetic identification and that motivational shame. Rogers writes that *Souls* "enacts and exemplifies" the "aim of rhetoric[:] to take the reader to the experiential source from which appropriate emotions and judgments spring."[60] But Du Bois's own sense of "appropriate emotions"—like that of most of his contemporaneous readers—was itself deeply patriarchal. As Carby writes, evoking Raymond Williams, "highly gendered structures of intellectual and political thought and feeling" permeate *Souls*.[61] Du Bois had absorbed gendered structures of feeling from his Victorian upbringing and education, which he would have shared with the majority of his readership. Supplementing Rogers's insights about *Souls'* rhetorical power with Carby's feminist critique, I argue that Du Bois's patriarchalism was in fact central to the efficacy of the essay "Of the Passing of the First Born."

Rogers observes that "the structure of *Souls* moves from attempting to cultivate sympathetic identification in several of the early chapters to eliciting shame in the reader by the end of the book."[62]

"Of the Passing" can be said to employ the same structure in miniature. By the time the funeral procession occurs, readers have been primed to feel the shock of shame: invited into an intimate tableau of maternal devotion and paternal dreams, precise embodiments of the defining norms of the proper family—perhaps even leading readers to identify Burghardt's angelic babyhood with that of one of their own. Thus positioned at close range, they have then witnessed the terrible loss, the baby's death and his parents' properly gendered anguish. Du Bois's carefully conventional characterizations invite elite white readers to feel the tragedy of Burghardt's death and the violence of the Jim Crow order. This is at the cost, however, of partially replicating the prevailing racial capitalist biopolitical/necropolitical ranking of life.

This ranking of life is presented most explicitly in the closing paragraph, in which Du Bois first wonders why he himself was not taken instead of his baby. He rails against the irony that such a nurtured and beloved life should have been taken, when "the wretched of my race that line the alleys of the nation sit fatherless and unmothered."[63] On the one hand, Du Bois's raw paternal grief is here poignantly expressed. Overcome with loss, he puts to paper his desperate and futile bargaining in the face of death's terrible finality. Why his son? Why this devastation for himself and his wife? Why not another whose passing might leave less sorrow in its wake? On the other hand, the contrast between golden Burghardt, cultivated in the most careful domesticity, and the Black wretches languishing in the streets, comes unsettlingly close to Hoffman's condemnations of the deficiencies of Black paupers, in their inadequate capacity for civilized affective responses like sorrow and thus unworthiness for life. Gomer Du Bois's maternal innocence, at the core of that domesticity, serves as a marker of unjust harm—while implicitly ratifying the relative worthlessness of indigent Black folks' lives.

And Yet—Du Bois's Maternal Ambivalence

The elegy thus depicts the Du Bois family as unimpeachably proper, over and against the "unmothered and unfathered" miserable Black masses. Nina Gomer Du Bois's figuration as a chaste, pious, and pure True Woman offers a bridge to educated white readers to see their own families as symmetrically situated. Following Rogers, this sympathy is part of the ground on which Du Bois's text can engender its motivating shame. Yet there are other features in the elegy, that militate against this exclusionary propriety. These are moments in which Du Bois rejects that symmetry, rejects the assimilability of white readers' situation and his own as a Black parent. In so doing, he rejects the moral metric of white innocence. He reveals the broader milieu of violence beyond the individual insult or action or behavior of overtly racist whites, signaling to white readers that the milieu in which they are raising their own precious children in safety is, for his own son and himself, incompatible with life. If the elegy's depiction of Nina engenders a shared horizon of experience, these moments of rage and ambivalence trouble this shared horizon, revealing the inadequacy of prevailing elite white-centric moral categories. Liberal white readers in the North, in particular, could comfortably condemn the N-word-slinging white Southerners. With regard to his indictments of the broader world and society as death-dealing, however, these same white readers are implicated. These moments thus counter *progressive* white innocence with a demand for accountability and radical transformation.

There are thus two levels of white innocence at play in the elegy and two corresponding indictments. One is the innocence of smug analysts like Hoffman and white citizens like the passers-by. Convinced of their scientifically- and culturally-ordained superiority, their "not knowing and not wanting to know" has an almost gleefully sadistic character. But then there is the innocence of Du Bois's sympathetic white readership, which has a different flavor. These might be thought of as the people, in the very opening of *Souls of Black Folk*, who "stutteringly" attempt to signal their sympathy with remarks about "fine colored men," Union partisanship, and shared rage against lynchings but can never come out and say "how does it feel to be a problem?" Du Bois says to them here that *you are yourselves the problem.* You too are among those who "do not want to know"—and this will divide us while the world remains as it is. As we have seen, the elegy in large part reproduces prevailing gender and class conventions. At the same time, however, the elegy's expression of raw ambivalence about Burghardt's death shares key elements of these maternal refusals of conditions that threaten Black children's present and future thriving—undercutting the elegy's patriarchalism in key ways.

Du Bois's ambivalence is most clearly expressed in his admission, after Burghardt's death, that "all that day and all that night there sat an awful gladness in [his] heart . . . my soul whispers ever to me saying, 'not dead, not dead, but escaped; not bond, but free.'"[64] This ambivalence jars with the elegy's more conventional depictions of late Victorian/Edwardian paternal bereavement. According with Rogers's theorization of political sympathy, the chapter's representations of the Du Bois's family's proper domestic bliss and devastating grief largely tend to emphasize the convergences between Du Bois's experiences and affects and the white reader's own. This passage, however, reveals an abyss at which that shared horizon stops. Du Bois signposts this asymmetry of his own and white readers' lifeworlds with the only second-person address in the elegy: "nay, blame me not if I see the world thus darkly through the Veil."[65] The temporality of this formulation is striking; Du Bois's "I see" suggests that this veiled vision persists into the narrative present. Likewise, while the "awful gladness" spans just one day and night, the fact that the soul whispers "ever" signals an ongoing time frame.

This passage thus departs from the prevailing conventions of fatherly grief—as the comparison with Ralph Waldo Emerson highlights at the end of the chapter. It evokes, rather, the moments of maternal refusal that thread through both slave narratives and Jim Crow-era Black political speech and writing. As Jennifer Morgan writes, it is important not to romanticize enslaved women's experiences of pregnancy and birth, as "ambivalence toward and distance from" enslaved children treated by law as violable commodities "would have been as logical an emotion as any."[66] At least some enslaved women's contraceptive practices—likely abetted in at least some cases by their community midwives—were a refusal to gestate and birth commodities.[67] The use of abortifacients may likewise have evinced this reproductive refusal. The very plant at the heart of the brutal machinery of nineteenth-century racial capitalism was in fact implicated in this exercise of constrained and tortured agency; cotton root bark is a powerful known abortifacient (it was later patented by whites as a tonic to "restore the menses") as well as a postpartum antihemorrhagic, as it causes the uterus to contract. The record also contains some cases of infanticide accompanied by maternal sentiments to this effect. Margaret Garner's case, fictionalized by Toni Morrison in *Beloved* (1987), is the most well-known of these.[68]

Discerning these practices of reproductive refusal within the official record from the high rates of infertility, pregnancy loss, and infant death caused by the hostile milieu of the plantation is vexed. Given the mythos of Black maternal deficiency by which enslavers justified their routinized rupturing and violation of kinship, accusations of infanticide in particular were rampant, especially accidental infanticide by "overlaying," or an adult's suffocation of a bedsharing infant by rolling over it during sleep.[69] In her history of Black experiences of infant loss from antebellum times through the Great Migration, Wangui Muigai attends to the complexities within Black political thought, cultural production, and praxis that navigated the conditions of Jim Crow necropolitics. Elements of uplift politics and eugenic notions of social and sexual hygiene animated some Black expert responses in the Progressive Era. At the same time, Black women commentators invoked the power of maternal refusal to bear children in the face of a polity bent on destroying them: "no more Black bodies to lynch." Muigai profiles Angelina Weld Grimké's 1916 play *Rachel*, about a Black woman who refuses to have children given the death-dealing conditions of the racial state.[70]

In an 1896 appeal made the year of Burghardt's birth to the white National Congress of Mothers, Du Bois's contemporary, Mary Church Terrell, expresses her anguish, as well as the limits of whites' sympathetic identification, in strikingly similar terms to Du Bois. Terrell, whose writings are the subject of chapter 3, herself lost three much-desired babies in the first five years of her marriage. As the Du Bois parents did with Burghardt, Terrell experienced inadequate and segregated medical care with her third loss in particular, which she speculated that racist neglect might have been the cause of her baby's death. In this speech, while not thematizing the threat of medical racism per se, Terrell underlines the incommensurability of experience between Black and white mothers:

Contrast, if you will, the feelings of hope and joy with thrill the heart of the white mothers with those which stir the soul of her colored sister. Put yourselves for one minute in her place (you could not endure the strain longer) and imagine, if you can, how you would feel if situated similarly—As a mother of the weaker race clasps to her bosom the babe which she loves as fondly as you do yours, her heart cannot thrill with the joyful anticipations of the future. For before her child she sees the thorny path of prejudice and proscription which his little feet must tread. . . . . So rough does the way of her infant appear to many a poor black mother that instead of thrilling with the joy which you feel, as you clasp your little ones to your breast, she trembles with apprehension and despair.[71]

Although she stops short of invoking death as a release from this grim destiny, Terrell's depiction of Black mothers' "apprehension and despair" about the future, where white mothers can "thrill with . . . joyful anticipations," reveals an unbridgeable distance between the experiences of motherhood within and without the Veil. Like Du Bois, she begins with the establishment of affective symmetry between Black and white parents, then dramatically emphasizes the nonidentity of these experiences. Also like Du Bois, Terrell simultaneously asks for white auditors' identification with her complex sentiments and acknowledges the impossibility of full identification. She asks the audience to "put yourselves . . . in her place," yet declares that they could never withstand the anguish.

In this articulation of the unarticulable, both Terrell and Du Bois partake in this politics of maternal ambivalence under enslavement. With regard to Du Bois, Cornel West makes this link explicitly: "Morrison's Sethe echoes Du Bois' own voice upon the painful passing of his First-Born."[72] But in its elegant formal register and rhetorical construction, it is Harriet Jacobs's autobiographical account of the anguish of enslaved motherhood that most closely prefigures Terrell's and Du Bois's ambivalence: "I loved to watch [my son's] infant slumbers; but always there was a dark cloud over my enjoyment. I could never forget that he was a slave. Sometimes I wished that he might die in infancy. God tried me. My darling became very ill. . . . I had prayed for his death, but never so earnestly as I now prayed for his life; and my prayer was heard. Alas, what mockery it is for a slave mother to try to pray back her dying child to life! Death is better than slavery."[73]

As Du Bois and Terrell would do four decades later, Jacobs reaches out to readers with rhetorical formulations that establish an affective symmetry—Madonna-like mother over sleeping babe—while simultaneously showing that the respective experiences of parenthood are utterly incomparable. Saidiya Hartman observes that Jacobs's narration, earlier in the narrative, of her sexual maneuverings under violent duress seems to concede moral superiority to her white readers but in fact demonstrates that "womanly" virtue is impossible under chattel enslavement, forcing readers to acknowledge "the situational ethics of the enslaved."[74] Similarly, in this passage Jacobs dramatizes the gap between the situational affects and expectations of free and enslaved motherhood. Under the living death of slavery, maternity is shown to present an agonizing paradox. Du Bois's directive to the reader not to judge him strikingly echoes Jacobs's denial of equivalence with whites' gendered moral compass.

In so closely paralleling Terrell, Jacobs, and the political and cultural iconography of Garner, this "awful gladness" evinces what Fred Moten terms "animateriality": the presence in Du Bois's writings of a "maternal mark that bourgeois respectability demands be relinquished."[75] This maternal presence disrupts Du Bois's respectable self-representations "most clearly after the fact of a deprivation."[76] It is thus unsurprising that it breaches the respectable surface of the elegy. Moten discerns this disruptive element in the sonic features of Du Bois's texts, especially the recurrent depiction of his enslaved African great-great-grandmother's song in his autobiographical writings.[77] The elegy similarly "both reveal[s] and repress[es]" this maternal mark through its lyrical components; even as the elegy invokes his "black fathers," the maternal is given a kind of encrypted priority in both the Sorrow Song that heads it—"I hope my mother will be there in that beautiful world on high"—and the accompanying Swinburne verse, which dramatizes maternal loss. It is perhaps most audible in his soul's whisper: "Not dead, not dead, but escaped; not bond, but free." Channeling a history of ambivalent losses and fugitive despair, Du Bois here insists on a more capacious notion of life than the white world can contain. For whites, he implies, are themselves souls "choked and deformed" who glory in the deliberate crushing of fellow human spirits. Life's duration under these conditions means at least some degree of spiritual death. Du Bois thus simultaneously grieves Burghardt's loss and celebrates his escape, his "wild pride of being" intact and free.

This fierce ambivalence prefigures the convention-defying characterizations, a quarter-century later, of Black maternity in *Darkwater*'s "The Damnation of Women."[78] In "Damnation," Du Bois forwards a vision of Black motherhood that departs strikingly from both the linkage of promiscuity with social pathology and from the late Progressive Era maternalism prevalent at the time.[79] Du Bois pays special homage to Black mothers past and present: from the hell of slavery, forced to "starv[e their] own wailing offspring to nurse to the world their swaggering masters" and subject to unimaginable sexual violence, to the defiant "future promise" of unmarried working-class Black women's motherhood.[80] For "this history of insult and degradation," while unforgivable, has also given rise to standards of strength and freedom unimaginable within a white patriarchal frame. In her reading of "Damnation," Lawrie Balfour argues that Du Bois "gestures toward what Hortense Spillers calls 'the insurgent ground' of an alternative female subjectivity."[81] Spillers—in whose work Moten's notion of animateriality is also rooted—theorizes *motherhood* in the white heteronuclear sense as impossible under the ongoing logic of enslavement; Black maternal practices are hence generative of modes of life, kinship, gender, and relations that cannot be contained by this logic.[82] "Damnation" does not thematize Black maternal ambivalence per se. But its laudation of Black women's enactments of freedom and care in violent exile from the conventions of motherhood extends the elegy's insurrectionary refusal of the white world's terms.

In so doing, it also accords with what Black women health organizers would name, decades later, as the core tenets of reproductive justice: the human right to have a child, not to have a child, and to raise children in safe and sustainable environments. Particularly relevant here are the first and third principles. The first principle calls attention to the colonial racial capitalism's institutionalized disruptions of maternity, parenthood, and kinship, especially among Black and Indigenous communities, and among poor and working-class Asian and Latinx immigrants, but also among poor and disabled people across racial classifications. As Dorothy Roberts traces with regard to Black families, these span English and colonial poor laws and the commodification of enslaved women's reproduction, to social worker surveillance and child removal, and the foster system under so-called child welfare programs.[83]

Both Du Bois and Terrell are forced to grieve the violation of this right under segregated health care; while it is not certain that access to the same quality health care that their white counterparts expected would have saved their respective children, it is certain that the inferior care that they received did not help to support their babies' survival. Both thinkers also prefigure the right to raise children in safe and healthy environments. Terrell's "thorny path of prejudice and proscription" bespeaks the hazards and harms that Black mothers and parents must witness, experience, and mourn as their beloved children grow up under white supremacy. Du Bois likewise describes a hostile milieu that depleted his own spark of life and blighted his boyhood and would inevitably assault his son's precious life as well. Attention to the "strangely red" earth and to the way that the insult of the white passers-by poisoned the "blithe morning" and white flowers of the burial link Du Bois's account particularly strongly with the third principle's expansive emphasis on how environments can support life—or fail to do so.

Reading elements of Du Bois's elegy as partaking in a tradition of Black maternal subversion, or as prefiguring the reproductive justice framework, raises thorny problems. James, Carby, and Balfour each caution readers that Du Bois's articulations of feminism are always incomplete and paradoxical, drawing attention to his propensity for ventriloquism of Black women's voices.[84] Du Bois's narration of his own "awful gladness" at his son's death in terms so similar to Terrell, Jacobs, and (public memory of) Garner could be read as ventriloquism, an uncited appropriation of Black maternal experiences and insights. Moreover, it remains true that his depiction of Burghardt's actual mother's grief is granted no such subversive complexity. It could be argued that, like West's parallel between Sethe and Du Bois, this reading of Du Bois's ambivalence as maternal elides the intergenerational horror of reproductive enslavement and its persistence in Jim Crow sexual terror, which looms large in Morrison's text as well as that of Jacobs's *Incidents* (even if not in the passage cited in this chapter). Finally, it could be argued that although the passage echoes both Terrell and Jacobs in depicting a baby boy, its emphasis on a masculine trajectory that so clearly evokes Du Bois's own life story counters its matrilinearity to some extent.

Yet the ambivalence of this passage nevertheless differs in crucial ways from roughly contemporary expressions of white paternal ambivalence, such as that which Shannon Mariotti discerns in Emerson's "Experience." Emerson laments that his son's loss ultimately left him unchanged; he "grieve[s] that grief can teach [him] nothing" about the true nature of things.[85] Near the end of this passage, he writes: "Nothing is left to us but death. We look to that with a grim satisfaction. . . . There at least is reality that will not dodge us."[86] For Emerson here, death is the ineluctable end of life, the fact of individual finitude. For Du Bois, however, these terms take on different and doubled meanings. Birth is entry into unfreedom and violence, a "living death" of the heart as well as the divine renewal of the world. And this violence is itself intersubjective and intergenerational, not merely individual. For Du Bois—as for Jacobs and Terrell—parenting meant in part reliving his own loss of innocence and the injuries of white innocence, anticipating their repetition on his child's body and soul, alongside the wonder and adoration. If Emerson's ambivalence issues from the fact that his son's death brings him no closer to the world as it truly is, Du Bois's ambivalence demands a different world altogether.

3 *Innocence and Inheritance*

Mary Church Terrell and the Reproduction
of the White World

In the fall of 1896, Mary Church Terrell suffered the devastating loss
of her beloved two-day-old son. This was her third infant loss in five
years. In their very first year of marriage, Terrell and her husband had
experienced the death of a premature infant, along with Terrell's
own near-fatal health crisis that precipitated it. A second full-term
pregnancy, birth, and neonatal death followed soon after. In public
life Terrell had begun her tireless work to contest the hardening Jim
Crow apartheid regime, lynch law, and convict lease labor. She was
elected the first president of the National Colored Women's Association in July 1896, just a few months before her third birth and loss.
She became the most visible spokesperson for Black women's voting
rights in the nation's capital—a "political celebrity," in Treva Lindsey's terms.[1] During most of her extraordinary career, Terrell would
be a working mother to two daughters—Phyllis, born in 1898, and
Mary, her biological niece, adopted in 1903. Yet Terrell's first years of
public struggle on behalf of Black Americans were joined three times
over with profound private grief.[2]

Terrell narrates these losses in her autobiography, *A Colored
Woman in a White World*, written over several decades and published
in 1940. While she mentions them briefly at a few points in the autobiography, she describes them most fully in chapter 11, "I Return to

America." As the title of the chapter suggests, these narrations are not contained within a standalone elegy like Du Bois's "Of the Passing of the First-Born" in *Souls of Black Folk*—although "Of the Passing" is likewise the eleventh chapter of its respective volume. Rather, these accounts of infant loss are embedded within a broader description of Terrell's painful reentry into the "white world" of the Jim Crow United States, as well as her return to the conventions of heterosexual courtship, marriage, and family among her circle of elite African Americans, after two years of travel abroad. Having experienced nearly unlimited freedom of movement and participation in European social and cultural life, she returns to the harsh constraints and everyday assaults of hardening Jim Crow segregation as well as the horrors of lynching. It is in this context that her first three pregnancies and bereavements occur.

And it is precisely the relation between the materialities of this context and experiences of maternal loss that Terrell illuminates. She begins the introduction to her autobiography with the following lines: "This is the story of a colored woman living in a white world. It could not possibly have been written by a white woman." In "I Return to America," Terrell connects her third and first experiences of bereavement—narrated in this reverse chronological order—to distinct settings and enactments of this white world's violence. With regard to her 1896 loss, she describes her agonizing conviction that medical neglect was responsible for her baby's demise: "Right after its birth the baby had been placed in an improvised incubator, and I was tormented by the thought that if the genuine article had been used, its little life might have been spared. I could not help feeling that some of the methods employed in caring for my baby had caused its untimely end."[3] Terrell writes that she was in a state of inconsolable despair for months in the wake of this withholding of lifesaving technology—a pattern of systematic withholding that, as Dána-Ain Davis shows in her work on the contemporary racial politics of

NICUs, persists to this day.[4] In describing the aftermath of her first loss, in 1892, in contrast, Terrell dwells less on the proximate causal factors at work in her infant's death. Rather, she highlights the emotional trajectory of her pregnancy and bereavement in the wake of a childhood friend's lynching and the embodied consequences of these experiences and feelings:

> While I was happily expecting [my baby's] arrival, the lynching of Tom Moss . . . occurred. The mob's murder of this friend affected me deeply, and for a long time I could think of nothing else.
>
> As I was grieving over the loss of my baby boy one day, it occurred to me that under the circumstances it might be a blessed dispensation of Providence that his precious life was not spared. The horror and resentment felt by the mother, coupled with the bitterness which filled her soul, might have seriously affected the unborn child. Who can tell how many desperadoes and murderers have been born to colored mothers who had been shocked and distracted before the birth of their babies by the news that some relative or friend had been burned alive or shot to death by a mob?

Earlier in the chapter, Terrell briefly links this first loss with a grave health crisis of her own the summer after her marriage. It is only here, however, that she explicitly reveals that her own illness and her child's death both took place in the immediate aftermath of the lynching of this friend, Thomas Moss, and his business partners. Terrell and Moss had grown up together in Memphis.[5]

As even these abbreviated selections make clear, Terrell's two narrations of loss encompass a broad range of the white world's harms: the agents, settings, scales, and material processes of these harms. If the third loss tracks the quotidian violence of medical neglect and its fatal failures to act, Terrell links the first loss with the murderous collective agency of the white mob. The hospital room signals Terrell's class status and urban milieu, as most US women, and the vast majority of Black women, still gave birth at home in 1896. With regard to her first loss, in 1892, Terrell figures herself as paradigmatic, her proximity to atrocity placing her alongside all Black mothers.[6] While Terrell describes the despair and torment of her ideations in the wake of the third loss, in her first loss she narrates the "horror and resentment" that characterized the pregnancy itself, sounding a note of ambivalence about mothering under white terror. Her third loss is private and interior, contained within the small space of the improvised incubator and the hospital room. In the first, in contrast, the violence is not only public and spectacular but extensive. It radiates outward beyond the horrors committed on the victims themselves to reach not only immediate witnesses but loved ones at a spatial remove. Terrell testifies to the hold of shock and grief not only on her own gestating body, with potential effects on the life growing inside of her, but on the untold harms that mob violence wreaks on literally countless other Black mothers and their children.

Terrell's narrations of infant death and maternal bereavement thus map the white world as a hostile environment for Black maternal and infant life—from the nation's white authorities who sanction lynching, to the murderous white citizenry that perpetrates these crimes, to subtle medical neglect in private hospital rooms, to impacts on very wombs of "shocked and distracted" mothers grieving their murdered loved ones. These narrations link the broader political milieu of racial capitalism, and the lynch law that enforced it, with systemic medical neglect and abuse of Black women and infants. In drawing these connections, Terrell's writings at once serve as a rejoinder to the gendered racism and white supremacist civilizational hierarchies that prevailed during the racial nadir, and prefigure recent and emerging accounts of racism, in our current political moment, as an environment of harm for Black mothers and infants from the systemic to the cellular.

Closely attending to the power of her material surroundings, Terrell's autobiography figures the white world itself as a milieu at once physiological, affective, and political. It highlights the objects and spaces that comprise the white world's threats to Black women and their children—from train cars to wedding gifts to the fatal improvised incubator—and tracks their harms to body and mind. It does not paint the white world as total environment; her writing catalogues the materialities, both exquisite and ordinary, of her activities and relationships. Terrell's narrative also links this attention to the material and spatial with a conceptualization of the white world's duration and reproduction over time. The autobiography as well as other relevant writings and speeches offer a political account of maternal feelings as key to this reproduction. These writings figure maternal feelings as not only responsive to their environments but as hereditary factors themselves, with the potential to become embodied and objective components of those environments. If Black maternal feelings can materialize harms under the conditions of the white world, white mothers' feelings (and lack thereof) reproduce that broader environment of harm itself, especially and including mob violence. Terrell's account of maternal feelings and infant loss are thus part of a broader theory of white world reproduction, entailing complex interactions of body and environment that both shift and endure over time.

White World's Material Environments: Mary Church (Terrell) Returns to America

As noted, Terrell's bereavements are situated within an account of her return to the United States from Europe. This return means not only her transition from relatively footloose young single woman and aspiring writer to married public activist. It reflects her reentry into a hardening Jim Crow regime, with its cruel constraints and the ever-present threat of deadly violence. At the close of chapter 10, Terrell narrates the latter part of her two-year sojourn in Europe. While she has faced a few ugly episodes of racism from white Americans, she has overall encountered warm interest and companionship among white Europeans, even having refused no fewer than four proposals of marriage. As her time in Europe comes to an end, Terrell considers her return to the white world of the United States, and what she knows will face her there. She reflects on her freedom of movement on European railways and ability to secure safe lodging, as well as her capacity to partake in the offerings of museums, theaters, architecture, and opera. Terrell looks back on the physical ease that accompanied her encounters with others: "My nerves were not on edge, neither was my heart in my mouth because I feared I would be the *persona non grata* to people . . . if perchance they happened to discover I was of African descent."[7] In contrast, as she considers the "return to my native land . . . my heart ached when I thought about it. . . . I knew that when I returned home I would face again the humiliations, discriminations, and hardships to which colored people are subjected all over the United States." She nevertheless decides to return for the sake of the higher happiness of "promot[ing] the welfare of my race."[8]

"I Return to America" more than bears out Terrell's trepidations. The chapter opens with a harrowing train journey that, as she had anticipated, stands in stark contrast to the ease of European railway travel. Terrell (at the time, still Church) is traveling from Ohio, where her brother has just graduated from college, to Memphis. On presenting her tickets, it becomes clear that the white train agent at the point of origin had scammed her, selling her a ticket for a Pullman sleeper that did not correspond to her rail ticket, which would require her to disembark at midnight and wait at a station overnight in Louisville. She is not carrying enough cash to purchase the correct rail fare on board. After much distress, a gentleman aboard who knows her father eventually lends her the difference for the new ticket. It is clear that as soon as she returns to her country, the white world's infrastructures immediately assail her intact well-being. She is "surprised and agitated" when the ticket scam is revealed; and "all the more wrought up because [she] suspected that [she] was being ejected from the Pullman car because of [her] race." This suspicion is grounded in the recent experiences of friends, including one who had been "seriously injured by a mob." She is not only displaced from her rest in the sleeping car, but she knows that she would not be able to obtain lodging in Louisville and would be extremely unsafe at a station overnight. Feeling that her "own doom had come," she is in "great distress."

If Du Bois dramatizes the color line in *Souls of Black Folk*, in part via a phenomenology of a Black male subject forced to ride in the Jim Crow car, Terrell narrates the terrifying raced/gendered particularities of being a lone Black woman at the mercy of white male train personnel. Moreover, she narrates precisely the bodily tolls of vigilance that she has forecast in the previous chapter. After having been able to move through Europe without her "nerves . . . on edge, heart in [her] mouth," her narration catalogs the spectrum of violence that comprises Jim Crow train travel—from these ever-present atmospheric worrying and wearying elements to outright interpersonal predation to serious injury or death by white mob.

This opening passage is particularly significant, as Terrell dedicated substantial writing beyond this chapter, both in the autobiography and in short fiction, to the perils of traveling by rail as a Black girl and woman. In the autobiography her devastating introduction to the color line occurs on a train. The five-year-old Terrell, smartly dressed and coiffed, is traveling with her father in a first-class coach; when he leaves her to go for a smoke, a white conductor tries to force her to move to the Jim Crow car and calls her a "little n———." Her father, empowered by wealth and connections, and with the pre–Jim Crow legal landscape on his side, eventually swoops in and forces the conductor to back down. Yet Terrell narrates her own and her mother's distress once she has returned home, as the bewildered child tries to make sense of the assault. She undertakes an inventory of her own behavior and appearance, trying to assess any possible fault in the neatness of her hair or clothing, the propriety of her comportment. Her mother tearfully reassures her daughter that she has done nothing wrong, and particularizes it in the moment to this white bad apple: "conductors are sometimes mean." Terrell, however, uses the anecdote to bring home to readers this particular toll that the white world's assaults on children takes for Black mothers: "seeing their children touched and seared and wounded by race prejudice is one of the heaviest crosses which colored women have to bear."[9]

As noted, however, trains hold further dangers for Black adolescent girls and women. While Terrell does not refer directly to these dangers in chapter 11, it is clear from other parts of the autobiography that the sleeping car itself would not have been only a matter of comfort and rest but a measure of reprieve from the assaults that were all too common for Black women passengers. As a public speaker, Terrell was forced to travel by rail frequently, and she dedicates an entire chapter to these dangers, titled simply "Travel Under Difficulties." She writes that "there are few experiences more embarrassing and painful than those through which a colored woman passes while traveling in the South."[10] She relates multiple harrowing experiences as a teenager and young woman. Traveling home from Oberlin College at sixteen, she is forced into the Jim Crow car despite her first-class ticket. She is "frightened and horrified" at the prospect of having to spend the night alone in that car, having "heard about awful tragedies which had overtaken colored girls" in these circumstances.[11] She describes the Jim Crow structure of the car itself, with the front serving as a white men's smoker and the back relegated to Black passengers. This carceral arrangement of space not only materializes of the suffocating atmosphere of White supremacy via the forced inhalation of white men's smoke. It also calculatedly renders Black women vulnerable to sexual assault at the hands of white men.

Although Terrell manages to protect herself in that incident, she relates that a few years later, she experienced even more threatening brutality from another white man, this time a fellow passenger. Once the other Black passengers have departed, this white man approaches and refuses to respect her request that he leave her in peace, instead making "ugly remarks" that left her "terror stricken"; when she tries to flee, "he seized me and threw me into a seat and then left the car." Terrell thus shows readers that "spending the night in a Jim Crow car is a real peril for a colored girl," even as she keeps the details of this assault and others she has suffered to herself.[12] In its design and spatial arrangements, this national infrastructure designedly threatens Terrell's health and life, as it does the health and life of other Black girls and women.[13] As she sums it up: "No pen can describe and no tongue portray the indignities, insults and assaults to which colored women and girls have been subjected in Jim Crow cars. If I should dare relate some of the things which have happened, many would not believe me."[14] Elizabeth McHenry argues that this reticence reflects the fact that stereotypes of Black women's lasciviousness were so ingrained in the white public imagination that even depictions of their sexual victimization could risk "unwanted attention"; thus Terrell "adopts an old strategy of fugitives from slavery, whose most devastating experiences remain shrouded in silence in their narratives."[15] It is also noteworthy that her phrasing here mirrors her assertion in the introduction that "even if I tried to tell the whole truth few people would believe me"—suggesting that this atmosphere of intimate bodily threat was central to that undisclosable "whole truth."

Terrell's descriptions often showcase Terrell and her family's elite status and at times starkly juxtapose the unusual affordances of this status with exposure to racist violence. At the same time, her narrative brings intimate objects into detailed focus as sites of sensuous, bodily, and relational life. These appreciations dovetail with what Brittney Cooper identifies in the text as a deliberate "insist[ence] on the importance of creating a space of pleasure in the midst of doing race work," through activities like swimming and dancing.[16] Sparing in description when it comes to most aspects of her personal life, Terrell describes her trousseau with fine-grained vividness. Her wedding dress is "white faille silk trimmed with a white chiffon embroidered scalloped edging instead of lace. There was a wide flounce of it across the bottom of the front gore, and a narrower width formed a bertha on the long-sleeved waist." She has also a "red cashmere dress and a maroon broadcloth made quite plain and tailored." Terrell narrates in detail her mother's insistence that her daughter have a hat to match the latter dress; a maroon hat not easily to be found, her mother spends an inordinate amount of money on the item on Fifth Avenue—$20, or about $655 in 2022 dollars. Terrell writes that she was "horrified and wretched"—not only at the extravagant price but at the fact that this costly item was nevertheless not even "becoming": it was "a little affair shaped something like a bonnet and made of velvet with two ball-shaped gilt ornaments stuck on each side of the front."

It is clear that—this divergence in taste and its possible class-related meanings notwithstanding—clothing holds a deep connecting significance for mother and daughter. This significance went beyond the pair's shopping together for the trousseau and the obvious importance that the gift of the matching hat held for Louisa Church. Church either did not wish to attend the Memphis wedding hosted by her estranged husband, or was not invited, and remained in New York during the nuptials. However, Church "dressed herself exactly as she would have done if she had actually attended the wedding, and at the hour she knew her daughter was being married she imagined she was listening to the ceremony and taking part in it."[17] Clothes here not only make the woman but link mother and daughter across space. Lindsey explores both the prominence of beauty culture, and hairdressing in particular, and the strategic hyperpropriety of Black clubwomen in dress and comportment.[18] In their respective attentiveness to the stage-setting power of attire and presentation, Terrell's hairdresser mother and Terrell herself link these two aspects of "reinvented" Black womanhood at the turn of the century. This appreciation for the material extends beyond the sartorial. Turning toward a catalog of their wedding gifts, Terrell makes explicit her particular affective relation to the things that honored her marriage and now lend themselves to elegant use within her home: "*I do not agree with those who say that one cannot love an inanimate object,* for I have a real affection for every wedding present I possess." The two objects that Terrell highlights, while exquisitely fine, are not objets d'art; like Pablo Neruda's "common things," they are functional: a silver cream pitcher and a set of oyster forks.[19] Moreover, as with Neruda, Terrell's love is not only for the objects themselves but for the relations that they encode. For Terrell it is particularly significant that these gifts were given to her and her husband by "people of both races." The silver pitcher was gifted by a grandson of Thomas Jefferson, a Northern white industrialist who had attended law school with Robert Terrell.

At the same time, even the most intimately beloved objects are not immune to the white world's weaponization. If the pitcher stands as material proof of the possibility of racial harmony, at least among elites, the oyster forks tell a different story, bringing Terrell's use of juxtaposition to a horrific culmination. In both their material (silver) and their intended use (eating oysters), the forks signal an elite social ambit most sumptuously. Yet as the next turn in the text reveals, these oyster forks are also a kind of portal into a living nightmare. They recall:

. . . the brutal murder of the donor, Tom Moss, one of my best friends. We were children together and he was always invited to the parties which my parents gave me . . . with several other colored men [he] opened a store in the suburbs of Memphis. Then the colored people . . . stopped trading at a store kept by a white man across the street, and began to patronize Tom Moss, because the supplies he sold were more reasonable and were exactly what they were represented to be, while the patrons themselves were treated right.

So angry did the white storekeeper and some of his friends . . . become that they decided to break up Tom Moss's store, and deliberately started a row. . . . They called in the police, who placed the owners of the colored store in jail, and the next night all three were taken out by a mob and shot to death. Thus Tom Moss, who left a wife and several children, and two others were murdered, because they were succeeding too well. They were guilty of no crime but that.[20]

In their class associations, the forks are a perfect allegory for the white world's deadly intolerance for Black economic success that was at the root of Moss's lynching. Not only were Moss's gift of forks literally sterling, but the common things that he dealt in were likewise solid in their qualities, reliably corresponding to their representation, as well as more reasonably priced—unlike the overpriced and shoddy goods that, as Terrell gives the reader to understand, were on offer from the white store. Terrell writes that she was shaken to the core by this murder of her childhood friend: "when a woman has been closely associated with the victim of a mob since childhood . . . the horror and anguish which rend her heart are undescribable." The horror precipitated a spiritual crisis as well; she narrates nearly losing her "faith in the Christian religion" given that white Christians in the United States "sinfully winked at" lynching, "making no protest loud enough to be heard."

Moss had gifted the forks to Terrell and her husband at their October 1891 wedding, fewer than five months before a mob lynched him and his partners, on March 2, 1892. Terrell does not assign dates in this part of the chapter, and the specific timeline of these events thus remains somewhat vague for the moment. It is nevertheless just after narrating this atrocity, and her own traumatization, that Terrell first describes her experiences of infant loss as well as her own ill health:

> The summer after my marriage I was desperately ill and my life was despaired of. My recovery was nothing short of a miracle, and my case is recorded in medical history. In five years we lost three babies, one after another, shortly after birth. This was a great blow to Mr. Terrell and me. The maternal instinct was always abnormally developed in me. As far back as I can remember I have always been very fond of children. I cannot recall that I have ever seen a baby, no matter what its class, color, or condition in life, no matter whether it was homely or beautiful according to recognized standards, no matter whether it was clad in rags or wore dainty raiment, that did not seem dear and cunning to me.

Wangui Muigai writes that Terrell's emphasis on the "abnormal development" of her "maternal instinct" pushed back on the prevailing notions of Black maternal deficiency, such as those so cruelly leveraged by Frederick Hoffman.[21]

As I describe below, however, Terrell can also be read as throwing into sharp relief the white maternal deficiency of feeling that attend the "cult of true babyhood." White mothers are hardened to all but their own white and propertied scions, whereas Terrell's maternal feelings are expansive, viewing all infants as equally "dear and cunning." If in Du Bois's "Of the Passing" Burghardt's unspoiled gaze dramatizes the unnaturalness of color hierarchy, Terrell here stages a mature version—aware of "recognized standards" yet dismissive of them and thus able to behold the humanity and promise of all infants. The passages detailing the third, unbearable loss are quoted above, with Terrell narrating her torment regarding the improvised incubator. She further describes her postpartum despondency: "When my third baby died two days after birth, I literally sank down into the very depths of despair. For months I could not divert my thoughts from the tragedy, however hard I tried. It was impossible for me to read understandingly or to fix my mind on anything I saw in print. When I reached the bottom of a page in a book, I knew no more about its contents than did someone who had never seen it."

The white world has thus also robbed the book of its power to console the ardently literary Terrell. The following passage relates a visit to Terrell's mother in New York, at the insistence of both her husband and her physician, and credits this visit with turning the tide of Terrell's postpartum anguish. Offering a sunny respite from the reminders of loss that surrounded her at home in Washington, DC, Louisa Church "scouted the idea that the baby could have been saved." Terrell testifies not only to the salvific power of Church's resolute cheerfulness but to the effects of being in her mother's space. She writes: "Many a human being has lost his reason . . . when a slight change of scene and companionship might have saved it." But this maternal reassurance and salutary change of setting also mirrors, in key ways, the episode of Terrell's terrifying awakening to the color line on the train. Church, twenty-eight years before, had insulated the five-year-old Terrell from the full horror of the white world by individualizing the meanness of the white conductor; here she "scout[s]" the murderous specter of Jim Crow medicine in response to her grown daughter's agony. There is thus a kind of through line in the text connecting geographies of anti-Black harm and death that underwrite white comfort and convenience, health and life: from that childhood train car, to the sleeping car at the beginning of the chapter and the Jim Crow cars where Terrell has faced threatened and actual assaults, to the segregated hospital ward and the ersatz incubator. As this scene of maternal care testifies, this "heaviest cros[s] which colored women have to bear," witnessing the suffering of their children under racism, constitutes both a lifelong burden and a repeating pattern across the generations.

In the closing paragraphs of the chapter, Terrell returns to her own painful experiences of maternity and loss. There is a temporal shift here; she has been narrating her third bereavement and the postpartum visit to her mother, in 1896, but this passage, with minimal signaling, casts her memory back to the first loss, in 1892, against the backdrop of Moss's lynching. This suggests the time-blurring impacts of trauma, of loss upon loss—as Jenny Edkins notes, "trauma time" "upsets . . . straightforward linear temporality."[22] A selection is quoted above; the entire passage reads as follows:

A few months after my baby's death a thought which came to me one day, while I was in a paroxysm of grief, helped to reconcile me to my loss. While I was happily expecting his arrival, the lynching of Tom Moss, to which I have already referred, occurred. The mob's murder of this friend affected me deeply, and for a long time I could think of nothing else.

As I was grieving over the loss of my baby boy one day, it occurred to me that under the circumstances it might be a blessed dispensation of Providence that his precious life was not spared. The horror and resentment felt by the mother, coupled with the bitterness which filled her soul, might have seriously affected the unborn child. Who can tell how many desperadoes and murderers have been born to colored mothers who had been shocked and distracted before the birth of their babies by the news that some relative or friend had been burned alive or shot to death by a mob?

I was greatly impressed by a statement made by one of my white friends who met me on the street one day shortly after I was bereaved. "I do not see," she said, "how any colored woman can make up her mind to become a mother under the existing conditions in the United States. Under the circumstances," she continued, "I should think a colored woman would feel that she was perpetrating a great injustice upon any helpless infant she would bring into the world." I had never heard that point of view so frankly and strongly expressed before, and while I could not agree with it entirely, it caused me much serious reflection. The more I thought how my depression which was caused by the lynching of Tom Moss and the horror of this awful crime might have injuriously affected my unborn child, if he had lived, the more I became reconciled to what had at first seemed a cruel fate.

"I Return to America" thus closes its arc—yet in so doing opens a number of tensions. The threat of mob violence that—so far from the ease of European travel—Terrell fears on her train journey is realized in murderous mob that lynched her dear friend. Her experiences of pregnancy, birth, and loss, as well as marriage, work, and everyday objects and pleasures, are nested within this environment of threat to life and limb.

Moreover, the looping timeline that frames the passage is of a piece with the nonlinear way that Terrell is conceptualizing mob violence itself. It is not only the murderous collective agency of the mob on their direct victims on that fateful day. Rather, the harm here extends outward both spatially and temporally. In the foregoing pages, she has described her horror, anguish, and spiritual crisis provoked by this lynching; the reader is now given to understand that all of these happened during her first pregnancy. The mob's violence, on this account, extends beyond the horrors committed on her friend and his comrades to her own gestating body, potentially affecting the life growing inside her. The inclusion of her white friend's commentary too is significant. In addition to its jarring insensitivity given the raw fact of Terrell's recent loss, it stages a kind of progressive white innocence vis-à-vis Black children's well-being under "current conditions." In other words, Terrell's closing narration of infant loss and maternal bereavement queries the connections between atrocity and ambivalence, heredity and environment, responsibility and reproduction. It is to these themes that we now turn.

Situating Terrell's Ambivalence

In the previous chapter I situated Du Bois's "Of the Passing of the First-Born" within a lineage of Black maternal ambivalence stretching back to Harriet Jacobs and Margaret Garner and forward to Terrell herself. This is not the only connection between Du Bois and Terrell. They would work together as founding members of the NAACP starting in 1909, and they were correspondents and collaborators on numerous occasions.[23] Even in this early period of their respective careers, however, they were navigating in parallel the paradoxes of simultaneous class privilege and profound vulnerability at a moment characterized, as Khalil Gibran Muhammad writes, by a blanket "condemnation of Blackness."[24] Both lose their first-borns during this time: Terrell in 1892, Du Bois in 1898, the year that Terrell's daughter, Phyllis, is born. They also evince similar tensions in their work and lives. Brittney Cooper calls attention to the trailblazing civil rights icon Pauli Murray's admiration for Terrell, and Murray's characterization of a signature polarity in Terrell's politics—both "a militant civil rights activist and longtime feminist who had fought for woman suffrage" and "the Essence of Victorian respectability."[25] Du Bois's writings likewise combine visionary militancy with—especially in this earlier period—deep adherence to Victorian class and gender norms.[26]

In chapter 2, I highlighted Terrell's speech to the National Congress of Mothers as an example of maternal ambivalence that foreshadows elements of Du Bois's elegy for his own son. The speech calls on the sympathies of white mothers, asking them to "contrast

... the feelings of hope and joy with thrill the heart of the white mothers with those which stir the soul of her colored sister. . . . So rough does the way of her infant appear to many a poor black mother that instead of thrilling with the joy which you feel . . . she trembles with apprehension and despair."[27] Like Du Bois's reflections on Burghardt's demise, Terrell here bemoans "the thorny path of prejudice and proscription" that is fated to wound her beloved offspring. In some ways Terrell's ambivalence about her 1892 loss in the autobiography hews even closer to Du Bois's text than this speech. Like Burghardt, this is Terrell's first child. While the framing of maternal ambivalence in the speech is prospective, looking ahead with trepidation to future perils, both "Of the Passing" and "I Return to America" are bereaved parents' retrospective reflections on known dangers foreclosed. Although in "Of the Passing," Du Bois does not explicitly mention the lynching of Sam Hose, in close proximity to his home in Atlanta, the white mob likewise carried out this unspeakable atrocity mere months before his own son's death. And like Du Bois, Terrell describes a kind of consolation amid paroxysmal grief. For both, a kind of innocence is preserved through early death.

Yet Terrell's narration of bereavement also diverges from that of Du Bois. This is not only in the striking reversal between Burghardt's unnamed and nearly silent mother, Nina Gomer Du Bois, in "Of the Passing" and the maternal grief that Terrell's autobiography actively voices, while Mr. Terrell's own mourning remains behind the scenes. Nor, along the same lines, is it the enclosure of Gomer Du Bois in the house—"writhing" in the chamber of death—in contrast to the bereaved Terrell's presence in public, as she is approached by the white friend in the street. There is also a key distinction between the two texts' respective conceptions of infant innocence. Du Bois's lines describing his own "awful gladness" at his beloved nineteen-month-old's death from diphtheria celebrate the preservation of Burghardt's innocence as an originary state of unhindered connection—a kind of existential belonging in the world that the assaults of racism had destroyed in Du Bois himself: "No bitter meanness now shall sicken his baby heart till it die a living death, no taunt shall madden his happy boyhood. Fool that I was to think or wish that this little soul should grow choked and deformed within the Veil! In the poise of his curl-crowned head did there not sit all the wild pride of being which his father had hardly crushed in his own heart?"[28]

Du Bois's words evince a conviction that had Burghardt lived to adulthood, he would have suffered the same destruction of this innocence as his father. Du Bois thus suggests that his own soul, under the cruelties of the color line, has itself grown "choked and deformed"; his own heart has died a "living death." Terrell likewise fears the deformation of her offspring's inner compass, but the dynamic that she describes is quite different. The assaultive "bitter meanness" for Du Bois comes from without the Veil, evoking Du Bois's memories of his own injuries at the hands of white peers and authorities. For Terrell, the bitterness with the potential to harm is her own, as the white mob's spectacular violence constitutes a less visible but wide-ranging attack on Black maternal bodies, potentially undercutting their lifegiving and protective capacities.

This notion of harm also distinguishes Terrell's formulation of ambivalence from works authored by New Negro intellectual women authors on Black maternity and mob violence.[29] As Muigai demonstrates, there are some strong resonances between Terrell's narration of her first loss and the literary formulations of Nella Larsen, Angelina Weld Grimké, Georgia Douglas, and others. Muigai notes the significance of Terrell's gendered formulation of loss—"my baby boy" in this passage—striking in its departure from the gender-neutral terms that she tends to use, like "my baby" or "the unborn child." This specificity, Muigai argues, links Terrell's account with works by these younger Black women writers that thematize Black mothers' refusal to bear or raise sons in a context ruled by lynch law, figuring childlessness or even infanticide as noble and preferable alternatives. These writings "depict characters that refused, as Larsen wrote in her 1928 novel *Quicksand*, to give birth to "more dark bodies for mobs to lynch"—with these bodies generally figured as male.[30]

Further bolstering this connection, it is likewise noteworthy that Terrell shifts into the third person when describing "the mother's" "horror . . . resentment . . . [and] bitterness," as well as eschewing the possessive with regard to the impacts of these intense effects on her fetus ("the unborn child"). On the one hand, it may align with her statement in the autobiography's introduction that she must titrate the truth for white ears; it may have seemed too confrontational to fully avow these hostile feelings. On the other hand, she may be employing this third-person formulation to reinforce the paradigmatic nature of her own experience of the white world's brutal antagonism toward Black maternity. In line with this, Terrell proceeds to more explicitly aver this shared experience, as she asks "how many colored mothers have been shocked and distracted" during pregnancy by the horrors of lynching—just as she herself had been.

Grimké's 1916 play *Rachel* is, as Koritha Mitchell notes, "the first black-authored, nonmusical drama to be executed by black actors for a broad audience."[31] The play is especially resonant with Terrell's narrative—the first full-length autobiography by a Black woman—for a variety of reasons.[32] The two texts share elements of what Nellie McKay names, with respect to *A Colored Woman in a White World*, a "missionary" character, "bent on convincing whites that if given the advantages of education and better economic opportunities . . . black people as a group would be as civilized in their behavior as their white counterparts, and to showing black people that whites will accept them when they acquire the accoutrements of Euro-American culture."[33] As Mitchell writes, "Grimké later explained that she had written the play to convince whites, especially white women, that lynching was wrong, as illustrated by the fact that even upstanding black citizens were vulnerable to it. The script therefore emphasizes the characters' propriety, education, and appreciation for European culture."[34] The family of the titular character is economically secure, if not elite like Terrell's. Moreover, Rachel is, like Terrell, likewise depicted as having an "abnormally developed" maternal instinct, wishing from a young age for many children to care for. Class privilege has not protected her family, however; she finds out during the course of the play that her journalist father and her brother, whose fates she had heretofore not known, had both been lynched by a vicious white mob. Rachel's mother, who had tried to protect her remaining children from the truth, reveals this fact with the deepest anguish. Rachel witnesses with great pain the racist slights and aggressions that a young boy from the neighborhood, with whom she has developed a kind of maternal relationship, experiences at school.

Rachel, like Terrell's autobiography, thus emphasizes Black maternal suffering at witnessing the white world's violence toward their children. Rachel's own shifting relationship to mothering, as well as the enduring agony of her mother, dramatizes this intergenerational anguish: having seen her joyful destiny to be a mother in a dream early on, Rachel begins to hear the begging of the unborn not to be brought into the world. By the end of the play, she has renounced her dream of motherhood, refusing a loving suitor and pledging to remain childless as a blessing to the unborn who would otherwise be fated to suffer. In fact, the closing scenes witness Rachel as experiencing both a loss of faith and deteriorating sanity as a legacy of her father and brothers' lynching. Facing a spiritual crisis, as Terrell represents herself as undergoing in her own narration, Rachel is, in Terrell's terms, "shocked and distracted," with these psychic states imparting dire effects even at the remove of ten years and the family's relocation to the North. Both accounts aim, as Mitchell writes about the play, "to show [their] audience the generational consequences of the nation's hypocrisy."[35]

At the same time, Terrell's narration of maternal ambivalence also departs from that of Grimké. As with *Rachel*, Terrell's account depicts mob violence as interrupting otherwise healthy intergenerational life. In Terrell's text this interruption does not engender Black women's refusal to become mothers; rather, it perpetrates a kind of moral harm on their fetuses, which might include a future propensity to violence and crime as "desperadoes and murderers." It is clear that the ultimate cause in this process is the murderous white citizenry, who either actively join in mob violence or passively sanction it by failing to protest and oppose it. Overall, Terrell's many writings and speeches against lynching, spanning decades, powerfully call the white nation to account for its atrocities, whether as active agents or passive consenters. Earlier in "I Return to America," Terrell's analysis of Tom Moss's lynching largely aligns with the radical vision of her contemporary Ida B. Wells, who was likewise a friend of Moss and deeply impacted by his mob murder. For Wells, as Megan Ming Francis writes, "the logic of lynching was not criminal; it was economic. Lynching and mob violence were tactics of economic subordination, used to protect white economic power and to ensure a captive black labor force."[36]

Wells in fact credits that atrocity with her political awakening to the deadly lie of lynching as a response to Black men's rape of white women, galvanizing her pathbreaking antilynching crusade. As Wells writes in her own autobiography, "Thomas Moss, Calvin McDowell, and Lee Stewart had . . . committed no crime against white women. This is what opened my eyes to what lynching really was. An excuse to get rid of Negroes who were acquiring wealth and property and thus keep the race terrorized and 'keep the n——— down.'"[37] At Frederick Douglass's request, Terrell had introduced Wells in 1893, at one of Wells's early speaking engagements in which she presented her paradigm-shifting findings. In "I Return to America," Terrell echoes Wells's analysis, writing that Moss and his colleagues had committed "no crime" but "succeeding too well," having established a grocery store whose quality goods and fair prices had attracted Black customers away from white businesses' inferior offerings.

In other writings from the turn of the twentieth century, however, as McHenry and Cooper both point out, Terrell ascribes criminality or low morals to impoverished and uneducated Black people, in ways that diverge from both Wells's analysis and *Rachel*'s plotlines. One striking instance of this is Terrell's 1904 essay on "Lynching from a Negro's Point of View" (her original title was "Lynching from a Colored Woman's Point of View"), which she writes of in her autobiography as one of her proudest achievements. "Lynching from a Negro's Point of View," published in the *North American Quarterly* was a rejoinder to well-known white author Thomas Page's sensationalistic essay on lynching in the same journal, which had luridly portrayed of Black masculine hypersexuality and predation.[38] As Wells does in *The Red Record* and *Southern Horrors*, Terrell's account opens with an unflinching description of the Inquisition-style public torture and lynching of a married couple, a man and woman. Drawing on Wells's data, Terrell backs up her arguments with statistical evidence, demonstrating the rarity even of charges of rape among lynching victims, as well as such charges' spuriousness in the vast majority of cases.[39]

At the same time, Terrell's account of lynching in this essay— unlike in her autobiography-- largely diverges from that of Wells's class analysis. Terrell writes that the two main causes of lynching are not economic but affective and institutional: "race hatred" and "lawlessness." Both Wells and Terrell emphasize white opposition to Black class advancement, but this takes on different meanings for each. Whereas Wells makes clear that lynching is a white response to Black economic gains, in this essay Terrell's analysis emphasizes white opposition to Black social and cultural development, understood both as more refined tastes and a bid for "social equality." Drawing a contrast between elite Blacks like her own circle and the uneducated Black populace, Terrell's account folds in elements of the racialized and elitist logic embedded in the notion of "criminal classes." McHenry notes that "in trying to be balanced"—a kind of "high road" rejoinder to Page's lurid account—Terrell ends up accepting a class-based distinction between law-abiding African American men and those she considers criminals, whom she describes in terms uncomfortably similar to Page's: "ignorant, repulsive in appearance and as near the brute creation as it is possible for a human being to be."[40] While the essay overall is a heroic defense of lynching victims, debunking the mythologies of Black men as rapists and lynching as the chivalrous defense of white women's endangered honor, her language here verges on recapitulating the predominant white representation of the Black poor as inherently criminal and irredeemably primitive—or at least leaving it undisturbed in the white public imagination.

Yet in her autobiography, and even in "Lynching from a Negro's Point of View" and other turn-of-the-century works, there are moments of this suggestive provocation with regard to maternity that militate against white norms. In that key passage detailing Terrell's first postpartum bereavement, despite the intergenerational perils of reproduction under white world conditions, Terrell nevertheless refuses her white friend's proposition that Black mothers themselves are agents of injustice. Although this anecdote does not elaborate on the reasons for Terrell's disagreement, other moments in the autobiography, as well as related writings, illuminate this conclusion. First, in line with the intimate relation that she describes between herself and her material surroundings throughout "I Return to America," Terrell's account of fetal harm itself presumes the exquisite sensitivity of Black mothers and infants to their environmental conditions. This layers her invocation of criminality in "I Return to America" with an additional significance that opposes dominant civilizationist and class hierarchies. Conversely, against the idealization of normative white maternity as the innocent apex of civilized sensitivity and feeling, Terrell brings into view white mothers' literal brutality. Partaking in a lineage of desensitization to cruelty engendered by slavery, they reproduce the environment that makes mob violence possible, at times actively participating in that violence. Both of these elements revolve around Terrell's conceptualizations of heredity and of the biopolitics of maternity and race.

Impressible Bodies: Black Maternal Sensitivities

In narrating her own brush with death during her first pregnancy, as well as her depression in the wake of Moss's lynching, Terrell in fact echoes the opening lines of the autobiography. These short lines detail her own mother's depression and suicide attempt while pregnant with Terrell herself: "To tell the truth, I came very near not being on this mundane sphere at all. In a fit of despondency my dear mother tried to end her life a few months before I was born. By a miracle she was saved, and I finally arrived on scheduled time none the worse for the prenatal experience which might have proved decidedly disagreeable, if not fatal, to my future." Terrell never discloses the details of her mother's gestational depression and attempted suicide, despite what may have been significant editorial pressure; in the foreword, British leftist author H. G. Wells expresses a wish that Terrell had been more forthcoming "in her opening pages," seeming to refer to that incident in particular.[41]

Yet precisely given her account's overarching discretion, as Brittney Cooper notes, it is significant that she nonetheless chooses to begin her book with this revelation: "the fact of her mother's suicide attempt, and her pointed mention of it, points to a history of Black women's pain and despair that remains largely unimagined and unnarrated or examined in the work of public Black women."[42] And although treading with lightness—the understated "decidedly disagreeable"—her opening also brings the reader into contemplation of Terrell's own brush with death and debility even before birth, her proximity to never having been born at all. Her own depression and despair while pregnant thus come clear as intergenerational patterns, reflecting the enduring environment of racism and sexism. As Muigai writes, "the 'fit of despondency' her mother experienced and the 'miracle' of her survival—foreshadowed Terrell's own struggles to become a mother"—Terrell names her own recovery, that summer of 1892, "a miracle" as well.[43] Imperiled maternity and infancy, as well as the saving hand of Providence, are thus throughlines in the text.

The fact the Terrell assures readers that she was "none the worse" for this incident also suggests concern that the opposite might just has well have been the case. In both the autobiography's opening passage and the closing paragraphs of chapter 11, Terrell evinces clear concern about the potential harms of prenatal exposure to maternal affects. Terrell's two narrations of infant loss both dwell intensely on her own maternal feelings in the face of these multiple forms of violence, from gestational horror and resentment to postpartum grief and anguish. Cooper argues for the importance of attending to the relatively rare moments of affective revelation in Terrell's writings, as they militate against a broad-brush characterization of "race women" like Terrell as wholly constrained by respectability's required dissemblances. For Cooper, Terrell's narration of maternal distress in particular in the autobiography—her mother's as well as her own—brings into view "a kind of affective archive that emerges in public Black women's works, and . . . gestures toward the debilitating emotional effects of racism and sexism on Black women's lives."[44]

The narration reflects conceptions of heredity and environment that prevailed from the 1890s until at least the 1920s. Reflecting on Terrell's narration of the 1892 loss, in the wake of Moss's lynching, Brittney Cooper writes that "invoking a belief in impressibility . . .

[Terrell] makes visible the uniquely volatile and unsafe conditions under which colored women gave birth to children. . . . The idea that racial traumas could create heritable traits related to social deviance reflected the deeply embodied sense through which Black women understood themselves and their experiences as racial beings."[45] Impressibility was the understanding of the human body's plasticity, responsiveness to its environment, and ability to pass on those responses intergenerationally—paradigmatically, through the pregnant body to its developing offspring. Within prevailing white supremacist understandings of human development and racial hierarchy at the turn of the century, higher levels of impressibility corresponded with higher civilizational status, with white, propertied, typically-abled Anglo-Saxon women cast as the pinnacle of exquisite sensitivity.[46] Terrell not only invokes this notion of impressibility but also reworks it in key ways.

The concept of impressibility in nineteenth-century science gridded long-standing notions of maternal impressions—the ancient and, while culturally variable, nearly universal understanding that maternal experiences during pregnancy can affect offspring in some way—into racialist and civilizationist frameworks and their "animacy hierarchies," as Mel Chen terms them.[47] As Kyla Schuller demonstrates, this became a core biopolitical principle in the latter half of the nineteenth century, as the white settler population came to experience its collective life as defined by a rarefied capacity for feeling, for receiving and responding to impressions from the surrounding world. As their constitutive biopolitical outside, in contrast, those racialized as nonwhite "were assigned the condition of unimpressibility . . . incapable of being affected by impressions themselves."[48] In contrast to white bodies, especially normative white feminine bodies, which were allegedly the most vulnerable, most in need of care and protection due to their lively responsiveness to environmental influences, impressibility posited Black, Indigenous, and Asian bodies as insensate *flesh*—as Schuller, drawing on Hortense Spillers's germinal distinction, schematizes it.[49]

This accorded with Hoffman's insistence that environmental influences were a negligible factor in Black ill health and high mortality, stemming instead from inherent "race traits." Moreover, according to the prevailing science, sexual difference was key to this biopolitical formation; whites posited themselves as embodying the apex of civilization by virtue of the most complete sexual dimorphism. If white men were, among all the races, the most active and upstanding, white women were the most sensitive, with exquisite faculties of sympathy. A key component of this sympathy was an appropriate response to others' suffering; in contrast, as Susan Lanzoni notes, some white experts of the day argued that a "savage would throw a crying baby to the ground because of 'torpid sympathy.'"[50] This lack of maternal responsiveness was an extension the lack of civilized sexual differentiation.

Impressibility underpinned a biopolitics of racial innocence in at least two ways. First, given the allegedly insensate nature of groups cast as uncivilized races, subjugation, harm, even violence toward their bodies itself had a different significance—a different ontology—than harm and violence toward sensitive white bodies. Harm, in fact, was not harm; what might have registered as violence for a white body might be ascribed any number of nonviolent meanings when visited on a member of a group cast as primitive. Merely enforcing nature's design, civilized whites were thus not culpable for this suffering, as it was in fact not suffering at all but, at best, a reflexive animal response. Second, white women's openness to inscription by environmental factors rendered them particularly vulnerable, mandating the careful guardianship of the purity of their sensitive organisms. Through their maternity, white women were also responsible for transmitting the untainted virtues of civilization to the next generation. White women, then, embodied innocence both synchronically (as the feminine avatars of fully realized civilization) and diachronically (as the assurance of the enduring supremacy of the race over time—the guardians of white settler reproductive futurity). Conversely, this biopolitics of impressibility rendered Black maternity as both insensible to environmental influence and as agents of degeneracy among their children; as both embodiments and reproductive guarantors of this exile from evolutionary and political time.

Yet the terms of impressibility could also be tuned to very different biopolitical frameworks and political meanings. Schuller tracks a counterdiscourse of impressibility in Frances Harper's writings that portrayed Black women as supremely responsive to the impressions of their environments, embodying all the hallmarks of civilized womanhood. She writes that "Harper articulated a negotiated biopolitics, one that worked within and modified structures of sentiment and sexualized racial difference to move the mass of African Americans toward civilization and thus toward life."[51] As Schuller shows, other Black women luminaries, including Pauline Hopkins and Anna Julia Cooper, likewise engaged with the science of heredity in their work. Portraying the most exquisite impressibility, Cooper, in her preface to A Voice from the South, characterizes Black women as "delicately sensitive at every pore to social atmospheric conditions."[52] As Schuller points out, Cooper highlights Black women's particular responsibility for the race's collective impressibility as a whole, which she characterized at the moment of her writing as "peculiarly sensitive to impressions. Not the photographer's sensitized plate is more delicately impressionable to outer influences than is this high strung people here on the threshold of a career. . . . Such is the colored woman's office. She must stamp weal or woe on the coming history of this people. May she see her opportunity and vindicate her high prerogative."[53] "Delicately sensitive" Black women, with their firsthand experience of the stakes of environmental influence, were charged with the "sole management" of the race's defining impressions, of ensuring the impress of noble characteristics within the collective as it rose to realize its destiny. Harper and Cooper thus countered not only the exclusion of Black women from civilized womanhood but the prevailing biopolitical figuration of African Americans as a moribund race outside of evolutionary time.

Terrell's narrative likewise reworks the racist biopolitics of impressibility. As observed earlier in this chapter, Terrell portrays herself as deeply responsive to the material objects and spaces of her environment as well as to the defining relationships in her life. Read within the framework of impressibility, the "affective archive" that Cooper emphasizes in Terrell's text takes on particular significance. For it not only reveals the emotional toll of Terrell's experiences with both racism and sexism—as Cooper points out, she articulates this as a "double handicap" in ways that prefigure later Black feminist accounts, like Kimberlé Crenshaw's intersectionality. It is, in addition, a political claim to the most fully evolved form of feminine human embodiment. Her representation of her anguished response to the suffering of others, and of Tom Moss in particular, paints her as overwhelmingly responsive on all levels—emotional, moral, and even spiritual. It is precisely because of the magnitude of her response to the unspeakable violence of the white mob that potential moral harm might come to her developing baby. Importantly, as well, she figures not only herself but Black mothers of all classes as vulnerable in this way, eminently impressible, open to the shock and horror that the white world as political environment entails.

Terrell's representation of these effects also encompassed the perils of moral degeneration for affected offspring. She was not alone in this thinking; as Muigai recounts, at an 1896 Atlanta University conference on "The Causes of Excess Negro Mortality," fellow NACW member and Tuskegee librarian Adella Hunt Logan, who like Terrell would lose three children of her own, sounded a strikingly similar note. Emphasizing that "the sensitive embryo receives the impressions made upon the mind of the mother," Logan stated: "If the pregnant woman is constantly wishing that her unborn child were dead . . . who can wonder that out of such murderous thought there come in truth a murderer!"[54] Such imagery conjures some of the prevalent racialized criminological categories, linked with class and civilizationist hierarchies. In view of the dominant fin de siècle notions of inheritance and maternal embodiment, however, there was at the same time a countervailing political valence to these figurations. Contra the prevailing white supremacist framework of impressibility, Terrell and Logan alike figured Black mothers as supremely sensitive and emotionally responsive to environmental influences.

This rejoinder with regard to Terrell's first bereavement dovetails with her imputation of medical neglect as the cause of her third. As Laura Briggs, Dána-Ain Davis, Deirdre Cooper Owens, and others have shown, in terms that closely align with Schuller's, the development of nineteenth-century obstetrics and gynecology figured Black women as what Owens terms "medical superbodies"—unlike civilized white women in their diminished sensitivity to pain and feeling, their endurance, yet nevertheless identical to white women in their physiology, making Black women the perfect experimental subjects for treatments that would be dedicated to white women's healing.[55] Davis terms this "obstetric hardiness," arguing that it continues to manifest in the pervasive refusal by medical practitioners to believe and to adequately treat Black women's pain. Davis argues that a derivative figuration of Black infants themselves as "hardy babies" attends this mythos and praxis of "obstetric hardiness," such that even premature Black infants are seen as less vulnerable than their white counterparts, less in need of lifesaving technologies, and thus less likely to receive the same quality of attention.

While Davis's study focuses on late twentieth- and early twenty-first-century experiences of middle-class Black parents in neonatal intensive care units, she cites Terrell's account as evidence of the "hardy baby" figure as having long shaped patterns in care. In line with her counternarrative of Black maternal sensitivity, against prevailing tropes of insensateness, Terrell likewise depicts her own newborn as particularly vulnerable in ways that medical staff failed to recognize or materially attend to. Terrell thus calls attention to the impressibility of Black mothers and infants alike, as well as to the range of hostilities to which the white world unjustly subjects them. This reconfiguration resonates in noteworthy ways in our own postgenomic era. Biographer Parker characterizes Terrell's account of her first loss in the wake of Moss's lynching as "reaching toward epigenetics."[56] Terrell's alignment with emerging contemporary understandings of environment-body interactions are, I argue, less augury than a reflection of the continuities between prevailing understandings then and now. As Schuller writes, the current "shift to epigenetics . . . harks back to the pregenetic era," casting mid- to late-twentieth-century genetic orthodoxy as a detour within a far longer continuum of understanding that our bodies (and all bodies) are shaped by our environments.[57] Nevertheless, Terrell's observations do bear some striking correspondences to key contemporary Black feminist engagements with research in the health sciences on racism, weathering, and epigenetics.

In arguing that Terrell's account of her own experience of gestational harm anticipates current-day epigenetic approaches, Parker invokes Black feminist and antiracist indictments of structural racism as a system of embodied harm with intergenerational consequences.[58] As described in this book's introduction, key recent Black feminist accounts have drawn on epigenetics to describe racism as an environmental hazard for Black women, particularly with regard to reproduction and intergenerational harms. For Shatema Threadcraft these findings underscore the importance of foregrounding the everyday forms of harm that often remain unseen and unaddressed.

Threadcraft calls attention to the ways in which a focus on spectacular Black deaths, such as police killings, can eclipse more quotidian
forms of violence. With coauthor Naa Oyo Kwate, Threadcraft invokes Arline Geronimus's notion of weathering—accelerated cellular
aging and inflammation due to the stresses of racism and sexism—as
an insidious form of assault linked to premature birth and low birthweight, the foremost proximate factors in infant mortality. Kwate
and Threadcraft track the harmful health impacts that ripple out
from direct incidents of state violence to the family members of direct victims.[59]

Terrell's account likewise makes clear that attention to spectacular atrocities alone can deflect attention from the distributed agency
that characterizes the white world as political environment. Threadcraft's emphasis on quotidian necropolitical dynamics, and especially sexual violence perpetrated by police, recalls the police function that Terrell's terrorizing train conductors play—the assaults that
the young Terrell experiences beginning at the age of five and whose
sexual nature she has learned to fear by age sixteen. Additionally,
while Terrell is not infertile, her grave health crisis during her first
pregnancy and her multiple bereavements resonate strongly with
Threadcraft's attention to "the sterile body [and] the unwell body."
Terrell's description of her anguish and depression in the wake of her
friend's murder resonate with Christen Smith's exhortation that
analyses of state violence (in Terrell's case, state-sanctioned vigilante violence) must pan out to include the sequelae suffered by
mothers, kin, and community members of those directly targeted.[60]

White Supremacist Maternity as Hereditary
Environmental Hazard

If Terrell reconfigures the predominant conception of impressibility
with regard to Black maternity, she undertakes a converse—and even

more pronounced—reconfiguration with regard to white maternity. Schuller argues that "heredity theory enabled Harper to point her finger at what she felt was the true origin of primitive tendencies lurking among African Americans: sexual abuse by white men, whose conduct violated the basic tenets of civilization."[61] Terrell's writings deploy heredity theory to complementary ends; she likewise posits an endemic violation of civilizational norms and virtues among whites, but for her it is white women, and white mothers in particular, who are the agents of violation and degeneration. Potentially answering why Terrell cannot "agree . . . entirely" with her white friend, this account nests the potential *proximate* intergenerational perils that Black mothers' feelings potentially present within a broader ecology of white violence, within which white supremacist maternity emerges as a prime mover.

There may be apparent elements of anachronism in positing that something published in 1940 rebuts the science of four decades earlier. There are two reasons for doing so nonetheless. First, Terrell wrote her autobiography over many years, she drew extensively on diaries and notes from each period of her life as she wrote each chapter, and—as in her narration of her first loss in "I Return to America"—she stages her own understandings in those particular historical moments. Second, Terrell's rhetorical invocations of heredity and environment over the course of the autobiography's production reflects the continued political utility of these conceptions for her opposition to lynching and Jim Crow, even as the genetic orthodoxy that would become dominant by midcentury was gaining prominence. In Terrell's autobiography "heredity" is a keyword that tracks her own shifting understanding of reproduction and responsibility. Early on in the text, Terrell narrates her distress, as a schoolchild, at the "iron law of heredity" as it was taught: "The injustice of the law of heredity stunned me. It seemed terrible to me that the children of drunkards should inherit a tendency to drink immoderately and the children of thieves might have a hard time to be honest, and so on."[62]

While this initial encounter is narrated in race-neutral terms, Terrell later recounts being particularly troubled by the ascription of a propensity to theft among Black people as a Lamarckian consequence of enslaved mothers' stealing food during pregnancy:

> From conversations which I heard in my childhood and youth I got the impression that practically all colored people would steal if they got a chance. Those who held this view declared that this tendency was easy to explain. Before the birth of their children slave women had to steal the food that appealed to their appetites. . . . Since this went on for nearly three hundred years, this tendency to steal was inherited, near-students of the problem declared. I was wretched. I did not want to steal, but I feared that I was doomed, since it was in every colored person's blood according to the theory just set forth.
>
> But after I went to Oberlin I ceased to worry on that score. During my college course I heard several missionaries state that in Africa theft is practically unknown, and that the natives do not learn to steal until they have come into close contact with other races. It was a great comfort to know that I would not be forced to steal, whether I wanted to or not. . . . It was a relief to be informed that I had inherited the strictest honesty from my African forebears, and if I developed a penchant for laying heavy hands on my neighbor's property, it would be an acquired rather than an inherited taste.[63]

Terrell thus describes the inner moral development of her child self, "wretched" at the prospect of having inherited criminal tendencies through no fault of her own. In this example, she is navigating two distinct notions of heritability with regard to crime—one through the maternal line, wherein enslaved women's deprivation-based theft during pregnancy impressed the next generation, in ways that were transmissible even after formal emancipation. The second is the knowledge—garnered secondhand from missionaries—about honesty as a kind of positive African "race trait," pushing against accounts like Hoffman's. Reversing civilizationist hierarchies and their evolutionary logic, the degenerative influences here are external and European. The first notion is framed as a mistaken childhood notion derived from hearsay and transmitted by those without real proximity to knowledge. In contrast, for Terrell the missionary status of those who introduced her to the counterpoint, as well as their firsthand experience in Africa, indicates the authoritative nature of this second and more reassuring position.

This reversal of white supremacist ascriptions of hereditary criminality reaches its culmination in the autobiography's account of Terrell's political activities in the 1930s. Here it is white mothers both committing crimes and transmitting this tendency to their own offspring:

> Several times in recent years I have appeared before committees in Congress to urge the necessity of passing the anti-lynching bill. "What effect do you think lynching will have upon the white women of the South?" somebody asked me. "We all believe in heredity," I replied. There is no escape from that. More than once white women in the South have applied the torch to burn colored men to death. Those women are being brutalized by the crimes in which they themselves participate. Their children will undoubtedly inherit the brutal instinct from their mothers and it will be more difficult to stop lynching on that account.[64]

Terrell here figures white women themselves as brutalized by these crimes, rendered less sensate as a result of their own actions, and passing this down to their children.

This figuration is quite similar to the deployments of heredity in her writings from the early twentieth century. While her figuration of the "brutes" of the Black criminal classes in 1904's "Lynching from a Negro's Point of View" is noted above, Terrell accompanies this ascription with allegations of brutality on the part of white women—a lack of civilized human feeling inherited from generations of white mothers who had learned not to feel:

> Lynching is the aftermath of slavery. The white men who shoot negroes to death and flay them alive, and the white women who apply flaming torches to their oil-soaked bodies to-day, are the sons and daughters of women who had but little, if any, compassion on the race when it was enslaved. The men who lynch negroes to-day are, as a rule, the children of women who sat by their firesides happy and proud in the possession and affection of their own children, while they looked with unpitying eye and adamantine heart upon the anguish of slave mothers. . . . In discussing the lynching of negroes at the present time, the heredity and the environment, past and present, of the white mobs are not taken sufficiently into account. It is as impossible to comprehend the cause of the ferocity and barbarity which attend the average lynching-bee without taking into account the brutalizing effect of slavery upon the people of the section where most of the lynchings occur, as it is to investigate the essence and nature of fire without considering the gases which cause the flame to ignite. It is too much to expect, perhaps, that the children of women who for generations looked upon the hardships and the degradations of their sisters of a darker hue with few if any protests, should have mercy and compassion upon the children of that oppressed race now.[65]

White mothers under the system of slavery, whether personally enslavers or not, had learned from the cradle not to feel. Inured through their own mothers' brutal pedagogy to the everyday horrors that enslavement visited upon their Black counterparts, they inculcated that concerted unresponsiveness to suffering in their own children in turn. Terrell's rhetoric here can be read as inheriting abolitionist accounts of slavery's brutalizing impacts on Black and white people alike, and white women in particular—with significant differences that mark shifting understandings of science. Terrell styled herself as an inheritor of Frederick Douglass's legacy; Douglass famously stages this dynamic, in *Narrative* as well as in *My Bondage and My Freedom*, in the fall from grace of his childhood mistress, Sophia Auld, a weaver by trade who had married into a family of enslavers.[66] At first inclined very kindly toward Douglass, Mrs. Auld is soon inducted into the discipline of callous apathy that enslaving requires and undergoes a dramatic transformation from heavenly sweetness and beauty to a demonic ugliness. This is reflected—in the *Narrative*, in her very visage, in vivid religious terms—as a transformation from angel to demon.[67]

As a political spokesperson of the succeeding generation, under Jim Crow and the rise of lynch law, Terrell likewise highlights the warping effects of slavery for whites as well as Blacks. As she writes in "Purity and the Negro," a speech given in 1905: "Morally speaking slavery was a weapon which shot both ways, wounding those who fired as well as those who were hit."[68] Parker writes that "Terrell saw herself as Douglass' protégé and intellectual compatriot, someone who could carry his legacy into the next generation."[69] Her account of harm, however, reflects the scientific understandings of the day; in "Lynching from a Negro's Point of View," Terrell might be read as positing a hereditary theory of the evils of slavery that Douglass couches in terms of the soul.[70] Terrell thus not only draws on Wells's statistical evidence to refute Page's apologia for lynching but also rebuts the white supremacist hereditarian science that underpins it. Far from embodying the highest possible degree of delicate impressibility, white women here are callous and indifferent; it is they who are characterized by the "torpid sympathy" as they in effect evince a primitive indifference to their "sisters of a darker hue" and their own "crying babes." This is not merely an individual trait; this affectively deficient mothering has taken collective intergenerational form as an environment of normalized "barbarity," marking an evolutionary retrogression across Southern white society.

These early twentieth-century writings thus anticipate Terrell's indictment of white women's heritable brutality before Congress decades later. She charges white mothers with shirking their responsibility to "arouse the conscience of the public toward the open and shameless debauchery of colored women by [white women's] husbands, fathers, and sons."[71] As Parker frames it: "Daring to shift the terms of the debate, Terrell moved from accusing white men to publicly charging white women with responsibility for perpetuating . . . assaults against black girls and women."[72] This responsibility was, again, a matter of heredity: "It is impossible to explain such hardness of heart . . . except on the ground of heredity. Descended from generations of mothers who were accustomed to look upon the wholesale debauchery of colored women without a protest and without . . . shock to their moral natures . . . their daughters have inherited this indifference to the degradation of colored women by the [white] men of the present day." This unshockable indifference to lynching among white women stands in direct opposition to the shock and horror of impressible Black mothers in "I Return to America."

For Terrell, then, in a stark reversal of the prevailing mythology of white femininity as the apex of civilized morality, purity, and innocence, white women's investments in white supremacy embody at once political culpability and evolutionary moral degeneration. Both culpability and degeneration may be transmitted across generations—a response to a brutalizing environment that gives rise to a brutalizing maternity, which in turn gives rise to another brutalizing environment. At the same time, Terrell's hereditarian rhetoric ultimately stops short of racial determinism. It serves as a cautionary mirror to white women readers, calling them into the authentic virtues of womanhood, not casting them as a lost cause. Terrell was a lifetime political collaborator with white women-led organizations— even as this sometimes yielded bitter disappointments.[73] Her 1904 essay holds out the possibility of redemption to even the morally blighted white women who foster racial terror: "But what a tremendous influence for law and order, and what a mighty foe to mob violence Southern white women might be, if they would arise in the purity and power of their womanhood to implore their fathers, husbands, and sons no longer stain their hands with the black man's blood!"[74] Terrell thus casts these unfeeling white daughters of unfeeling white mothers as falling short of civilizational ideal of womanhood— but also suggests that fulfillment of this ideal is a matter of political will.

Moreover, Terrell's persistent emphasis on the responsibility of white mothers for an environment of racial violence pushes against the long-standing blame of Black mothers themselves for inequitable health outcomes. It militates against the implicit presumption—still predominant today—that the normative white maternal body is the politically *and* biologically innocent standard. Against that presumption, Terrell's writings firmly locate white maternity and heredity as key elements of an environment of violent threat to Black life. They thus anticipate critiques of ways that epigenetic approaches can smuggle in "race traits" logics that pathologize Black maternity and infancy, rather than the environment of racism and collective responsibility for that environment. Stephanie Jones-Rogers has called attention to the plantation as a "school" for young white girls who would be future enslavers as well as future mothers of white children. Recounting many instances of this ghastly education, including a three-year-old white girl's demand for the mutilation and replacement of her enslaved caretaker, as well as a white mother's destruction of an enslaved woman's face with a rocking chair, Jones-Rogers highlights the pedagogical function of exposing white children to routine atrocities.[75] Decades later, Ida B. Wells recounts in her autobiography a chilling anecdote in the wake of an 1893 lynching in Paris, Texas:

> Miss Laura Dainty-Pelham was traveling through Texas a year later and she often told how the wife of the hotel keeper kept talking about it as if it were something to be proud of. While she talked, her eight-year-old daughter, who was playing about the room, came up to her mother and shaking her by the arm said, "I saw them burn the n____, didn't I Mamma?" "Yes, darling, you saw them burn the n____," said the complacent mother, as matter-of-factly as if she had said she saw them burn a pile of trash.[76]

As Elizabeth McRea demonstrates, white mothers were central to the maintenance of twentieth-century Jim Crow as well. She tracks the ways that white mothers served as "segregation's constant gardeners," as they "guaranteed that racial segregation seeped into the nooks and crannies of public life and private matters . . . being a good white mother . . . meant teaching and enforcing racial distance in their homes and in the larger public sphere."[77] This included organizing against both school integration and anti-lynching legislation. White supremacist maternity, in Terrell's telling, is both a hereditary and an environmental factor—absorbed and passed down via maternal lessons in aggression and desensitization, it creates the "climatic" conditions for acute racial violence to ignite.

Terrell's Maternal Meanings

Terrell's theorization of heredity, from these early twentieth-century writings to the autobiography, is not a textbook scientific notion, entailing definite and consistent relations between embodied heritable traits, cultural practices, individual will, and environmental influence. Her figurations of maternity and heredity over several decades are, rather, political claims about reproduction under white world conditions—as well as about the reproduction of the white world itself. As I have argued, these engagements with the scientific paradigm of impressibility rebutted race traits–oriented approaches to infant mortality, reversing the prevailing civilizational hierarchy between Black and white maternity.

Terrell's rhetorics of maternity and heredity at times partially re-tain, even as they recast, prevailing understandings of civilizational and evolutionary hierarchy. They are thus, in certain moments, in-tertwined with elitist characterizations of poor Black people as prim-itive, ignorant, and criminal. Reflecting on Terrell's 1904 essay, Ha-zel Carby makes an additional critique of Terrell's assertion that "lynching is the aftermath of slavery." In contrast to what she casts as the more internationalist and anticolonial visions of Du Bois and Anna Julia Cooper, Carby argues Terrell and like-minded thinkers at the dawn of the twentieth century "used the term 'aftermath' to make the point that their own era was contiguous with the three hun-dred years during which people of African descent had been en-slaved in America."[78] For Carby this assertion of linear continuity made for a US-centric and often ahistorical frame of reference, one that excluded Indigenous genocide and US imperialism—and hence also the complex and specific historical links between these distinct fronts of colonial racial capitalism and the specific forms of Jim Crow racial violence. Terrell's 1904 essay indeed falls short of Carby's call for an integrated analysis of imperialism, settler colonialism, and ra-cial capitalism. As discussed, the essay's explanation for lynching, unlike that of Wells, does not entail a full-throated indictment of these atrocities in terms of their maintenance of capitalist class power alongside white supremacy or of racialized class hierarchies. It is also true, underscoring Carby's critique, that her autobiography refers to Native dispossession as "benign appropriation."[79] At the same time, Terrell's theory of that "aftermath of slavery" as a matter of maternity nevertheless reconfigured the biopolitics of racial innocence in important ways.

Terrell's analysis itself was necessarily complex and dynamic, shifting over her incredibly long and multifaceted political life. Noaquia Callahan shows that she was a leading figure in international women's antiwar organizing from at least the 1910s.[80] And her framings of both lynching and its racist and gendered harms in the United States were likewise dynamic. As sketched earlier, Terrell highlighted white women's cultivation of an intergenerational environment of racism, through both everyday feminine and maternal routines of white supremacy and active participation in mob violence. Furthermore, Terrell's final political campaign, undertaken when she was nearly ninety years old, likewise shifted the horizon of her analysis, bringing together a more radical economic critique with additional elaborations of the reproductive harms of lynching and the broader environment of white terror.

Communist Party organizer Claudia Jones's foundational 1949 essay, "An End to the Neglect of the Problems of the Negro Woman," highlights Terrell's leadership in the political coalition that arose in defense of Rosa Lee Ingram.[81] Ingram, a widowed Black mother of fourteen children—twelve living, two whom had passed—was a sharecropper who had been condemned to death, along with two of her sons, for defending herself against the violent attack of a white neighbor. Also a sharecropper, this neighbor had previously attempted to sexually assault Ingram. In this subsequent attack, the neighbor had wielded a gun and struck Ingram first. After the conflict the assailant later died, and a Georgia court tried and convicted Ingram of murder, along with two of her sons: Wallace, sixteen years old, and Sammie Lee, fourteen. Although the Ingrams' lawyers argued that the act had been in self-defense, the court condemned mother and sons to death by electric chair.[82] The case galvanized public protest at a national scale; as Dayo Gore writes, there was "immediate protest from black communities throughout Georgia" that "soon spread nationally," thanks to the Black press, and "such overwhelming grassroots support for this black woman's right to self-defense spurred into action the leading civil rights organizations of the period."[83] The NAACP and the Communist Party-associated Civil Rights Congress formed an "uneasy alliance" in response to the death sentences; Terrell was part of a women's delegation that met with President Truman and his attorney general. While, under national pressure, the judge quickly commuted the sentences to life in prison, political organizing to free the family continued, and Terrell played a key role.[84]

In an unusually close collaboration with radical organizers in the Civil Rights Congress, Terrell agreed to take leadership of the National Committee to Free the Ingram Family. As part of that role, she delivered an address in September 1949 to the United Nations Economic and Social Council's Human Rights Commission. Terrell and her fellow organizers recruited W.E.B. Du Bois to pen the petition to the commission; Terrell authored a substantial extension of Du Bois's text.[85] The address comprised both sections. The text of Du Bois's petition situates the miscarriage of justice for Mrs. Ingram and her sons, and the federal government's failure to intervene, as a test case for the UN to exercise its authority regarding "the relation of democracy in the United States of America, to its citizens of Negro descent."[86] Terrell's appeal puts a finer point on the gendered, as well as racial, violence at the heart of the case. She characterizes the neighbor's assault and the criminalization of Mrs. Ingram and her children's self-defense as paradigmatic of the country's systemic anti-Black sexual and reproductive violence. She emphasizes the fact that, with near-total impunity, white citizens and authorities pervasively target Black women for sexual assault and even lynching—in some cases while pregnant.

Generally speaking, a colored woman who is the victim of a white man's advances or violence has no redress in the courts. The brutal and shocking manner in which colored people are lynched in the United States . . . causes the world either to doubt or to sneer at our claim of being a Democracy. The world's condemnation of such lawlessness and cruelty is increased because it is generally known that the perpetrators of these crimes are rarely punished. On several occasions the bodies of colored women have been ripped open their babies snatched out and thrown into a river nearby or on the ground.[87]

Terrell thus extends her previous accounts of white terror as a reproductive harm to encompass not only the indirect impacts of lynching on Black mothers and their children and white men's sexual predation but the vulnerability of Black women and their offspring—even before birth—to the direct violence of lynching as well. Her speech further highlights the interconnections of gender-based violence, racial terror, and white legal impunity with unjust educational, housing, and labor conditions, and legally enforced poverty: "The money spent for the education of colored children in the public schools is often only half or less than half of that spent on the education of white children . . . because of prejudice against their race thousands of well trained colored people are unable to secure employment, so that they can earn a living and help support their families."

Terrell continued to organize for Ingram's freedom with leftist organizers of the Civil Rights Congress; she served as chairman of the Women's Committee for Equal Justice (WCEJ) in 1951, while radical left organizer Yvonne Gregory, who had worked on the *We Charge Genocide* document, was the WCEJ's executive secretary. As Gore writes, not only were Black women in leadership of this multiracial national organization; "its brand of interracial solidarity pushed beyond leftist-inspired calls to 'unite and fight' to demand that white women actively participate in dismantling white supremacy."[88]

Terrell's testimony to Congress in the 1930s had held up a damning mirror to Southern white women's collusions—not innocent victims in need of chivalrous protection but brutalized and brutalizing perpetrators, enacting physical violence on their fellow Black citizens and moral violence on their own white children.

As part of the Women's Committee for Equal Justice, Terrell, then in her late eighties, partook in a political appeal to progressive white women, to recognize the ways that the interconnections of racial domination, sexual violence, and economic oppression also harmed white women themselves: a rigorous invitation to transform their common ground. Natali Valdez writes: "Pregnancy and reproduction are not individual processes. We all encompass the maternal environment. We all collectively participate in reproduction, regardless of sex, race, gender, orientation, ability, or fertility. We all contribute to the social, institutional, and environmental circumstances that shape each pregnancy, birth, and child."[89] Terrell's figurations of white maternity and heredity summon a closer look at the maternal environments of Jim Crow racism and its wake, alongside the more spectacular forms of racial terror that these environments have enabled and perpetuated. Terrell's attention to white maternity and its reproduction of white world conditions looks to the collective that constitutes the person's context: not only maternal responsiveness to, but collective responsibility for, the material environment and its political effects.

Terrell's attention to these material conditions spanned writings across her political life. Her dedication to Rosa Lee Ingram's case, however, brought special attention to the conditions of poor rural Black women who mothered, labored, experienced pregnancy, experienced loss, and gave birth under conditions very different than Terrell herself had, in her elite urban East Coast milieu. At midcentury, when organizing for Ingram was at its peak, many rural Black women across the South still looked to community-based midwives for their care. Both medical segregation and the laws regulating—and some-times criminalizing—these midwives' care marked yet further perils to and encroachments upon the reproductive lives and freedom of Black women and the wellness of their children and kin. Under these conditions midwives carried out crucial practices of care and protec-tion. It is to these midwives that the next chapter turns.

4   *The Midwife's Bag*

The disappearance hypothesis began to lose its grip in the 1910s, only to give way to new, statistically grounded convictions about the alleged threat that Blacks posed to the morals and health of the white citizenry. David McBride shows that "by the end of World War I a crescendo of statistics grew supporting the idea that blacks posed a public health menace," above all, as allegedly disproportionate carriers of TB and venereal diseases like syphilis; hence "mainstream [white] American society through the World War I decade generally viewed black Americans more as a source of contagion than as fellow victims."[1] As Shaka McGlotten writes, Black people have been "hailed by big data" in a race toward a variety of objectifying ends; "technes of race and racism reduce our lives to mere numbers . . . as commodities, revenue streams, statistical deviations, or vectors of risk."[2] Given that Black infant mortality did not constitute a direct threat to the white population, it gained no increased visibility during the 1910s as a problem to be contained. Scattered local programs in Northern cities did attempt to prevent Black infant mortality in the later 1910s.[3] The biopolitics of racial innocence, however, still guided patterns of response once Black infant death finally emerged as a white public health concern in the 1920s. A new Black community pathology came into view: the midwife.

The landmark 1921 Promotion of the Welfare and Hygiene of Maternity and Infancy Act, more commonly known as the Sheppard-Towner Act for its congressional sponsors, was the United States' first federal social welfare legislation. Initiating the provision of federal funds to states for maternal and infant care, it marked a sea change in the official status of Black infant life and death. Overseen by the federal Children's Bureau, whose official aim was comprehensive medical and nursing care for every birthing mother, the Sheppard-Towner Act articulated a mandate for "the promotion of the welfare and hygiene of maternity and infancy" among all citizens.[4] The legislation nominally included Black infants and their mothers within its biopolitical ambit. In practice, however, the entrenched racial hierarchy in the South largely prevented the act's programs from addressing Black infant mortality's determining factors. Following the previously established bifurcation, Sheppard-Towner funds in the North, Midwest, and West augmented and coordinated efforts at the local level to support maternal and infant health among poor white and immigrant populations through environmental, educational, and expert care interventions. Officials in the South concentrated on the alleged ignorance, unhygienic practices, and superstitions of Black midwives as the primary cause of high infant mortality rates. "Midwife control"—surveillance, regulation, and ultimately elimination—was hence the primary target of Southern reform.[5]

Black midwives had been crucial healers and key authorities in their communities since slavery times. Often called to the vocation through divine revelation, as well as learning through apprenticeship to older midwives, they cared for men and women across the lifespan, often attending both births and deaths, and maintained a broad repertoire of knowledge about herbs and other medicines.[6] They still attended the majority of births in rural Black communities.[7] While the text of the act confirmed the biopolitical inclusion of Black infants, the Southern emphasis on midwife control served to deflect attention from enforced poverty and racial terror, the true causes of infant and maternal mortality. It figured the mechanisms of infant mortality as a sort of shadow play against a blank screen, in which the midwife, the mother, and the infant were the only characters. All emphasis was thus placed on the midwife's observation of—or failure to observe—what public health authorities deemed proper procedure during the birth event itself.

At the heart of proper procedure was the midwife's bag. As a key element of what Alicia Bonaparte calls "rounding up midwives," community midwives were required to surrender their own home-made satchels, equipped with herbal remedies, vernacular and sometimes commercially prepared medicines, and other tools of the trade.[8] These were replaced with standard-issue bags: usually black leather tote bags with metal clasp and two handles, washable linings, they contained a small inventory of permitted items, including a safety razor, sterile gown, antiseptic, soap, scissors, and silver nitrate eyedrops for infants. This chapter homes in on the bag as a key material signifier of racial innocence. Reflecting the "true babyhood"-inflected apprehension of Black infants as less deserving of care and attention than their white counterparts, the exchange of "primitive" for standardized bags served as a substitute for substantive, time-consuming transformations of the conditions affecting maternal and infant health. Midwifery training in South Carolina, for example, showed that the first several years "largely focused on bag and birth certificate checks and permit renewal" rather than on instruction in care.[9]

While subject to intensive surveillance, criminalization, and labor exploitation that rendered practice impossible for many, thousands of Black midwives combined the rudimentary tools offered by the state with lineages of reproductive knowledge and practices to offer crucial care to mothers and infants. Moreover, this punishing regime did not define all points of contact between midwives and the state.

As Wangui Muigai shows, Black physician Ionia Rollin Whipper, in the employ of the Children's Bureau, worked with midwives across the South, developing a training curriculum addressing the actual conditions of Black infant health and midwives' vital roles.[10] As Muigai writes: "African Americans knew that highly publicized campaigns to 'save the babies'. . . failed to address. . . broader sociopolitical concerns of Black well-being."[11] Whipper was thus one of many Black physicians who, along with nurses and health reformers as well as pastors and churches, concertedly addressed these concerns.[12]

Yet the "standardized, surveilled" bags and the meanings that they encoded were pervasive. Declaring Southern states and their segregated medical and public health apparatuses innocent of any role in Black infant mortality, they figured the vernacular knowledge and expertise of the community midwife as itself the main threat to Black babies' lives. Without this constant surveillance, the implication was these midwives would revert to their default state of primitive superstition, unhygienic practices, and criminal tendencies. The supposedly heroic effort to transform and maintain midwives, from this malignant natural state to benign carriers of modern medical protocols, both demonstrated that Southern states did care for Black infants; yet this always-present specter of anachronism and dangerous carelessness remained a convenient excuse for high infant mortality rates.

Bags as Surveillance Objects

Alabama midwife Onnie Lee Logan, active between 1936 and 1976, participated in her state's registration and training programs; her mother, also a midwife, practiced in the years before the inception of these programs. In her autobiography Logan marks the difference between these two generations through the difference in their bags: "The midwives would always make them a sack. They didn't have bags naturally like [the bag] that I have. But they would make them a

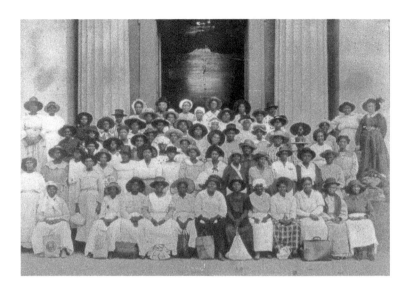

FIGURE 1. Midwives in Canton County, Mississippi, 1920s. *Source*: Courtesy of the Archives and Records Services Division, Mississippi Department of Archives and History.

sack and they would put their stuff in there and put a drawstring on it."[13] As a photo from the 1920s taken in Mississippi shows, at the outset of the midwife registration effort, African American community midwives used a wide variety of materials to contain their birth equipment, as evidenced by the distinct shapes and sizes of satchels that the midwives are holding or have set at their feet (figure 1). The photo is captioned: "A group of midwives in Madison County before any instruction."[14]

This photograph of "untrained" midwives presents a striking contrast with the photograph taken at a weeklong 1934 "midwife institute," or training course, in Saint Augustine, Florida. Dressed in identical white gowns and headbands, each midwife holds one of two standardized Black leather bag models on her lap. The last line written at the top of figure 2 reads: "Largest per cent complete equipment."

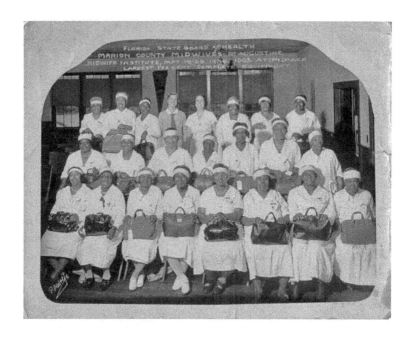

FIGURE 2. Florida Midwife Institute. *Source*: Courtesy of the State Archives of Florida.

Besides location, date, and the 100 percent attendance rate, this positive grade awarded to the midwives' bags (though the temporal and geographical reference points for "largest per cent" remain unclear) was the only datum deemed worth preserving in the written record. Moreover, on at least two of the bags, tags are visible; up close, these tags were likely very similar, if not identical to, the bag tag in figure 3. Both of these images are from Florida, but similar tags were used throughout the South, listing the equipment that midwives were officially required to keep in their bags, accompanied by a hortatory slogan, such as this one: "The Safe Midwife keeps her bag clean and ready at all times." Potentially useful as checklists for busy practitioners, the tag's exhortation also served as a reminder that the midwife was to maintain her bag in a state of constant readiness for display.

MIDWIFE'S EQUIPMENT

This bag should contain a clean
washable lining.
Safety Razor - with new blades.
Sterile Gown.   Nail brush.
Bottle of Synol Soap.
1 per cent Silver Nitrate Solution.
2 Sterile sets of cord dressings.
1 Sterile set of wipes.
Mask for nose and mouth.
Sterile cap.   Orange stick.
Bottle of Lysol.   Blunt Scissors.
Sterile tape to tie cord.

The **Safe Midwife** keeps her bag
clean and **ready** at all times.
                    (OVER)

FIGURE 3. Midwife bag tag. *Source*: Courtesy of the State
Archives of Florida.

Both contemporary and historical sources, from midwives' oral narratives to public health officials' accounts, are strikingly unanimous in their depiction of the ritual of the bag inspection.[15] Nurse supervisors or public health officials, usually white, performed inspections at each midwives' meeting and training course, evaluating each midwife's bag for cleanliness and the completeness of its equipment, as well as ascertaining that it contained no prohibited items such as herbs or surgical gloves. If midwives refused, if the equipment were found incomplete, or if prohibited items were found in the bags, midwives faced harsh sanctions, including fines and the loss of their permits, without which it might be illegal for them to practice.[16]

As Gertrude Fraser notes in her ethnography *African American Midwifery in the South*, the state midwife training apparatus can be usefully understood as a Foucaultian technique of discipline, aimed at inciting an attachment to the priorities and criteria of the public health agency.[17] Using Foucault's schema of disciplinary procedures, the bag inspection can be characterized as an instantiation of the ritualized *examination*. The examination "imposes on those whom it subjects a principle of compulsory visibility"; as a record of this continual surveillance, it creates an archive of written documentation that makes of each subject an individual "case" comparable to others.[18] Combining "hierarchical observation" with "normalizing judgment," for Foucault the examination is the core mechanism of the disciplinary apparatus.

> The examination . . . makes it possible to qualify, to classify, and to punish. It establishes over individuals a visibility through which one differentiates them and judges them. That is why, in the all the mechanisms of discipline, the examination is highly ritualized. In it are combined the ceremony of power and the form of the experiment, the deployment of force and the establishment of truth. At the heart of the procedures of discipline, it manifests the subjection of those who are perceived as objects and the objectification of those who are subjected.[19]

The ritual of the bag inspection indeed imposed a relentless visibility upon the examined midwives; one Southern public health doctor asserted that the key characteristic of the bag was its "easily scrutinized contents."[20]

The bag inspection was a ceremony not just of institutional but of racial power. Fraser outlines this form of racial-disciplinary power, observing that midwives were conscripted into "a 'unified' field of observation in which not only midwives but also physicians, pregnant women, births, deaths, 'health conditions of the races,' marital patterns, and sexuality could be systematically monitored and studied and the racial and economic hierarchy of the society reproduced and maintained."[21] Drawing on the linkage made by David Brion Davis between Bentham's Panopticon—Foucault's model of disciplinary power—and slave plantation management, Saidiya Hartman argues that it is "necessary to consider the way discipline itself bears the trace of what Foucault would describe as premodern forms of power but which perhaps are more aptly described as 'discipline with its clothes off.'"[22] Simone Browne pushes this line of argumentation further; for Browne this "naked" aspect is better described as the anti-Blackness that has been constitutive to modern discipline from the beginning. Browne writes that "an understanding of the ontological conditions of blackness is integral to a general theory of . . . racializing surveillance—when enactments of surveillance reify boundaries along racial lines."[23]

Accounts of midwife meetings convened by state and county boards of health are nearly unanimous in depicting the bag inspection as the opening and often focal activity of each gathering, each time reasserting the power and propriety of the white gaze and disciplinary apparatus.[24] Fraser writes that "inspections of midwives' bags formed part of the routine of the relationship between public health nurses and African American women." Kelena Reid Maxwell concurs that the new regime of inspections exposed midwives to unprecedented scrutiny: "Aspects of their lives and their work, which were previously hidden from the gaze of white medical officials, were routinely examined."[25] Even accounts that aim to portray a happy co-operation between nurses and midwives cannot but acknowledge the unidirectionality of the gaze. Edna Roberts and Rene Reeb's retro-spective account describes the two groups in rural Mississippi as hav-ing created "a partnership that worked." And yet, in their description of a typical midwife meeting, they write that "the nurse prepared her set-up and the midwives began to arrive. *It was a bit tense as bags were inspected.*"[26] Their passive formulation does not specify the subjects of this tension—nor, for that matter, who was doing the inspection—but it was midwives, not the nurse, who were on the spot.

Bag inspections could never render the midwives' practices en-tirely visible, however. Even where regular midwife assemblies were required, the bags could not always be counted on to reliably testify to midwives' actual practices. The group bag inspections were thus supplemented by the one-on-one extension of the ritual into mid-wives' homes, through the technique of (often unannounced) home visits. As a pair of white nurses in Mississippi reported in the 1930s: "We . . . never miss an opportunity to stop at their homes and inspect bags whenever we are in the neighborhood."[27] Maxwell affirms that it was common practice for public health nurses throughout the South to conduct random bag inspections in the homes of the mid-wives under their supervision.[28]

Assessing the state of the bag was the putative reason for these visits, but the bag also served as a kind of warrant for the nurse supervisors—usually white women—to inspect the hygiene of mid-wives' homes as well. For instance, white educator Marie Campbell's 1946 account of Georgia midwives, which narrates accompanying a nurse supervisor on a home visit, includes a detailed assessment of the domestic scene: "Martha's house was beautifully clean throughout. The bed coverings were fresh and clean, the window curtains were newly laundered, and the bare pine floors were scrubbed white."[29] While indisputably positive (an affirmation signaled, as in the snowy garb of the "reformed" midwives, by the whiteness of the scrubbed pine floor), this description reveals the casual entitlement of nurse and author to inspect the midwife's five-room home "throughout." The house served as an extension of the bag's space, equally open to unclasping and scrutiny by white observers, its condition grounds for judgment in the continuous trial of the midwife's fitness in the eyes of state officials.

The bag as an instrument of racial discipline thus situated the nurse supervisors within the venerable lineage of white women as philanthropic visitors to the homes of people of color, from Reconstruction-era Northern "friends of the race" to social workers. Hartman notes that the "genre of the philanthropic visit" comprises the benign-sounding components of "the evaluation of progress, the inspection of order, an examination of proper domestic hygiene, and the dispensation of advice." But, in fact, she argues that during Reconstruction "the domestic was the ultimate scene of surveillance: a fence in need of whitewashing, a dusty house . . . invited punitive judgments. The description of the [domestic] good life . . . actually authorized the normative gaze, which, by detailed observation of all areas of life, judged the suitedness of the formerly enslaved to freedom."[30] Decades later, a similar dynamic characterized social workers' surprise visits to welfare recipients, assessing the domestic virtues and vices (such as the presence of a man in the house) as grounds for approving or denying continued assistance.[31] As Evelyn Higginbotham writes, the racial regime in the US has historically "rendered [Blacks] powerless against the intrusion of the state into their innermost private lives."[32] Following this pattern, the bag-cum-home inspection subjected the midwife's private domain to the discretionary judgment of the public health nurse, serving as a ritual reinforcement of racial domination as well as potentially affecting the former's continued eligibility to practice.

"Surveillance," Browne writes succinctly, "is the fact of anti-blackness."[33] The bag inspection as both signifier of racial innocence and technique of racial discipline thus joined the patterns of visibility common across disciplinary regimes with the hypervisibility specific to the Black female body. In prioritizing the bag's (and the midwives' own) orderly appearance as the primary sign of competence, above less visually evaluable criteria of skill and experience, it devalued midwives' expertise and short-circuited the potential for respect for and responsiveness to communities' own needs and preferences. And as a "gateway object" for home hygiene inspections, the bag affirmed white authorities' implicit right to the intimate spaces of African American life, as its perpetual openness to scrutiny was seen as necessary to the health of the social body.

In accordance with Foucault's account, this regime of visibility was accompanied by a proliferation of written documents—but, in line with Hartman's and Browne's assertions, this record-keeping entailed harshly punitive dimensions. In addition to bag tags, midwife manuals, permission slips to attend patients, syphilis test results, and assessments of personal hygiene, public health officials maintained an ongoing written record of the bag evaluations on midwives' permits, which had to be renewed annually in most places.[34] Compounding midwives' presumed a priori guilt for infant deaths, in the eyes of white medicine and public health, this permit system gave white people in a range of positions—Fraser names "public health officials, physicians, [and] local registrars"—authority to rescind a midwife's permit, making it illegal for her to practice.[35] This system of legal sanctions, at least in some states, was linked to the new "racial integrity" laws. Midwives were responsible for recording the race of each child on the birth certificate; in Virginia, for example, Fraser notes that "failure to accurately report a newborn's race brought down the full wrath of the state," as it was a felony punishable by a year in prison.[36]

Given these new bureaucratic restrictions and the climate of fear that they entailed, it is perhaps unsurprising that the most significant effect of the Sheppard-Towner Act in the South was a reduction the number of midwives serving African American communities: "In 1922 Florida had over four thousand midwives; by 1929, the state claimed that three thousand women considered 'physically unfit or . . . incapable of receiving instruction' had left the business . . . the number of midwives dropped from over 6,000 to 4,339 in Virginia and from 4,209 to 3,040 in Mississippi."[37] Yet white physicians were no more willing to serve poor African American women by the end of the 1920s than they had been prior to the act's implementation, a fact Toni Morrison dramatizes in the first pages of *Song of Solomon*.[38] Thus Black women in the South had a new barrier to access to experienced birth attendants, which necessarily raised their risk of complications. Moreover, new associations of criminality and deviance with midwifery led Black women into an impossible situation; physicians and public health personnel increasingly depicted choosing the care of a midwife as a sign of maternal indifference, breathing new life into long-standing stereotypes of pathological mothering. While European immigrant midwives were also stigmatized, the communities that they served were in fact were targeted by the Children's Bureau and other agents of Progressive Era reform for both sanitary improvements and assimilation into the emerging standards of obstetrical care—even, as in the case of some Italian immigrants, as they resisted the latter.[39] Sheppard-Towner programs had institutionalized official inattention to Black infant mortality, and the numbers reflected this: mortality among white infants nationwide declined from 72 to 64 per 1,000 births by 1928, whereas the Black infant mortality rate per 1,000 births declined only very slightly, from 108 to 106.[40]

Although the Sheppard-Towner Act was only officially in effect until 1929, the pattern that it established lasted at least until the New Deal took effect, and in many places far longer; in the most rural parts of the South, programs such as midwife assemblies constituted the main form of infant mortality (non)intervention until the early 1960s.[41] The midwife's bag and its attendant procedures were thus a key everyday instantiation of Browne's racializing surveillance, wherein "enactments of surveillance reify boundaries, borders, and bodies along racial lines."[42]

Midwifery as Persistent Danger

The caption in figure 1 ("midwives before any instruction") presents a paradox. Had these women in fact never received *any* instruction, they could not be called midwives in the first place. Yet it captures the white public health regime's epistemological commitments, which excluded midwives' often extensive empirical training from the categories of instruction or knowledge. In contrast, figure 2 and its commentary reflect white public health officials' sense of pride and accomplishment at putting things in their proper arrangement. A white public health physician's words depict this transformation from his perspective: "The old Negress in dirty nondescript dress, a pipe stuck in her mouth, and a few odds and ends of equipment thrown into a paper shopping bag or a drawstring cloth sack began to be replaced by a cleaner woman in a white starched dress and a white cap carrying a black leather bag which contained a carefully scrutinized set of supplies."[43]

For white public health personnel the new bag and vestments worked an almost magical transformation of the midwife from Black "Negress" to whitened (via dress and cap) woman, from dirty to "cleaner" (though still not *clean*).[44] Far from concerning themselves with substantive improvements in Black infant mortality and morbidity, the transformation to which these writings attend most vividly is that of the palatability of the midwife's bodily habitus to a white observer. Constance Van Blarcom, a nurse reformer, wrote a similar appraisal: "The rows of pupils with tidy heads and hands, immaculate in their wash uniforms, might have been the staff of any visiting nurse association. There were no leathery, rheumy-eyed old crones. . . . Their bags with washable linings and appropriate contents, conformed to State Department of Health requirements. They were evidently put to practical use and were not merely for exhibition."[45] Van Blarcom's insistence on the bags as tools of "practical use" rather than objects for show arguably testifies to some anxiety about the authenticity of this transformation. Nevertheless, the revolting specter of "leathery, rheumy-eyed crones"—the civilized white reader cannot but recoil—against the "immaculate" backdrop of the white uniforms showcases the bag's importance as a container not only of equipment but of the unruly and abject corporeality of African American midwives in the their "natural" state. Oozing contamination has given way to "washable linings" and "appropriate contents."

Sara Ahmed, drawing on Frantz Fanon's phenomenological account "The Fact of Blackness" in *Black Skin, White Masks*, writes that "racism 'stops' black bodies inhabiting space by extending through objects and others."[46] The transformation of midwives from vernacular experts drawing from a long legacy of multifarious knowledge traditions into auxiliary instruments was just such a grand project of extension and disorientation. The bags' dazzling uniformity served to homogenize the midwives in the eyes of public health and medical experts, obscuring potentially important differences between them; as a sign of (relative and limited, good-enough-for-Black-folk) competence, it preempted any acknowledgment of the broad variety of knowledge and experience midwives brought to their work. Returning again to the contrast between the photographs earlier in this chapter, the second photo's portrayal of the institute's attendees as proud graduates, with their proper and "complete" bags as the sine qua non of their expertise, negates the knowledge of the empirically trained midwives in the first photo.

Alabama midwife Margaret Charles Smith, empirically trained with an experienced elder midwife as well as a veteran of numerous state midwifery classes, points out in her autobiography: "I took training courses, but the midwife had already trained me, Ella Anderson. . . . [E]verything, everything I learned, I learned from Miss Anderson."[47] As oral historian Linda Janet Holmes observes in her commentary on Smith's narrative, "no matter how short or disparate the formal training program," it conferred "favor with professional health care providers" on midwives who received it.[48] A weeklong training institute, accompanied by the proper appearance and a complete and sterile bag, counted for more than the decades of experiential knowledge that many midwives brought to childbearing women. As Ahmed writes, "even bodies that might not appear white still have to inhabit 'whiteness'"—in this case, white instruction, however inappropriate to their function—"if they are to get 'in.'"[49]

In addition to compulsory compliance with the optics of white public health, midwives were permitted to carry only the items listed on their bag tags (see figure 3) or similar official inventory lists. As Fraser writes about the case of Virginia, "midwifery programs intended to clean up the midwife, strip away her superfluous rituals and beliefs, and make her, so far as was possible, a creature of science."[50] This list showcases the extremely narrow scope of practice within which the disciplined midwife was expected to confine herself; her tasks focused on cleanliness, and she was expected to eschew both practices deemed "unscientific" and those considered overly advanced for her allegedly limited intellectual and moral faculties. Thus substances and practical objects deemed insufficiently medico-scientific for a (semi-) trained (semi-) professional were banned.

Primary among these prohibited items was the midwife's extensive *materia medica*, rooted in Native American, African, enslaved African American, and southern Euro-American herbal knowledge. Passed on over many generations, it included remedies for pain relief, management of labor, breastfeeding problems, diseases of infancy, and emergencies such as hemorrhages. For example, Holmes names castor oil, ginger tea, black pepper tea, and May apple root as commonly employed labor stimulants.[51] Midwife Smith recalls the health officials' prohibitions: "'No more pepper tea, no dirt dauber [a kind of insect with medicinal properties apparently salutary for birth], no kind of root or nothing.'"[52] Any items related to folk practices deemed "superstitious" or unnecessary for the rationalized procedures of birth and postpartum care were also prohibited.[53] "The white world," Ahmed writes, "'disorients' black bodies such that they cease to know where to find things—reduced as they are to things among things."[54] Under the Sheppard-Towner programs, midwives found themselves unanchored from the repertoire of efficacious remedies central to their role as healers. The racial disciplinary aspect of midwife control, of course, was closely intertwined with this process of instrumentalizing disorientation. Midwife Smith continues: "They said, 'They better not catch nobody giving no tea of no kind. If they do, she was going to jail and then the pen.'"[55]

At the other extreme, the rules also prohibited equipment deemed overly medico-scientific for these midwives. Gloves, in particular, used to perform vaginal examinations during labor, and sometimes to reposition the fetus' head or body, were strictly prohibited, as vaginal examinations were the exclusive province of physicians—nearly all of whom were white men. The vaginal exam was a highly charged locus of struggle in the ascendancy of obstetrics over midwifery in the United States more generally.[56] In a context of poor rural Black communities, however, this prohibition reveals the extreme vulnerability of Black women's bodies under the regime of Jim Crow apartheid. Like the nurse supervisor's surprise home inspections, the definition of Black women's birth canals as the exclusive domain of white physicians reflects the broad prerogative of white authorities to enter the most intimate spaces of African American lives. But it also reflects the power relationship that inhered in what Hazel Carby calls "the institutionalized rape of black women," even if it did not entail the act itself.[57] Since most white physicians refused to treat Black women under most circumstances, the violence of this white male prerogative thus manifested through omission as well as commission. Given that at least some midwives had learned lifesaving techniques that entailed manual contact with the birth canal during their apprenticeships, the prohibition on gloves almost certainly cost the lives of Black mothers and babies, who either could not receive these techniques or had to face a risk of infection from them.

The double prohibition on herbs and gloves makes clear that Southern public health's midwife control efforts were an *agnotological* project—that is, a project of deliberate unknowing—backed by the threat of state violence.[58] If as Fraser asserts, "southern public health officials had to confront the African American midwife as a privileged knower and knowing subject," their reform procedures rendered much of this knowledge impracticable, if not criminal.[59] These efforts can thus be situated in a long lineage of forced forgetting among Black people reaching back to the Middle Passage.[60] Midwives' knowledge was inextricable from material practices: laying of hands, medicinal preparation and administration, food recommendations and restrictions. Ahmed writes that "the 'matter' of race is very much about embodied reality . . . what is and is not within reach."[61] As a racializing project, Southern white public health reconfigured what was within reach, and for whom. It severely limited midwives' own reach, providing a bare minimum of hygienic equipment while prohibiting vital techniques for birth and postpartum support. However, public health extended its own institutional reach: it put "reformed" midwives to work as prostheses, allowing the nominal extension of its concern into Black homes without requiring white physicians to offer services across the color line, addressing poverty or white supremacist terror, or in any other way disturbing the racial order.

Tensions of Innocence and Failed Orientations

Under this disciplinary regime, the metonymy of the bag was arguably supposed to work two ways: in the presence of nurse supervisors and public health officers, it stood in for the midwife, its cleanliness and compliance continuous with and substitutable for her own personal hygiene, its easy unclaspability continuous with her mandatory openness to scrutiny. But in the field, at births, where nurses and public health personnel rarely ventured, it seems also to have been meant to serve as a kind of supervisory proxy, the bag tag's admonitions echoing those of the instructors, its stern official outlines evoking the implacable observational presence of the public health officers even there. At the same time, the record of midwifery control is in fact replete with evidence of midwives' refusals of these techniques of objectification: using the bag and its contents in the service of care that defied the standardized privations of segregationist public health, and laid bare this regime's lies of racial innocence.

George Stoney's film *All My Babies: A Midwife's Own Story* dramatizes some of these tensions. *All My Babies* is an instructional film for the education of empirically trained midwives made for the Georgia State Board of Health. Its selection for inclusion in the National Film Registry of the Library of Congress for "historical, cultural, or aesthetic merits" in 2002, however, bears witness to its transcendence of the instructional film genre. Stoney noted in an essay he wrote about the film in 1959 that most film schools required its students to watch it, just as medical schools did.[62] Shot in 1952 in the small segregated town of Albany, Georgia—less than a decade later, this was the setting of the Albany Movement of 1961-62, a coalition of the Ministerial Alliance, the NAACP, the Federation of Women's Clubs, the Negro Voters League, SNCC, and the Southern Christian Leadership Congress, and Dr. King was jailed for leading a 1961 march—the film communicates far more than proper procedures for maternity care.[63] Georgia Health Department physician William Mason recalled that at the time the film was made, Albany was experiencing "an almost reign of terror inimical to the emotional and to some extent the physical health of blacks."[64]

Notwithstanding this climate of everyday violence, the Georgia public health officials who hired Stoney told him that there could be "no intention of even suggesting an unhappy relationship between whites and blacks existed, nor in any way promoting a change in black-white relationships."[65] The film reflects these paradoxes. Scripted as a sort of morality tale, it is at once a moving homage to the expertise and ingenuity of an African American midwife and an apparent endorsement of the innocence and benignity of Jim Crow white medical and public health authorities. As one of the producers recalled, the film was a "glorification of a figure [the midwife] . . . whom the southern medical establishment wasn't at all anxious to glorify, although it was highly dependent on her."[66] As Wangui Muigai writes: "*All My Babies* is a remarkable portrait of a midwife who is proud of her work and respected in her community. At the same time, it lays bare the conditions of rural black health care in the Jim Crow South and the fraught relationship between black midwives and white medical professionals in the mid-twentieth century."[67]

Accordingly, in the film Mary Frances Hill Coley's bag both signals her expertise and marks a key site of tension. The film is fully scripted but uses nonactors in all of the roles and several health care practitioners play themselves. Coley, a highly experienced Black midwife in Albany, plays herself in the film's starring role, and the bag that she carries in nearly every scene is her own. Dialogue was based on real-life dialogue Stoney had recorded over months that he spent shadowing Coley through her attendance at labors and checkups, and it was finalized in intensive collaboration with Coley. It was shot on location in Coley's actual house and the public health clinic, and showed Coley attending patients in actual homes in Albany.[68] Intended to depict childbirth authentically in both good and miserable conditions among Southern African Americans, the film features two contrasting characters as patients of Coley. Ida Flemming, played by Martha Sapp, an actual pregnant patient of Coley, has a supportive husband (played by Coley's son) and two beautiful young children (played Coley's grandchildren) and a comfortable, relatively spacious home in town.[69] In contrast, Marybelle Dudley, troubled and underfed, is childless, having previously suffered a stillbirth and a miscarriage. Already seven months pregnant, she has drifted into town with her husband and lives in an isolated, squalid shack.

The storyline follows Coley's exemplary attendance upon the pregnancies and births of these contrasting characters. It depicts her as an expert in her own right but also as a faithful subordinate to the doctor and nurses who run the public health clinic. Coley's bag, featured in nearly every scene, constitutes a key element in each of these plotlines. After a white-sounding male voice-over introduces the characters, the very first scene shows Coley preparing her bag (figure 4). She is ironing while chatting with Ida, who is admiring the photographs that cover Coley's wall. She affirms that the photographs are "all my babies—I've delivered over fourteen hundred." Coley carefully folds the gown and places it in the bag. Her deft movements in preparing her bag, as she confirms the number of babies she has delivered, project professional accomplishment and competence. The camera then pans down, leaving Coley's face out of the frame; in a kind of virtual bag-cum-home inspection, the film lingers over the spotless approved equipment arrayed on Coley's parlor table (figure 5).

After a home visit Coley is filmed among several rows of other Black midwives in a meeting or class at the clinic (figure 6). This meeting has been convened after a newborn in the care of one of the midwives has recently died from a cord infection. Bags in their laps, the midwives listen gravely to the doctor standing before them.

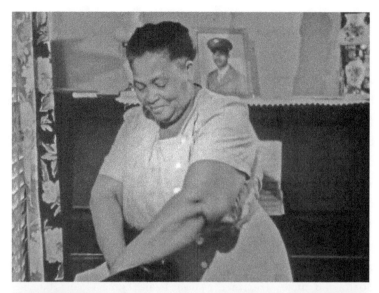

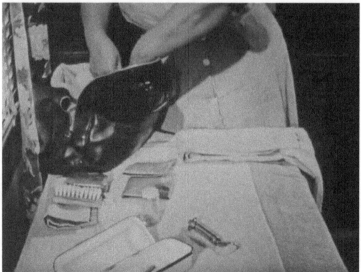

FIGURE 4. Midwife Mary Coley appearing in *All My Babies. Source*: Library of Congress, Motion Picture, Broadcasting, and Recorded Sound Division.

FIGURE 5. Midwife bag contents, in *All My Babies. Source*: Library of Congress, Motion Picture, Broadcasting, and Recorded Sound Division.

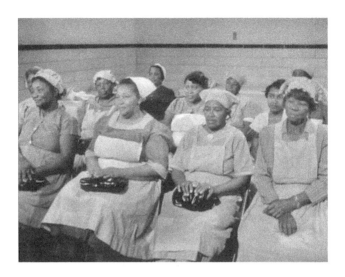

FIGURE 6. Midwife meeting, in *All My Babies*. *Source*: Library of Congress, Motion Picture, Broadcasting, and Recorded Sound Division.

While acknowledging that it can be "hard to keep clean in some the homes where you have to go," and that, despite this difficulty, the midwives have done a "wonderful job," he gravely states that the infection occurred because "something wasn't clean." Brandishing one by one the pieces of equipment that stock the midwife's bag, he speculates: "Maybe they didn't boil scissors long enough, or use sterile dressing."

The doctor's conclusion that a midwife's unclean equipment is to blame showcases the bag's enactment of racial innocence, deflecting attention from the structural causes of high infant mortality among Blacks in the South implied by the many other possible explanations. Offering the bag as a stand-in for more expensive measures in official efforts to prevent these deaths (figure 7), the persistence of death becomes the failure of midwives to properly deploy the bag's sanitizing powers—and, secondarily, the inability of the households that

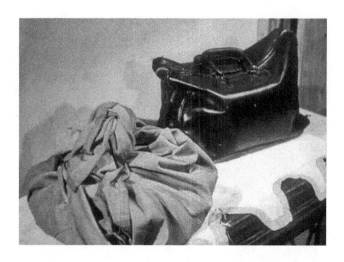

FIGURE 7. Black bag and laundry bundle, in *All My Babies*. *Source*:
Library of Congress, Motion Picture, Broadcasting, and Recorded
Sound Division.

they serve to "keep clean." Thus the death was allegedly the outcome
of the midwives' incompetence even after training: ignorance, failures of hygiene, self-neglect. Fraser discusses a similar dynamic at
work in a medical report from Virginia in the 1940s that explained
the circumstances of a young mother's death from postpartum hem-
orrhage after doctors waited eleven hours before initiating a transfu-
sion. Although the report acknowledged a grave mistake on the part
of the doctors, it concluded that in fact the death was the fault of the
patient herself, as she was to blame for "the absence of prenatal care,
the failure to seek medical attention at the onset of the bleeding [the
sign of danger]. These failures were due to neglect or ignorance on
the part of the patient and her family."[70] Like the fetish object of the
"clean, complete and sterile" bag, the notion of available care—the
actual availability of which may reasonably be doubted, and which in
any case would have comprised the very doctors who let the woman
bleed for several hours—makes it possible to exclude both structural

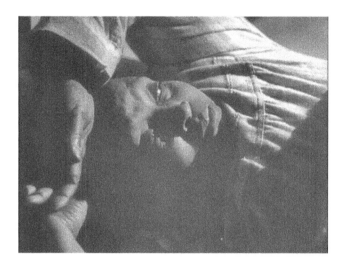

FIGURE 8. Midwife Coley closeup, in *All My Babies*. *Source*: Library of Congress, Motion Picture, Broadcasting, and Recorded Sound Division.

and proximate factors from considerations of causation, and blame African Americans for their own demise.

Coley's bag is put to use in accordance with public health protocols at Ida's birth. As she empties her bag to set up for the birth, it dwells on the details of her equipment—her scrub brush and scissors, sterile gauze in a basin on a table—and her scrubbing and gowning routine as well. All goes well with Ida's birth in the film—though her live delivery, captured by a white film crew in that social and political context, bespeaks elements of extraction, if not outright exploitation; Martha Sapp also reported being cruelly shamed by a white nurse at the clinic during the process.[71] Coley arrives home from the birth at five in the morning. Exhausted, she sits on the bed and puts the bag and the bundled laundry from the birth on a night table saying to herself: "Too wore out to fix a clean bag tonight. I'll fix it in the morning."

The screen darkens. The camera cuts to a close-up of Coley's face as she tosses and turns in bed (figure 8). Her eyes are closed, but a forehead creased with worry tells us that all is not well. A voice-over of the white doctor's admonition reveals what is echoing in her head, like God's call to Samuel, as she tries to sleep: "something wasn't clean," he says, and repeats: "Something wasn't clean. Something wasn't clean." Coley opens her eyes: "Can't sleep . . . thoughts preying on my mind," she mutters. The bag materializes both surveillance and innocence in this sequence. Given the biblical, or at least ghostly, resonance of the doctor's echoing admonition, the bag channels official disapprobation, reproaching Coley for her neglect from its perch on the table. Even the exemplary Coley, it suggests, requires an external spur to optimal hygienic practices. Coley cannot let this stand; she gets up in her nightgown to sterilize her instruments and restock the bag with clean linens. Coley's sacrifice of sleep for hygiene's sake turns out to be providential. No sooner has she gotten back into bed for a well-deserved rest when Adam, Marybelle's husband, roars up in his truck: Marybelle is in premature labor. The denouement reveals that Adam Jr., thanks to Coley's expert delivery, clean bag inventory, and the timely arrival of an incubator, is thriving at four months of age, just like Ida's baby.

The specter of infant mortality as reflective of Black community pathology, filth, and backwardness both opens and closes the film. Coley's compliance with the disciplinary protocols of bag hygiene is clearly shown to have allowed her to help save Marybelle's baby. To some extent, her virtues rely on the extent to which she has internalized the relationship of surveillance congealed in the bag. Nevertheless, Stoney's film also shows that the bag could never have served its purpose without its skillful deployment in Coley's expert hands. It pays tribute to Coley's power to make a place where Black mothers and infants were cherished and protected, for a little while, from a hostile and indifferent social world. And it also evinces the burdens that accompanied her role as expert caregiver. As dramatized by this film, attention to the shifting and simultaneous roles reveals lines of tension and contradiction within the biopolitics of racial innocence that governed the midwife control programs.

Sousveillance and the Bag

Many of the texts produced by and about midwives during the period of the state campaigns to reform them suggest that the midwives also defied the protocols of surveillance. In making a case for the key role of anti-Blackness in surveillance practices, Browne coins the term "dark sousveillance" to denote practices of "critique of racializing surveillance." Such practices include "antisurveillance, countersurveillance, and other freedom practices" that "appropriat[e], co-op[t], repurpos[e], and challeng[e]" "the tools of social control" "in order to facilitate survival and escape."[72] Significant evidence indicates the bag itself facilitated sousveillance practices among midwives. Stoney reports observing such a practice as he accompanied rural Georgia midwives for several months in the course of his preparatory research for *All My Babies:* "One county health officer pridefully had me observe his monthly inspection of the midwives' bags and equipment. I never saw cleaner scissors or whiter towels. Two hours later I was sitting in the kitchen of one of his midwives when she explained without a trace of guile: 'Yes, the Doctor, he likes our things to look nice and clean at the inspection. So all us ladies keeps one bag to show and one to carry.'"[73] Midwife Margaret Charles Smith describes this practice as well.[74] A powerful disciplinary object in some settings, the bag opened onto an array of oppositional possibilities in other contexts, acting as a cover for the continuation of prohibited expert practices. Valerie Lee notes that midwives persisted in carrying herbal remedies in their bags for use, arguing that they therefore "attested more to ingenuity and rebellion" more than compliance.[75]

Disciplinary notes also mention the presence of gloves, suggesting that midwives continued to conduct internal exams in spite of public health personnel and physicians' prohibitions.[76]

Browne's link between sousveillance and survival is particularly pertinent here. Midwives did not refuse the official tools and tasks of hygiene; rather, they offered something beyond the official vision of substandard care. The inclusion of herbal remedies and gloves, in addition to the officially approved bag contents, affirmed midwives' capabilities, the forms of expertise that they had learned through apprenticeship and their own experiences as practitioners. But this was not merely an act of individual self-affirmation. As these practices had been developed and preserved in the context of Black communities over time, it was also an expression of solidarity, a responsiveness to the needs and expectations of the women that midwives served. Smith quotes one of her clients as saying that she had heard from other women "about what good stuff [Smith] had. Why don't you give me some? Fix some for me so I can get through with this baby."[77] Although Smith narrates this episode as part of her own ultimate relinquishing of herbal remedies in the face of threats of incarceration from public health officials, she judges the official system, not her own, as an insufficient repertoire of care, representing its restrictions on herbal remedies as a mandate "not to try to help" those in need of care. Moreover, relating her experiences after having retired from practice, and therefore out of the reach of sanctions, Smith reveals that although she eventually acquiesced to the official restrictions, she "had been working a good while" before she complied.[78]

Under the cover of the bag, midwives carried their officially forbidden tools to work in the service of the lives and health, as well as the comfort, of the women and babies that they served. For at least some midwives, complying with the imposed regime of practice would have been incompatible with the fulfillment of their calling, and this may be one reason their ranks thinned. Smith recalls that one midwife at a meeting, when told that she could not employ herbal remedies, replied defiantly: "I think I'll bring my bag in and give it to you all because you all are not there when this labor is going on. You don't know how it goes. Rubbing helps and teas help. If I can't give them some hot teas which I know will help, I just as well ought to give it [midwifery] up." Outright challenges to the authoritative knowledge of the nurse supervisors appear to have been rare, but Smith prefaces this episode by commenting on public health officials' unjustified fears of herbal remedies' effects and makes no critical commentary of these remarks—seeming, if anything, to affirm them.[79]

Moreover, disciplinary hierarchy, so effective in the classroom, did not travel so well. Stoney reports that several Georgia nurse supervisors confessed that fear of exposing their own inexperience with labor and delivery prevented their ever accompanying midwives on deliveries. They feared their authority would crumble if a midwife asked them "to do something they knew nothing about."[80] As Browne writes, "dark sousveillance . . . speaks to black epistemologies of contending with antiblack surveillance."[81] The defiant midwife's charge that the nurses really "don't know how it goes" very likely struck a nerve, exposing a void behind the disciplinary regime's claims to authority.

Praxes of Care against Racial Innocence

Ahmed writes of the potentials of "failed orientations," wherein "bodies inhabit spaces that do not extend their shape" and "something happens other than the reproduction of matter."[82] Southern public health positioned itself as transmogrifying midwives from unruly vernacular experts to scientized instruments for the transmission of basic principles of hygiene. Yet it would be more accurate to say that many midwives appropriated this hygienic repertoire into what remained a radically different ethos and set of practices. One of these was noncommodified care. Doctors refused to serve women who could not pay their fees, which were considerably higher than those of midwives.[83] Most midwives, in contrast, were emphatically not profit-driven. Often invoking service to God, and midwifery as a sacred calling, midwives' narratives testify to their service to families regardless of ability to pay, despite the financial hardship that this usually entailed.[84] A fourth-generation Virginia midwife in Fraser's account states that she had "never known a midwife to refuse a case, no indeed, even if they owed her from the last baby she would go."[85] Moreover, they often stayed with families for multiple days, depending on the needs of the mother and baby, sometimes performing the cooking and domestic tasks that would otherwise have fallen to the mother, and even sewing clothes for the infants of the very poor.[86]

One of the responses to a 1925 midwife survey in rural Texas explained why women chose midwives over physicians thus: "Midwife does more for you, gives tea etc., and helps with her hands."[87] Ahmed writes that "it is the hands that emerge as crucial sites in stories of disorientation."[88] Over the first half of the twentieth century, in addition to becoming more and more expensive, obstetrical care in the United States was an increasingly rationalized affair, requiring the women in its ambit to conform to a standard time-scale of "normal" labor, or else submit to interventions, creating quasi-Taylorist routines for processing parturients—the rise of what Robbie Davis-Floyd terms the "high-tech, low touch" model of hospital birth.[89] In contrast, Black midwives' hands enacted care that combined the scientific with herbal remedies and lineages of practical knowledge. This creative and pragmatic approach, which Fraser terms midwives' "philosophy of praxis," was responsive to the needs of individual women and infants in their particular situations: the opposite of objectification.[90] These trajectories together shaped the terrain of gendered racial domination and its pervasive impacts on life and health, as well as Black midwives and their communities' strivings to foster life in the face—and behind the back—of these daily assaults.

Midwifery Care in the Broader Ecology of Harm

It is vital to acknowledge Black midwives' practices of antisurveillance and creative appropriation in response to the Southern medical establishment's regime of midwife control and the racial innocence that underpinned it. At the same time, such acknowledgment should not obscure the everyday violence and enduring efficacy of these objectifications. Midwives' sousveillance could not displace the hardship, nearly universal for Black women under Jim Crow, of tremendous work for very little pay. In fact, it often added to these women's burdens. Many, if not most, midwives attended births in addition to full-time jobs as domestic servants, cleaners, or fieldworkers. Moreover, midwives' extensive knowledge, creative innovations, and responsive modes of caring, the fact remains that their practices—including subversions of the disciplinary regime—thrived to the extent that they did in part because the white medical establishment did not consider Black mothers worth its attention. The new obstetrical imperatives to manage labor scientifically, including intrapartum anesthesia, simply did not apply to Black women, at least in the rural South.[91]

Nor did public health bureaucrats object to the broader necropolitical conditions of Black pregnancy and birth, innocently refusing to consider socioeconomic status, nutrition, or access to quality medical care for the great majority of Southern Black people. Yet they nearly succeeded in discrediting and eliminating Southern Black community midwifery: an important site of Black women's authority and expertise, a whole domain of practical knowledge of the body and of herbal medicine, and a rare site where African American birthing was cherished and protected.[92] Gertrude Fraser implies that perhaps the greatest loss was that of a collaborative path untaken, in which the protected spaces, affirming relationships, and effective knowledge of African American midwifery care could have been respectfully combined with the advantages of obstetrical medicine. Technical improvements in care for Southern African American women and infants that (all too slowly) did eventually succeed did not require the midwife's eradication.[93] In fact, growing evidence points to the optimal situation of maternity care depending on the integration of midwives—not their exclusion.[94]

Ahmed characterizes whiteness as a habit that persists over time; "the habitual," she argues, "can be thought of as a bodily and spatial form of inheritance."[95] Public health habits have persisted in refusing to see—or, more recently, to materially support—effective care practices rooted in Black communities themselves. I would argue that this failure is at least partially an effect of public health habits established through the processes of objectification at work under the Sheppard-Towner programs. In chapter 5 I foreground the paradigm-shifting work of Black-led reproductive care and justice projects—some led by Black midwives and doulas who, with reference to the sousveillance practices sketched in this chapter, locate themselves in the radical lineage of Black Southern midwives—that are supporting healthy Black maternity and infancy. In a stunning reversal of the demonization of Black midwives a century ago, much mainstream public discourse now posits Black birthworkers as a key solution to what the White House itself has named the "maternal health crisis."[96] At the same time, I ask whether certain habits of racial innocence that subtended the midwife control programs—including failure to address the everyday reproductive necropolitics that US racial capitalism entails and the exploitation of Black women's caring labors—may nevertheless persist.

5 From Infants in Crisis to Maternal Health Crisis: Birth Justice against Racial Innocence

In June 2022 the Biden-Harris administration released its "White House Blueprint for Addressing the Maternal Health Crisis." Like the statements issued by so many major health organizations, institutions, and government agencies since the summer of 2020, the Blueprint excoriates racism as the underlying cause of health inequities. The achievement of optimal pregnancy health for all, it asserts, "is only possible if we address the systemic racism that is entrenched not only in our health care system—but also . . . in our laws and public policies, and in our public and private institutions."[1] For the Blueprint, maternal mortality among Black and Alaska Native/American Indian communities, as well as for people in rural areas, is at the heart of the crisis, and racism—which the Blueprint names but predominantly operationalizes as *bias*—is largely to blame. But the Blueprint is also noteworthy for what it does *not* highlight. If maternal mortality is the crisis here, infant mortality is almost nowhere to be found. Out of seventy-four instances of "mortality" in the text and citations of the Blueprint, only four refer to infant mortality. It is mothers, even more than their infants, who are spotlighted as the subjects of crisis, danger, and death.

Only a decade ago, the reverse was true. Around 2012, when I began work on the dissertation project that would be the springboard for this book, concern about Black infant mortality seemed to be everywhere. I had been a midwife before graduate school, and I was still moving between the worlds of midwifery and academia. This project itself was spurred in part by indictments by midwives of color of the national white-dominant midwifery organizations' own long-standing racism—including these organizations' studied inattention to Black infant and maternal outcomes.[2] While white midwives were not paying attention to Black infant mortality, however, researchers, government agencies, and journalists were vehement that Black infants were in crisis.

There are continuities between these two moments. Materially speaking, the disproportionate vulnerability to death for US Black infants has not changed, even as their mothers' precarity is now framed as the site of crisis.[3] Moreover, at least some of the scholarship that shaped the discourse around Black infant mortality still informs current indictments of racism as a threat to health. Yet the framings are markedly distinct. This chapter briefly tracks some key features of this shift. I sketch the previous moment, arguing that the preceding approach to Black infant mortality as a crisis entailed a paradoxical dynamic. It was informed by a wave of research on the physiological harms of racism from the 1990s and 2000s—some of which was quite radical in its conclusions, attended closely to the material interplay of racism, sexism, and class exploitation, and called for sweeping societal transformations. The related national campaign targeting Black infant mortality, however, nonetheless framed individual Black mothers' behaviors and choices as the primary cause of their infants' demise, and related programming did not address systemic factors. In other words, this campaign followed the familiar pattern of the biopolitics of racial innocence.

Moving to the current conjuncture, I note three significant shifts. The first is this move to maternal mortality, rather than infant mortality, as the site of crisis. The second is the focus on medical racism, in particular what anthropologist Dána-Ain Davis terms "obstetric racism."[4] The Blueprint highlights medical provider bias as a key danger to maternal health, especially for Black mothers. Previously, the main issues with pregnancy and birth care tended to be framed as its accessibility, or—when accessible—its inability to mitigate the harms wreaked by systemic oppression. With some exceptions the character of this care tended to be represented as benign, or at worst ineffective. In the current moment, however, mainstream obstetrical care is itself often framed as a site of harm and violence. Finally, and relatedly, is the third shift: the naming of Black midwives and doulas as key actors in solving the maternal health crisis departs from the previous moment.

The Blueprint places unprecedented emphasis on the benefits of midwifery and doula care, with an accent on culturally congruent doula care in Black and Indigenous communities. In all of these and many more elements the Blueprint takes a cue from the organizing and advocacy for birth justice and equity that have gained momentum over the past decade. This new framing disallows some of the elements that made recourse to racial innocence possible with regard to framing of the infant mortality as a crisis. At the same time, given the long-standing entrenchment of the biopolitics of racial innocence, I query whether its mandates might be taken up in ways that allow the patterns of fatal deflection to persist.

Stress and "A Healthy Baby Begins with You"

In May 2007 the Office of Minority Health (OMH) of the US Department of Health and Social Services launched an initiative, "A Healthy Baby Begins with You."[5] Designed to "targe[t] the African American community, to combat its disproportionately high rates of infant deaths," the campaign's brochure makes clear who this "you" is: the individual Black mother herself (figure 9).[6] The front of the brochure features the campaign title, in pale blue sans serif font against a terra cotta background with a scrolling motif. Below the text is a photograph picturing the head and upper shoulder of a wide-awake, chubby-cheeked, open-mouthed baby with light brown skin, looking to be just a few weeks old, cradled in a pair of hands a few shades darker brown. The shapely fingernails on the hands are unpolished, neatly manicured into a rounded oval that meets the tip of the thumb and finger, communicating understated femininity. Underneath the statement that "A Healthy Baby Begins with You," this little life literally rests in her hands. The background color of the back and in-fold is mostly orange; the division between the two colors describes a curve that suggests a pregnant belly. The back of the brochure is much smaller text, with the heading "African American Infant Mortality" (figure 10). It informs readers that "celebrating a baby's birth should be a joyous and momentous time for a family. Unfortunately, the celebration ends too soon when a baby doesn't live to see his first birthday. Infant mortality rates among African Americans are more than double that of the United States as a whole. That's more than 7,500 infant deaths per year."

After this assertion that African American babies are "unfortunately" prone to disproportionate death, the brochure repeats its appeal, this time as an exclamation: "A Healthy Baby Begins with You!" The second-person address continues: "The Office of Minority Health of the U.S. Department of Health and Human Services wants you to know that infant mortality is preventable. Step up and help end infant mortality!" If there were any doubt about the "you" who is supposed to "step up," the brochure's inside flap—under the heading "Contributing Factors," makes it unmistakable. Although it states that "an infant's survival and long-term health is influenced by many factors," this introductory sentence concludes with naming only "the mother's age, health status and behavior during and after pregnancy." In text printed over the stylized image of a very slender

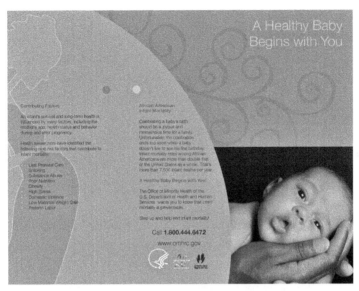

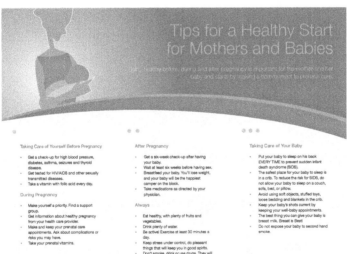

FIGURE 9. "A Healthy Baby Begins with You" brochure front. *Source*: Office of Minority Health of the US Department of Health and Human Services.

FIGURE 10. "Healthy Baby" brochure back. *Source*: Office of Minority Health of the US Department of Health and Human Services.

pregnant woman in profile, looking downward with her hand resting atop her belly, the brochure informs the reader that "health researchers have identified the following nine risk factors that contribute to infant mortality." These risk factors appear in a bulleted list on the figure's belly: "Late Prenatal Care, Smoking, Substance Abuse, Poor Nutrition, Obesity, High Stress, Domestic Violence, Low Maternal Weight Gain, [and] Preterm Labor." Of these nine factors, all but three—high stress, domestic violence, and preterm labor—are clearly linked to behaviors deemed irresponsible or pathological, including eating too much or not enough, smoking, use of drugs and/or alcohol, and failing to seek prenatal care. None of them suggests a link between infant survival, maternal well-being, and the broader social and political environment.

Both the appearance of stress as a risk factor identified by "health researchers" and the way in which it appears are significant here. The 1990s and early 2000s witnessed a growing body of research positing a link between anti-Black racism and health inequities, and infant mortality in particular. While "stress" may seem to be an overly anodyne term for these assaults, it became a keyword in research positing a connection between the assaults of what Fleda Mask Jackson termed "gendered racism" on Black women and their reproductive outcomes.[7] Often grounded in explicitly antiracist, feminist, and redistributive approaches, this research explicitly opposed the pathologizing emphasis of individual maternal behaviors. I briefly sketch three key lines of this research here: stress and resilience, weathering, and the life course approach.

From 1993 to 1997, Black feminist anthropologist Leith Mullings, along with an interdisciplinary cohort of scholars, carried out the Harlem Birth Right Project, an ethnographic participatory action research project. This project collaborated with communities to study what Mullings and coinvestigator Alaka Wali would term, in the title of their 2001 book *Stress and Resistance*, the stress and resilience that characterized the reproductive lives, experiences, and outcomes of middle-class, working-class, and poor Black women in that setting.[8] Funded by the CDC's National Center for Chronic Disease Control and Prevention, through its Division of Reproductive Health, the study looked in-depth at the contexts of women's lives, embedded within community networks, in Central Harlem. This setting, as Mullings, Wali, Diane McLean, Janet Mitchell, Sabiyha Prince, Deborah Thomas, and Patricia Tovar, highlight, was both vibrant, with deeply rooted community and cultural institutions, and deeply shaped by the harms of long-standing systemic racism. During decades before as well as during the study itself, the community sat at the nexus of some of the harshest dynamics of neoliberal disinvestment, which manifested as job losses, especially of unionized jobs, displacement from housing, and high poverty.[9]

The study examined the complexity of women's lives, attending to all of these features—the context of housing, of employment, of kin, and community networks. This yielded a more complete picture of what "stress" entailed as well as highlighting the crucial supports that Black women themselves forged and sustained. While sometimes entailing additional stressors, these practices of resilience helped to foster collective life in the face of the many sources of strain undercutting Black maternal well-being. The researchers concluded that effective public health interventions "must confront . . . the ways in which gender inequity, racial discrimination, and class inequality impose limitations on access to health care and, perhaps more important, on secure jobs, adequate housing, good nutrition, adequate child care, a safe and healthy environment, and necessary social services" as well as building on already existing and effective "individual and collective coping strategies around housing, family, and community."[10]

Drawing out this dual emphasis, in related writings Mullings coined the term "Sojourner Syndrome" "in order to incorporate and conceptualize the multiplicative effects of class, race, and gender on health, as well as to integrate a history of resistance and allow for an exploration of agency."[11] Invoking Sojourner Truth's powerful illumination of "the contradiction between ideal models of gender and the lives of Black women," as well as Black women's individual and collective labors for community survival and liberation, this framework situated stress as expressing not individual risk factors but as an indicator mapping "the relationships among groups defined by their positions in race, class, and gender hierarchies."[12] Importantly, Mullings links Sojourner Truth's legacy of persuading US whites of their own material stakes in ending the system of racism, classism, and sexism that enslaved African Americans with the political potential of this framework. In the present day, the structural transformations needed to address the root causes of stress that endanger Black infants—"a living wage and full employment, restoration of full civil rights for former prisoners . . . free quality public education for all, and universal health care" for all—would benefit all people in the United States.[13]

Mullings writes that, as the team was analyzing the findings in the late 1990s, "stress" was coming to the fore in research on the physiological processes implicated in adverse pregnancy and birth outcomes.[14] A key concept in this wave of research on the physiological impacts of stress and racism was health researcher Arline Geronimus's "weathering hypothesis," first put forward in an article published in 1992, a year before the initiation of Mullings's study. The weathering hypothesis posits that "Blacks experience early health deterioration as a consequence of the cumulative impact of repeated experience with social or economic adversity and political marginalization."[15] Accelerated cellular aging, the wear and tear of dysregulated inflammatory, metabolic, immune, and endocrine processes, the hypothesis posited, at least partially explained the gaping inequities in Black-white life infant mortality, life expectancy, and overall health. Geronimus thus called for "addressing the larger structural relationships that produce inequality."[16] Other researchers in this vein have taken up this hypothesis and expressed the cumulative impact as the body's *allostatic load*, or chemical elements, such as adrenaline and cortisol, that respond to crisis conditions. Allostatic load, they argued, becomes an allostatic *overload* when triggers are frequent and pervasive, potentially leading to sustained inflammatory processes and cellular aging. The psychological, emotional, ecological, and physical aggressions and deprivations targeting Black women's existence in the United States over the entire lifetime issues in a persistently elevated allostatic load, predisposing Black women to myriad chronic and life-shortening health conditions.[17]

Meanwhile, some researchers were positing that these harms have intergenerational reach through "fetal programming" via epigenetic pathways, or processes that can cause heritable changes in gene expression. Departing from the genetic determinism that dominated much of the twentieth century, leading up to the Human Genome Project, epigenetics tracks the ways that experiences, environments, and exposures alter gene expression, in ways that can be intergenerationally heritable, without changing the genetic code.[18] This research argues that the persistent Black-white inequities in infant mortality in the United States is rooted in the profound persistent assaults of white supremacy over Black women's entire lifetimes, not only affecting the endocrine and inflammatory processes that cause low birthweight and premature birth but effecting potentially harmful changes in the fetal epigenome itself. While weathering impacts two generations—the gestating body directly, the fetal body indirectly—epigenetic inheritance can endure over multiple generations. The same elevated stress hormones thought to cause inflammation in the uterus, for instance, also impact the epigenetic markers relevant to the fetus's own physiological stress response. High levels of cortisol in the gestating body overtax the fetus's HPA (hippocampus-pituitary-adrenal) axis, also known as the "stress axis," predisposing it to higher-than-average levels of cortisol in response to stressful events over its own lifetime. If that fetus is born and grows up to gestate another fetus in turn, this stress/inflammation pattern may repeat—even if the environment undergoes significant transformation.[19]

Zaneta Thayer and Christopher Kuzawa write that "there is evidence that psychosocial stress can have transgenerational effects on epigenetic profiles and related physiologic and health outcomes . . . parental experience of psychosocial stress can be transmitted across generations through epigenetic modifications that affect the germline, and are therefore not limited to direct maternal-offspring transfer."[20] In pregnant people this can occur through processes like methylation (molecular groups attaching to genes, hindering their expression—positive in the case of genes for heart disease or diabetes—or detaching from them, allowing expression), where the fetus is not only subject to the outcome of the gestating body's stress (which can lead to premature birth and/or restricted uterine growth) but to alterations in its own chemical determinants of gene expression, or epigenetic markers, potentially from several generations back.[21]

On the one hand, such an approach compellingly demonstrates the literal materialization of racism in the form of disproportionately vulnerable embodiments within the US polity. As philosopher Shannon Sullivan argues, "epigenetics . . . can be part of a critical race and feminist arsenal for combating racism by fully comprehending [how] . . . the social often becomes durable and transgenerationally biological."[22] Yet, on the other hand, Sullivan cautions that the deployment of epigenetic research as evidence of intergenerational damage can lend support to long-standing racist, sexist, and ableist hierarchies of normative maternity. The presumption of irreversible physiological harm among marginalized groups replicates long-standing ascriptions of doomed and biologically inferior forms of reproductive embodiment—framed as a tragic, but nonetheless accurate, affirmation of white normativity. This dovetails with concerns voiced by legal scholar Dorothy Roberts to ask whether public health, policy, and popular conceptions of intergenerational harm might give rise to more pernicious new modes of biopolitical governance for "intergenerationally disadvantaged" populations.[23]

Anthropologist Natali Valdez terms such moves a kind of "epigenetic foreclosure." Such uncritical uses of epigenetic research illuminate a measure of racial innocence animating the comparative approach to race and health more broadly, in its assimilative impulse toward white bourgeois standards of life, reckoning neither with past harms (that are not even past) nor with the ongoing class, racial, gender, and ability hierarchies that underpin those standards. As Valdez shows, such hierarchies can shape not only interpretations of epigenetic research but research agendas themselves. For instance, there is evidence of epigenetic transfer via *patrilineal* pathways, as well as evidence of epigenetic changes that can occur across the lifespan. Yet applications of epigenetic science to birth outcomes focus almost exclusively on pregnant women's behaviors, construing the fetal "environment" as limited to the maternal body.[24] Paradoxically, then, the science of environmental influences can nevertheless bolster longstanding patterns of mother-blame and ineffective, as well as often racist, ableist, fatphobic, and classist interventions that emphasize individual behavior modification.[25]

Moreover, uncritical deployments of the notion of intergenerational trauma can cause the phantoms of civilizationist hierarchy and race traits thinking to resurface. As Valdez writes: "A foreclosed interpretation of transgenerational inheritance is the assumption that Black and Indigenous communities might already be predisposed to adverse health outcomes, regardless of medical interventions." Thus the notion of heritable trauma might even be used "to justify high maternal and infant mortality rates among Black communities," disregarding "the fact that epigenetic modifications are malleable, unpredictable, nonlinear, and potentially reversible."[26] This critique resonates with Unganax scholar Eve Tuck's refusal of what she terms "damage-based research" among communities harmed by colonialism, racism, militarism, and resource extraction.[27] Instead, Valdez argues, as these processes are brought to light, it is crucial to continually emphasize the collective agency at work in creating and sustaining the social and political environments that can engender these epigenetic changes. "Instead of focusing on how to change individual bodies to make them better fit . . . or be 'resilient' in toxic, racist environments, we should ask, 'what kinds of environments promote healthy beings and relations?'"[28] Keeping the notion of racism, class exploitation, and sexism as collectively maintained political environments front and center, as well as a nondeterministic and dynamic understanding of epigenetic processes, is vital.

The "Life Course" Approach

The "life course" approach, introduced in 2003 by doctors Michael Lu and Neal Halfon, extends both weathering and epigenetics research; in focusing on structural factors, in both its diagnoses and prescriptions, it largely avoids the pitfalls of epigenetic foreclosure. The life course approach "conceptualizes birth outcomes as the end product of not only the nine months of pregnancy but the entire life course of the gestating person before the pregnancy, including fetal life."[29] Lu and Halfon argue that early fetal programming dovetails with weathering, or the "cumulative pathway mechanism," such that at each successive generation, the gestating body may have inherited a disproportionate vulnerability to the very physiological stress processes that are most implicated in premature birth and low birthweight, the primary proximate causes of infant mortality.

While the life course approach addresses racism, gender-based oppression, and poverty, it ascribes distinct power to racism, since the gap in infant mortality rates in fact widens at higher socioeconomic levels. Positing that each pregnancy is shaped by a social context that presents harmful "risk factors" and mitigating "protective factors," however, this research interprets the gap between Black and White infant mortality as reflecting the fact that the white maternal body is cushioned by far more protective factors, while fewer risk factors bear down upon it, while Black mothers face the converse situation. Lu and Halfon dedicate a section of the article to pointing out the limits of prevailing approaches to studying stress and maternal health, which are often limited to "acute, individual psychological stressors that occurred immediately before or during pregnancy" and self-reports of stress. Instead, they argue, it is "chronic social stressors . . . factors in the community, social relationships, economics, discrimination, politics, housing, etc. . . . that over time cause wear and tear on the body's allostatic systems, and that underlie racial disparities in birth and other health outcomes."[30]

In conceptualizing racism as a factor within this more systemic and chronic account of stress, Lu and Halfon point to limitations of studies relying on self-reports of experiences of racial discrimination, indicating the need to link residential segregation and other material factors with adverse birth outcomes. In language that reflects the uptake of Geronimus's concept, Lu and Halfon note that "exposure to racial discrimination is not limited to pregnancy, but extends across the life span . . . this weathering of racism and racial discrimination over the life course."[31] They thus argue that the short span of prenatal care is insufficient to address the lifelong exposures to the harms of systemic racism for the pregnant person, although they stress its potential importance for fetal programming and intergenerational health. They emphasize the importance of good lifelong health care, including family planning, "preconceptional, interconceptional, preventive, and primary cares for women," and argue that ultimately universal health coverage is needed. In addition, Lu and Halfon argue, the broader social contexts of reproduction must be addressed, stressing community health supported by "investments in infrastructure . . . affordable and decent housing . . . clean air and water" in terms "decided by and with the community"—citing Mullings and colleagues as an example of such collaboration. They call as well for European-style labor protections and paid leave for pregnant and parenting people.

The ascendancy of the life course approach as an explanatory paradigm for the Black-white gap in infant mortality was the PBS documentary *Unnatural Causes*, aired in 2008, dedicating one of four hourlong segments to the Black-white disproportion in infant mortality. The documentary's narration presents the link between racism and stress as a new consensus. Over graphics of internal reproductive organs inside the outline of a slim feminine torso, the narrator intones: "Stress can . . . constrict blood flow to the placenta, which could limit fetal growth and may lead to premature delivery. Chronic stress may also contribute to serious inflammation inside the uterus, which can trigger premature labor. Research suggests it's not so much stress during pregnancy that may determine the health of a mother's baby, but the cumulative experiences of the mother over the course of her entire life, regardless of race. Dr. Lu calls this hypothesis the 'life-course perspective.'" The segment prominently features Lu, along with Camara Phyllis Jones, eminent scholar of racism and health, and other physicians and scholars positing connections between the stresses of racism and inequitable pregnancy outcomes.[32]

All three of these conceptualizations of stress as bearing on reproductive health caution against a focus on individual behaviors, instead framing these harms as arising through complex, multifaceted, interconnected dynamics of oppression. Mullings states most pointedly that stress and resilience, framed through the Sojourner Syndrome, "challenges the concept of individual risk, which has the potential to move the emphasis from social reform to personal behavior . . . as well as research emphasizing dysfunctional cultural and individual behaviors. . . . Instead, by directing attention to the structural constraints and the ways in which people resist them, it points to the need for large-scale changes that provide access to employment, shelter, education, and healthcare."[33] The biomedical paradigms of weathering and the life course are not as attuned to the complexity and dynamism of stress and resilience alike, arising in people's negotiations of material environments shaped by racism, sexism, economic disinvestment, class exploitation, individual and collective agency, kinship, and community networks and institutions. For example, Lu and Halfon's dualism between "risk factors" and "protective factors" as a matter of quantity—white women have more of the latter, Black women bear more of the former—do not get at the ways that protection and risk interact and may not translate across contexts: for instance, as Mullings writes, in the ways that "race dilutes the protections of class."[34] Yet these approaches also largely concurred that addressing the harms of stress called for such broad systemic transformations.

"A Healthy Baby Begins with YOU": Stress as Individual Maternal Pathology

Nevertheless, even as these analyses were circulating and *Unnatural Causes* was about to debut, the "Healthy Baby Begins with You" campaign enacted precisely the opposite: namely, the reduction of "stress" to a matter of individual behavior. I note above that "high stress" is enumerated in the campaign brochure as one of the "nine risk factors" identified by "health researchers." Presumably, given its increasing prominence, this refers to the paradigm anchored, at least in part, by the research sketched above. Yet the interior sections of the brochure offer advice to the individual mother only on how to "step up": not only during pregnancy but before pregnancy and after the birth, framing "high stress" itself as a behavioral choice that excludes contextual factors entirely. Alongside familiar recommendations to "eat healthy, with plenty of fruits and vegetables" and to "exercise at least 30 minutes a day," is the newer incitement to *"keep stress under control, do pleasant things that will keep you in good spirits."* This framing of stress, in 2007, as a risk factor best addressed through maternal behavior modification is simply of a piece with the abovementioned recommendations about nutrition and exercise. This emphasis on individual responsibility and risk-management without regard to context evinces the neoliberal mode of population governance. Neoliberal reproductive regimes' punishing incitements to individual health operate with tyrannical disregard for the racist, sexist, classist, and ableist stratifications of access to those choices deemed proper.[35]

These directives are thus made without reference to pregnant people's access to quality foods, safe environments to exercise in, or time and space for exercise. Likewise, the directive to "do pleasant things" and to "keep stress under control" leaves any and all stress-inducing structural conditions and environmental factors outside the frame, placing full responsibility on the Black mother herself. This was also the case with the campaign's directive to "tak[e] care of yourself before pregnancy." As Miranda Waggoner observes, while the notion of "preconception care" was in circulation at least since the 1980s, US federal health agencies' emphasis on preconception as a target for intervention dates from 2004 to 2006—just before the launch of "A Healthy Baby Begins with You." Waggoner writes that "in 2004, the Centers for Disease Control and Prevention launched the Preconception Health and Health Care Initiative . . .

mov[ing] the temporality of pregnancy health risk and maternal responsibility to actions taken in the months—or sometimes even years—before pregnancy, thus situating essentially any body of reproductive age as posing risk to healthy reproduction."[36] In 2006 the CDC's *Mortality and Morbidity Weekly Report* ratified this preconception paradigm with a set of recommendations for preconception health optimization. Yet as Waggoner notes, "while the pre-pregnancy care framework attempts to address persistent and dramatic racial and ethnic health disparities," it has instead "reinscribed racialized notions of reproduction" while failing to address the actual causes of these inequities.[37] What Waggoner calls the "temporal (bio)politics of health risk" thus bolsters the biopolitics of racial innocence.

This emphasis on preconception risk management was not only incorporated into the "Healthy Baby Begins with You" campaign through the brochure's directives to "get a check-up for high blood pressure, diabetes, asthma, seizures and thyroid disease. Get tested for HIV/AIDS and other sexually transmitted diseases. [And t]ake a vitamin with folic acid every day." An additional arm of the campaign targeted "preconception health management," teaming up with historically black colleges and universities, as well as other college campuses, to create peer health educator programs. After a brief training, "preconception peer educators" (PPEs) were deputized to encourage healthy behaviors among Black high school and college-age students, as well as within communities identified as suffering significant rates of infant mortality.[38] The characterization of the young peer educators as biopolitical missionaries is evident in a 2013 article profiling the program in *Minority Nurse*: "Aim for a healthy weight. Get enough folic acid in your diet. Find effective ways to manage stress. Talk to your doctor about your family history. All very important information to maintain good preconception health, but as nurses know all too well, people don't always follow good advice.

But how about when the message is coming from someone you can relate to and trust [?] . . . PPEs serve as messengers—drawing attention to the critical link between healthy behaviors in youth and improved maternal and overall health in adulthood."[39] This focus on individual behaviors is underscored by a characterization of "people" as generally reluctant to do the responsible thing. It extends the burden of individual responsibility and self-surveillance backward in time, to include not only pregnant bodies but potentially pregnant bodies.[40]

The years following the initiation of "A Healthy Baby Begins with You" witnessed a proliferation of both policy discourse and journalistic coverage labeling Black infant mortality as a *crisis*. Many cities, including Milwaukee and Cincinnati, were also featured in long-form journalism using the idiom of *crisis*.[41] In 2009 the Office of Minority Health released *Crisis in the Crib*, produced, written by, and featuring Tonya Lewis Lee, whom the OMH had appointed spokesperson of the "A Healthy Baby Begins with You" campaign. Focusing on the more recent discursive turn toward framing Black maternal mortality as a crisis, Jennifer Nash cautions that "the discursive explosion marked by temporalities of urgency often stands in for political work designed to ameliorate the very conditions that produce the 'crisis.'" In fact, Nash suggests, such "outpouring of attention alongside political stasis [is] actually constitutive of the crisis frame."[42] *Crisis in the Crib* enacted precisely such a dynamic.

The film opens at a Memphis cemetery, as a community in grief commemorates more than four hundred babies who had died before age one in the previous two years—the highest rate in the United States among cities of a certain size. The film follows Lewis Lee, a delegation of PPEs from Spelman, Morgan State University, and other campuses, Office of Minority Health personnel, and Memphis city officials over a week of action. In a speech early in the film, Lewis Lee states that infant mortality "is not just a matter of individual responsibility." Moreover, racism and poverty- and gender-related stress make an appearance, both in the segment featuring national experts on racial inequities in health Fleda Mask Jackson and Camara Phyllis Jones, and in the wake of a civil rights–themed tour, for the visiting delegation, that profiles the MLK assassination. An Asian American nursing student who is part of the delegation observes afterward that "all the struggles and the consequential stresses that African Americans have to face ... that's part of the reason why infant mortality is a problem."

Nevertheless, as in the brochure, despite these emphases on the broader context, the overarching message centers on maternal—and to some extent paternal—responsibility. One bereaved older sister narrates the story of her sister, Katina, who was born very premature, over an album that lovingly photographed and documented her few months of life. When the camera returns to her face, she reasons, "maybe my mom wasn't on a healthy diet ... maybe she wasn't getting enough exercise." The "Healthy Baby Begins with You" campaign on the ground instilled a narrative for this teenage girl that her own mother's behaviors were responsible for her little sister's demise. The only bereaved parent featured in the film is a young father, whose testimony is met with the PPEs' advice to tell his wife or girlfriend to get healthy *now*—before another pregnancy, it is implied—as well as his own responsibility for bringing the right energy to the environment of this hypothetical future pregnancy. The NICU doctor featured in the film, while stressing compassion, understanding, and even collective responsibility, also invokes the stereotype of the "high-risk" mother; in conversation with the PPEs, he describes the figure of the pregnant "fifteen-year-old" who has "made a mistake." Even as it gestures to some extent toward structural causes, the film puts a primary emphasis on the labors of PPEs as a solution. As the PPEs fan out over the neighborhood, representing themselves from door to door as "from the Office of Minority Health," they spread the message of *awareness* and *behavior* as the solution to the "crisis in the crib."

The film calls urgent attention to racial disparities as preventable and gestures toward racism as implicated in these deaths. Yet it largely casts Black mothers and potential mothers—and, to a lesser extent, fathers and potential fathers—themselves as individually responsible for their own pregnancy outcomes. As one young PPE from Morgan State asserts, the "campaign has illustrated what people can do at a grassroots level, how powerful social marketing is . . . if we can just brand the idea that these are the behaviors that bring about a healthy lifestyle, or healthy birth outcomes." While a Memphis public health program is credited as part of the background, the film focuses not on these efforts nor on the responsibilities of hospitals, city officials, urban planners, industrial polluters, police, or other bodies whose actions materially determine the environments of gestation and birth in Memphis. Nor does it highlight the community institutions and networks through which Black mothers and parents in the city live and negotiate those environments, experience and respond to systemic vulnerability, exercise individual and collective agency, and bear and raise their children. Rather, the film showcases these young Black volunteers as they spread the message of Black maternal responsibility—extending, through "preconception," to encompass all potentially pregnant girls and women—for healthy choices.

"A Healthy Baby Begins with You" thus enacted all three key features of the biopolitics of racial innocence. The imprint of the new research paradigm is evident in the fact that "high stress" is counted as a factor. Yet *willful ignorance* stymies the translation of the considerable body of evidence pointing to systemic factors into appropriately systemic responses, many of which are spelled out within that research itself. Rather, in a move congruent with Valdez's epigenetic foreclosure, the campaign stressed individual maternal responsibility: the singular "you"—taking recourse to the familiar *displacement of blame* onto Black mothers themselves. It emphasized responsibility for seeking preconception health management, for eating well, and even for controlling one's own stress levels for the sake of the fetus. Local-level campaigns in the following years tended to emphasize individual parental risk factors, including maternal obesity, smoking, and co-sleeping with infants.[43] Moreover, while terms of these interventions bear a neoliberal inflection, they also manifest the disjuncture between research and practice that, as evidenced throughout this book, has long characterized the biopolitics of Black infant mortality—scientific knowledge about preventing infant death, on the one hand, and actual public health interventions among Black infants on the other. Meanwhile, *liberal reforms* like the peer preconception educator program, while proclaiming a commitment to addressing root causes of health inequities across the lifespan, including infant mortality, in fact left structural factors entirely unaddressed.

The individual pathologization of "A Healthy Baby Begins with You," and its enabling of racial innocence, has also underpinned physician practices. Khiara Bridges's ethnography of pregnancy care at a New York public hospital showed that both overtly racist lore about patients of color as well as their biopolitical classification as "risky bodies" threatened these mothers' well-being in myriad ways—yet also functioned to displace blame from physicians and hospital personnel and harmful protocols onto mothers themselves.[44] During research in the 2010s on the ways that racism shapes premature birth, as well as NICU protocols and practices, anthropologist Dána-Ain Davis remarks on parallel sleights-of-hand among four white neonatal intensive care unit physicians. Premature birth is one of the primary proximate causes of infant mortality—not a root cause but a closely associated condition and a primary way, in Davis's reading, that the legacies of slavery persist in the health impacts of anti-Black racism.[45]

Referring both to a robust research literature and to the visible demographics of the babies in these physicians' care, Davis asked neonatologists what factors might explain Black infants' overrepresentation in the NICUs—why might, for instance, rates of premature rupture of membranes be more common among Black women? Why do Black women with advanced degrees give birth prematurely at higher rates than white women with the lowest educational status? The physicians were forthcoming, even loquacious, on other topics. But Davis describes them as deflecting the question.[46] They acknowledged the demographics but refused to explicitly name race—let alone racism—as a factor in premature birth, insisting that poverty is the decisive element. At the same time, they consistently couched their class analyses in the racially loaded idioms of "broken families," lack of education, substance abuse, and inner cities.[47] Timeworn racist ascriptions of ignorance and familial pathology lurk just under the surface. And as in that report, Davis's interviewees refuse to countenance the racism that—in entanglements with economic hierarchies far more complex than their analyses allow—manifestly shapes NICU demographics. They thus insulate themselves from consideration of their own institutional participation or structural implication in Black infants' heightened vulnerability to prematurity and death.[48]

The Maternal Health Crisis

The White House Blueprint for Addressing the Maternal Health Crisis marks a very different moment. The opening paragraph of its executive summary proclaims:

> The United States is facing a maternal health crisis. Our country's maternal mortality rate is the highest of any developed nation in the world and more than double the rate of peer countries, and most

pregnancy-related deaths are considered preventable. Beyond maternal mortality, severe maternal morbidity impacts far too many families. . . . Systemic barriers, together with a failure to recognize, respect and listen to patients of color, has meant that Black and American Indian/Alaska Native (AI/AN) women, regardless of income or education, experience a greater share of these grave outcomes, as do rural women.[49]

Not only is the subject of crisis distinct from "A Healthy Baby Begins with You": from not infants but their mothers. The Blueprint's framing of responsibility and harm is different as well, as the emphasis has shifted away from the individual and toward the systemic. The need for adequate support for behavioral health needs is emphasized throughout; maternal *behavior* is mentioned just once, in relation to data gathered on mental health and substance abuse—the latter framed sympathetically rather than punitively.[50] In contrast, maternal *experiences* are central to the discussion, occurring at least twelve times in the text of the document. In contrast to the previous translation of stress into an individually controllable risk factor, Geronimus's notions of weathering and stress are cited directly: "Experts also believe that the chronic stress of discrimination—a process known as 'weathering'—takes a toll on Black and AI/AN people in ways that result in higher rates of perinatal depression hypertension, preterm birth, and infant mortality."[51] The executive summary closes with a ringing indictment, quoted above, of systemic racism as the ultimate problem to be addressed.

In its avowal of racism as a the ultimate cause of inequitable pregnancy outcomes, the Blueprint is of a piece with the many statements, declarations, and plans of action recently issued by national and local health organizations, institutions, and journals as well as municipalities and states.[52] Like the policy proposals at the federal level, these statements and plans evince a sea change in the prevailing discourse around race, racism, and health inequities in the United States. The notions of "structural racism" and "systemic racism" have gained far wider purchase than ever before, particularly during and after the summer 2020 uprisings demanding a stop to normalized state violence targeting Black communities. Just for some examples, the American Psychological Association, the American Medical Association, the American College of Obstetricians and Gynecologists, the American Public Health Association, and the National Institutes of Health have all made such statements.[53]

But while harmonizing with these recent avowals, the Blueprint also reflects significant and specific shifts in the framings of racism, capitalism, reproductive health, and pregnancy outcomes in scholarship, public discourse, policy work, and advocacy as well as in coalescing praxes of care. The Blueprint builds on a wave of legislative efforts, including the Black Maternal Health Momnibus Act of 2021, introduced by Congresswoman Lauren Underwood, Congresswoman Alma Adams, Senator Cory Booker, and members of the Black Maternal Health Caucus. The act was stunning not only in its breadth of vison, its depth of engagement with critical research on the social determinants of health and the impacts of racial discrimination, and the ambition of its reach but also in its unprecedented engagement with transformative community-based work. The act reads: "In the richest nation on earth, moms are dying at the highest rate in the developed world—and the rate is rising. For as dire as the situation is for all women and birthing people, the crisis is most severe for Black moms, who are dying at 3 to 4 times the rate of their white counterparts. Native Americans are more than twice as likely to die from pregnancy-related causes." While the mere repetition of mortality statistics can have ambivalent effects, the act embeds them in a thoroughgoing indictment of structural racism's impacts on health. The act names "racism" no less than sixteen times and includes support for midwives and doulas of color in its proposals. Additional recommendations call for broad-based social transforma-tions, including investments in housing, transportation, and nutrition, funding community-based organizations that are already transforming maternal health outcomes, funding midwives and dou-las of color, and ending shackling of pregnant people in prisons.

Media representations have also signaled this shift. Linda Villa-rosa's 2018 cover story in the *New York Times Magazine*, "Why Amer-ica's Black Mothers and Babies Are in a Life-or-Death Crisis," marked a pivotal moment in this turn toward Black maternal precarity. Not only does the article focus on mothers *and* babies, but it names the former first and focuses its narrative through the experiences of a Black mother. Villarosa encapsulates the growing acceptance of re-search on racism and stress within the medical field and exemplifies its increasing circulation in public discourse. She writes: "For black women in America, an inescapable atmosphere of societal and sys-temic racism can create a kind of toxic physiological stress, resulting in conditions—including hypertension and pre-eclampsia—that lead directly to higher rates of infant and maternal death. And that soci-etal racism is further expressed in a pervasive, longstanding racial bias in health care—including the dismissal of legitimate concerns and symptoms—that can help explain poor birth outcomes even in the case of black women with the most advantages."[54]

Villarosa's article profiles a young Black mother based in New Or-leans, Simone Landrum, who had lost her third child—and nearly died herself—due to preeclampsia, a condition of organ malfunction during late pregnancy that first manifests as dangerously elevated blood pressure. A survivor of both Hurricane Katrina and the white male physician who fatally ignored her symptoms, Landrum experi-enced a life that exemplifies elements that Villarosa identifies as threatening the lives of Black mothers and infants. Villarosa also pro-files the pivotal role that a Black doula, Latona Giwa, plays in helping to ensure an optimal outcome for Landrum's fourth pregnancy.

While querying the political ramifications of the crisis framing for Black mothers, Jennifer Nash notes the broad impact of Villarosa's story; not only was it "picked up by Public Broadcasting Service (PBS), National Public Radio (PBS), *Truthout, Mother Jones,* and *Democracy Now,*" but it was "cited by state legislatures as they formed task forces to respond to the crisis of Black maternal health; and also inaugurated a year of significant coverage of Black maternal health in every major US newspaper."[55]

Tonya Lewis Lee's second film on pregnancy outcomes, the documentary *Aftershock*, released in 2022, underscores the fact that the center of political gravity has shifted from infant to maternal mortality. Also covered in major news outlets, *Aftershock* profiles the preventable deaths of two healthy Black mothers due to medical negligence, and the film could not be more different than *Crisis in the Crib.*[56] It follows the mourning and activism of these mothers' families in the wake of these deaths. Like Villarosa's article, it uplifts Black birthworkers—a term that encompasses midwives and doulas alike—and the midwifery model of care as offering crucial lifesaving alternatives to a racist obstetrical care system.[57] Leading midwife and advocate Jennie Joseph, founder of Commonsense Childbirth, the only Black-owned midwifery school in the United States, was named a Woman of the Year by *Time Magazine* in 2022.[58]

Although it may seem sudden, the attention to medical racism and the emphasis on Black birthwork in legislative proposals and public discourse is grounded in more long-standing practices, scholarship, advocacy, and organizing. I offer just two examples here. Midwife Joseph has for decades operated prenatal care clinics that have defied prevailing patterns of racial inequity in birth outcomes. Operating on what Joseph names the "easy access" model, no one is turned away or forced to wait for insurance or payment, and every encounter with staff entails dignified and unhurried care attentive to the whole person from the time they walk in the door—from receptionist to medical assistant to nurse to midwife or physician.[59] This departs starkly from many standard prenatal clinical sites, where receptionists often serve as hostile gatekeepers to care that is often perfunctory and impersonal, if not overtly racist; those people on Medicaid or uninsured are often made to wait for care.[60]

The Birthing Project USA, a network led by Black doulas, birthworkers, and community advocates, works to support Black infancy and maternity in the face of a racist health-care system and society.[61] Public health scholar and birth advocate Kathryn Hall-Trujillo founded The Birthing Project—which claims the designation "the underground railroad for new life"—in 1988 in response to high rates of Black infant mortality in her California community, and over the years it has operated in approximately a hundred sites nationwide and internationally. It entails one-on-one support for pregnant people from members of the same community, who help them navigate prenatal care, resources, postpartum wellness, and the first years of motherhood.[62] Not a one-size-fits-all model, Birthing Project sites "operat[e] from homes, churches . . . clinics, health departments and hospitals—any place where a group of ten women can commit to being conductors on The Underground Railroad for 18 months," and center the conditions, needs, and visions particular to each site.[63] While these grassroots efforts often do not have infrastructure or funding for formal evaluation, existing assessments demonstrate striking improvements in infant survival across multiple settings. In its Nashville site from 2003 to 2008, for example, participants' infant mortality rate of zero was significantly better than that of their white counterparts locally and nationwide.[64] The project continues to expand, even as mainstream public health literature and interventions combating racial reproductive health inequities have largely failed to give the project due attention.[65]

This shift in official emphasis toward acknowledgment of medical racism and Black birthwork as a solution in part reflects the force of Black feminist and critical race scholarship on reproductive health injustices. Across fields including medical anthropology, the history of medicine, the health sciences, and beyond, this scholarship clarifies the connections between racism, capitalism, sexism, and reproductive oppression targeting Black women. Villarosa quotes Dána-Ain Davis, whose account of neonatologists' deflections is profiled earlier in this chapter. In her 2019 book, *Reproductive Injustice: Racism, Pregnancy, and Premature Birth*, Davis situates the actions of individual providers within historically rooted protocols of white supremacy that structure contemporary maternal and infant health care—from medical education to labor and delivery units and NICUs. In the book she offers a trenchant four-part schema of these protocols of medical racism: (1) the potentially fatal *diagnostic lapse*: the rampant tendency to minimize and/or ignore Black women's symptoms, often in the face of Black women's own insistence that something is wrong. Davis's interviewees recount an outrageous range of ways that such lapses endangered their own and their babies' lives.[66] This in turn is linked to the governing tropes of (2) *obstetrical hardiness* and its derivative, (3) *hardy babies*—remnants of nineteenth-century obstetrics' founding mythologies of effortless birth and fecundity among "primitive" peoples and related to the still-pervasive medical myth that Black people feel pain less acutely than white people. Finally, (4) *menacing mothers* denotes a maternity cast as deviant, threatening, and deserving of punishment for any and all reasons, from not being present enough—"neglectful," no matter what the circumstances—to being too present and thus "demanding"—as if Black women themselves, and not a racist, sexist, and profit-driven maternity care system, are the agents of harm.[67] The persistence of these tropes in view of the staggeringly disproportionate rates of infertility, miscarriage, premature birth, and mortality is not only cruelly ironic. It also bespeaks the long-standing figuration of the typically-abled, cisgender, and slim white woman's body as the default obstetrical norm (as illustrations from the very first obstetrical textbooks to the present testify). As historian Deirdre Cooper Owens shows, this genteel depiction of the white lady patient is a key move to racial innocence, as it effaces the origins of the field of obstetrics itself in institutionalized experimentation on enslaved Black women's bodies as well as extraction of their knowledge.[68]

In additional work, under the rubric of "obstetric racism," which "lies at the intersection between obstetric violence and medical racism," Davis has elaborated this schema, in ways that offer patients language for their experiences and institutions themselves a reflection of their own harmful protocols. Moreover, Davis's concept, and collaboration with radical OB Karen Scott, has in fact grounded the first-ever patient-reported measure of obstetric racism.[69] The analytical and practical purchase of Davis's concept signals the efflorescence of transformative work that—across scholarly journals, policy analyses and advocacy documents, and toolkits—centers the voices and experiences of Black women themselves in tracking key ways that racism deeply shapes maternity care and in proposing and leading the implementation of solutions grounded in this research.[70]

This assemblage of work and praxis demonstrates that longstanding, historically-rooted racist health-care institutions and practices in fact amplify and compound an environment of everyday racism, sexism, and economic deprivation and exploitation.[71] By the same token, these scholars, advocates, organizer, and practitioners point to lineages of care, contestation, and refuge within this context. Much of this work explicitly invokes *reproductive justice* and *birth justice*, frameworks for theory, practice, and movement building that has arisen from these life-fostering legacies. Rooted in Black feminism, and originally formulated by Black women who were longtime reproductive health organizers, reproductive justice puts those most directly impacted by reproductive oppression at the center of its analysis and visions.[72] As leading reproductive justice scholar, organizer, and public intellectual Loretta Ross, cofounder of the reproductive justice movement, writes: "Reproductive justice is based on the human right to make personal decisions about one's life, and the obligations of government and society to ensure that the conditions are suitable for implementing one's decisions."[73] It centers the human rights (1) to have a child, (2) not to have a child, (3) to parent children in healthy and safe environments, (4) to gender freedom, and (5) to sexual autonomy.[74]

Reproductive justice is central to this book's concerns with a political environment that threatens Black infant life as well the ways that the US racial state has directly targeted and impeded the right for Black parents to have children. Reproductive justice forwards a collective rather than individualist understanding of health and emphasizes storytelling as a central practice of building community power and coalitions. Reproductive justice offers a vision of liberation, grounded in sites of struggle where transformative modes of relation and care are already taking place. As Ross makes clear, reproductive justice scholarship also highlights and rejects white complicity in this ongoing history of violence and injustice—especially the persistent failures of whitestream reproductive politics to apprehend and actively oppose the racism that is intertwined with sexism and heterosexism to the very core—a particularly persistent brand of racial innocence.[75]

The reproductive justice approach departs definitively from a liberal individualist notion of human rights, insisting that any individual's health or illness manifests the conditions of that person's community and environment and that children are a collective societal responsibility. This aspect of the framework offers a potent critique of the prevailing notion that reproductive outcomes are a matter of "choice."[76] Furthermore, it is particularly well poised to oppose the decontextualizing and individualizing operations that have long cast the Black maternal body as pathogenic, rather than the interlocking violences of a white supremacy, heteropatriarchy, and capitalism. Founders of the Black Feminist Health Science Studies Collective Moya Bailey and Whitney Peoples offer a lineage of Black health organizers and advocates who have "reclaim[ed] health from a strictly medical context and rearticulate[ed] it to better reflect the specificities of Black women's histories, experiences, and needs." Along with Loretta Ross, one of the generators of the term "reproductive justice," and SisterSong, a reproductive justice organization that she cofounded, Bailey and Peoples include the Black Panther Party in its medical activism, particularly the sickle-cell detection and prevention program; Fannie Lou Hamer, in her linking of embodied structural violence, reproductive violence, and direct state violence; Audre Lorde, in her conception of self-care as a political practice, and Byllye Avery's promotion of "self-help" as simultaneously a principle of individual and collective health. Like these forbears, reproductive justice advocates powerfully posit, in Bailey and Peoples's terms, "Black women as subjects of health and wellness rather than as objects that mark its antithesis"—not only as an ethic but also as a material realization.[77] Rooted in legacies of on-the-ground work by and for Black women's health, labor, and care, reproductive justice invites all who support its tenets into a broad vision of bodily autonomy, interdependence, and collective wholeness for all—calling as well for land return to Indigenous peoples and climate justice.[78]

The reproductive justice framework illuminates the context of Black infant mortality with a view to fundamentally transforming structures of racial capitalist violence from the root level up. Legal scholar Dorothy Roberts highlights the work of leading Black doula Chanel Porchia-Albert, founder of Brooklyn's Ancient Song Doula Services, as "a form of mutual aid that advances reproductive justice."[79] As the foregoing suggests, Black community-based birthworkers like Joseph and Porchia-Albert are playing a key role in this new framing. The movement for birth justice—also comprising

Indigenous doulas and midwives, Latinx and immigrant doulas and midwives, queer and transgender birthworkers—is an extension of the reproductive justice movement and framework. California-based Black Women Birthing Justice Collective states:

> Birth Justice exists when women and transfolks are empowered during pregnancy, labor, childbirth and postpartum to make healthy decisions for themselves and their babies. Birth Justice is part of a wider movement against reproductive oppression. It aims to dismantle inequalities of race, class, gender and sexuality that lead to negative birth experiences, especially for women of color, low-income women, survivors of violence, immigrant women, queer and transfolks, and women in the Global South. Working for Birth Justice involves educating the community, and challenging abuses by medical personnel and overuse of medical interventions. It also involves advocating for universal access to culturally appropriate, women-centered health care. It includes the right to choose whether or not to carry a pregnancy, to choose when, where, how, and with whom to birth, including access to traditional and indigenous birth-workers, such as midwives and doulas, and the right to breastfeeding support.[80]

The Southern Birth Justice Network defines birth justice in similar terms:

> Birth Justice recognizes that all peoples can birth and be parents; People of color, immigrant peoples, and LGBTQ+ communities in particular have survived a history of trauma and oppression around our decisions to have and not have babies. We know that when we, mothers and parents, are empowered, our community is transformed. If we bring our babies into the world, with justice, in the natural way, without anyone telling us how to do it, then it nurtures our

innate power as mothers and parents to create a free world for our children to play and learn and grow.

Birth Justice includes access to health care during the childbearing year that is holistic, humanistic, and culturally centered. This health care is across the pregnancy spectrum including: abortion, miscarriage, prenatal, birth, and postpartum care. Birth Justice includes the right to choose whether or not to carry a pregnancy, to choose when, where how, and with whom to birth, including access to traditional and indigenous healers, such as midwives and other birth workers, and the right to breastfeeding support. The complete range of pregnancy, labor, and birth options should be available to everyone as an integral part of reproductive justice. These are our rights as mothers and parents.[81]

Birth justice advocates offer a different genealogy of obstetrical violence than the white-dominant alternative birth movement has historically done, situating its critique of obstetrics within histories of enslavement, colonization, medical experimentation, segregation, and policing and incarceration—illuminating the ways that obstetrical violence reaches far beyond the delivery room. In terms that resonate with James Baldwin's suggestive spatial analysis—as sketched in the introduction—of racial-capitalist violence as a threat to Black birth, midwife Joseph, in a recent report coauthored with Paula X. Rojas and Haile Eshe Cole, brings the differential geographies of maternal and infant health into particularly sharp focus. She defines "materno-toxic areas" as "any area where it is unsafe to be pregnant or parenting . . . fac[ing] birth outcomes that are worse than those in adjacent zip codes and suffer[ing] an increased risk for premature birth, low-birth weight, and infant and maternal morbidity."[82]

Writing as part of the National Perinatal Task Force, Joseph highlights the spatial converse to these "materno-toxic zones."

"Perinatal Safe Spots"—community-based clinical sites and birth care practices where Black, Indigenous, and/or Latina mothers and infants thrive, led by birthworkers who center justice and largely hail from the communities that they serve.[83] Reflecting a close engagement with the research highlighted above, as well as alignment with the broader movement for reproductive justice, Perinatal Safe Spots model "an understanding of systemic power differentials; a popular education methodology for learning that emphasizes the power of personal stories in collective work . . . a focus on the allostatic load and the Social Determinants of Health."[84] Joseph's own long-standing Florida clinical sites have demonstrated the efficacy of this alternate approach, fostering excellent outcomes among Black and Latine birthing people that meet or surpass parity with their white counterparts—unlike births in the surrounding county and state levels.[85] And in the hospital setting itself, doula care has been linked to numerous improvements in outcomes, and data seems to point to particular efficacy when doula care is culturally congruent.[86] These responsive community-based forms of care thus appear not only to shelter Black pregnant and birthing people and their infants from the harms of environmental but also to create localized shifts in the atmosphere itself.

The Blueprint reflects the turn toward birthwork as a keystone solution to the maternal health crisis, acknowledging that "a larger role for midwives in the perinatal experience . . . [achieves] significantly better results on key measures of maternal and neonatal health. Midwifery can also play a particularly important role in understanding a community's traditions and providing culturally appropriate care."[87] The Blueprint also cites research showing that "doulas are associated with lower rates of maternal and infant health complications, lower rates of preterm birth and low birth weight infants," the leading proximate factors in infant mortality. Moreover, it names the fact that "both the midwife and doula professions remain overwhelmingly

White. . . . The lack of diversity in clinical providers and non-clinical workers is troubling, especially given studies that show how beneficial care from diverse providers can be, especially for women of color."[88]

Thus, almost exactly a century the Sheppard-Towner Act passed, initiating the era of state surveillance and control of Black midwives in the South, midwives are again featuring prominently in federal health policy. Unlike in 1921, however, these midwives are not figured as responsible for infant mortality or other poor pregnancy outcomes. In fact, it is quite the opposite. Along with doulas, emerging public and policy discourse now spotlights midwives, especially Black and Indigenous midwives and midwives of color, as offering key solutions. Moreover, alongside key organizations like the Black Mamas Matter Alliance, birth practitioners themselves, including midwives, doulas, and physicians, have taken center stage as a public advocates on these issues.[89] Midwife Joseph herself is a member of the Advisory Council of the Congressional Black Maternal Health Caucus founded by Congresswomen Alma Adams and Lauren Underwood, and has offered powerful testimony in that capacity.[90] A 2021 congressional hearing in support of the Momnibus and related Acts, "Birthing While Black: Examining America's Black Maternal Health Crisis," spotlighted Black-led birthwork. The power of Black midwives and doulas to improve Black birthing people's experiences and outcomes is a central theme of the hearing, articulated by providers, lawmakers, and witnesses alike. Dr. Joia Crear-Perry, founder of the National Birth Equity Collaborative, was one of the expert witnesses, and advocates for support for nurse-midwifery tracks at historically Black colleges and universities. She also uplifts the current work of Black midwives and doulas, calling attention to the historical attacks on Black community midwifery. Actress Tatyana Ali testifies to the difference that a Black midwife made in her second birth, as compared to her traumatic first birth under OB care. Midwives themselves offered written testimony for this hearing, including

Bronx-based Afro-Latina midwife, birth justice advocate and mutual aid organizer Carmen Mojica, in addition to two hospital-based nurse-midwives.[91]

This hearing—along with the Momnibus Act and the Blueprint—is starkly different from previous federal efforts. For example, in one of the first congressional hearings on health disparities, centering Black infant mortality, in 1984, Reagan administration representatives left before the sole practicing physician serving Black families and the only Black woman called as expert witness, obstetrician and Third World Women's Alliance organizer Dr. Vicki Alexander, offered her scalding testimony.[92] In its emphasis on obstetric racism and the physiological toll of societal racism and sexism, framing also differs significantly from that characterized in "A Healthy Baby Begins with You." As birth justice advocates, providers, and patients alike demand transformations in institutional, policy, and practice—and testify to power of existing Black-led care models—the ruses of innocence indeed seem to be losing purchase.

Potential Pitfalls: Persistent Claims to Innocence

In this book I have tracked the biopolitics of racial innocence across a century and more of interventions, institutionalized mechanisms, habits, and techniques of practiced blamelessness that have enabled and obscured racial capitalism's fatal impacts on Black gestation, birth, and infancy. The Blueprint thus emerges in a moment very different from 2007, wherein the biopolitics of racial innocence can no longer find such firm purchase. In the translation between the scholarship, advocacy, and praxis, however, the Blueprint exemplifies how their partial uptake, if leaving the necropolitical status quo overall undisturbed, nevertheless presents some potential pitfalls. *Displacement of blame* from economically exploitative and white supremacist structures, as well as medical and other forms of institutional racism, onto Black women, families, and communities themselves is a central feature of the biopolitics of racial innocence. As Jennifer Nash suggests, this displacement of responsibility might manifest in new forms in the governmental and institutional turn to Black midwives and doulas, if the considerable infrastructure necessary to actually support the sustainability of these roles and labors is not robustly supplied. Nash observes that, in the course of the politicization of Black maternal mortality as crisis over the past few years, "black mothers have been increasingly sutured to crisis discourse," entering public view as tragic subjects bound to suffering and fatal peril.[93]

While this may be considered an improvement over earlier paradigms construing Black mothers as promiscuous or pathological, Nash argues that it nevertheless perpetuates the pattern of symbolically overloading Black maternity and constraining the potentials of Black mothers' political subjectivity—in essence rendering them legible only in their proximity to death. This highly cathected representation could in fact draw political will away from the practical steps needed to transform US institutional protocols and predatory structural conditions that actually threaten the lives of Black birthing people and their infants most acutely, but in fact threaten reproductive life and well-being across the country and around the world. In addition, even as public discourse increasingly construes Black maternity as heroically tragic, long-standing characterizations of Black mothers as deviant and dangerous remain potent and continue to undergird racist maternity care practices. Keisha Goode highlights the long-standing racism and economic exclusion that Black midwives and aspiring midwives have faced within midwifery education and organizations—no small factor in explaining the overwhelming whiteness of the field to this day.[94] The Blueprint laments these numbers, but it is not clear that any of its recommended actions, which include increased funding for doula training only, will substantially shift these patterns.

This is in no way to refute the incredible lifesaving work that these birthworkers do. But history offers a cautionary tale: as detailed in chapter 4, under the Sheppard-Towner Act, Southern health officials simultaneously surveilled and scapegoated Black midwives for poor infant health outcomes, rather than the racial terror and enforced poverty actually at the root. They offered them little or no compensation for their crucial caregiving. In the present moment state- and city-sponsored programs providing "culturally congruent" doula services risk carrying forward the legacy of undervaluing—and in fact stealing—the caring labors of Black birthworkers. Reimbursement rates in these state and city programs have tended to be meager and sometimes extremely difficult to collect.[95] Moreover, institutions may be *outsourcing* the labors of saving Black maternal and infant life, at great cost to doulas themselves. Without changing their own racist protocols, doulas become shock-absorbers for the racism that their pregnant and birthing clients face—which itself can take a major toll on these caregivers' health—many, if not most, of whom are themselves Black mothers. As doula Tia Murray, based in Madison, Wisconsin, observes:

> This is something that has been really a recurring theme amongst sessions with our doulas—this idea of caring for others and also caring for ourselves, because we're still embedded within the various systems that are working to our demise. So that I think is one of the most challenging aspects of this work. And, again, also sort of protecting the space to do the work and meet the needs. It is important that our doula work not be regulated by the same systems that are causing so much harm. We are working uphill in a lot of ways, because we are producing and seeing really good outcomes and impacts, yet are still working within the systems that are contributing in real time and historically to our demise, as I said, and it's tough. It's really tough to continue the care work in the face of that sort of monstrous hold.[96] Julia Chinyere Oparah and colleagues have charted the

ways that Black birthworkers experienced high levels of stress and burnout during COVID-19, witnessing medical racism as well as experiencing it as targets themselves.[97]

Even given doulas' demonstrated efficiancy, mainstream public health by and large has failed to robustly support long-standing practices of Black-led community-based doula care, in terms of a living wage or integration into birth care teams. These life-fostering practices may thus also be another way that a white supremacist state and health-care system is relying yet again on Black women's uncompensated labor. Commemorating the mentorship of late Black feminist scholar Nellie Y. McKay, Cherene Sherrard-Johnson extends Christina Sharpe's notion of racism as *the weather*, positing that, in the context of a thoroughly racist campus, McKay created "microclimates" for younger Black women scholars. Sherrard-Jones makes clear that this sheltering work came at a clear cost for McKay and many other Black women academics who have died young.[98] The most common form of Black birthwork, care by Black doulas in the hospital, and community caregivers might be said to constitute similar "microclimates" within the broader hostile environment—while likewise taking a toll on the health and lives of the doulas themselves.

This cycle of institutional violence is not inevitable. In fact, there are alternate care models already in place that sustain the well-being of both Black birthing people and their birthworkers. For just one example, Joseph's "easy access" model explicitly values each clinical role as crucial to the well-being of the pregnant person and their family—not only refusing the medical hierarchy of roles but preempting the harms that arise when the onus is on Black providers' individual labors. More recently, flagship reproductive justice organization Sister Song created a COVID birth justice care fund that worked directly with Black midwives and doulas to determine sustainable and equitable reimbursement rates.[99] If they truly aim to empower Black birthwork as a transformative intervention into the necropolitical conditions of Black maternity and infancy, state and federal governments should take a cue from these sustainable models.

A second pitfall entails the risk of resurgent liberal reformism. The Blueprint does not emphasize individual maternal responsibility for pregnancy outcomes. However, the slippage from racism to bias risks individualizing harms that in fact must be addressed at the institutional level. Health economist Tiffany Green and coauthors call our attention to the increasingly pervasive emphasis on implicit bias among individual physicians. In the realm of criminal punishment, Naomi Murakawa notes that "the habit of blaming implicit bias . . . equating racism with psychological error—risks exonerating institutional arrangements that incentivize and legitimize racist harm."[100] Analogously, as Green and coauthors argue about the medical setting, emphasis on "treating implicit bias as an individual-level problem decouples bias from social context and ignores the ways in which medical training and health care institutions embed prejudice and stereotyping into medical practice."[101] Implicit bias can actually stand in for—and hence obstruct—the identification, accountability for, and transformation of racist institutional protocols.

Moreover, a focus on individual bias deflects attention from the endemic patterns of structural racism in both medical education and health-care institutions: "greater numbers of Black physicians in training, education, and practice can result in more 'learning opportunities' for non-Black students and colleagues to correct their false beliefs—but only if Black physicians are able to voice concerns about racial stereotypes and other inappropriate norms." It is, to begin with, unjust that the is onus on individual Black medical students and Black physicians to teach and correct their colleagues. Compounding this is the fact that those same racial stereotypes, racist hostility from patients, professors, and other providers, and inappropriate norms continue to systematically marginalize and harm Black medical students and physicians themselves at every turn: obstructing entry into the field (reflected by disproportionately low numbers), undermining their education, and squeezing them out of academic medicine completely.[102] While the Blueprint calls for ongoing antibias training within a broader agenda of institutional transformations, it remains to be seen whether and how hospitals and medical schools themselves will undertake the deeper work.

Every new human being, the human being that carries it, and the beings that sustain this miraculous and unique unfolding of life, are part of a vast and delicate ecology, at once exquisitely responsive to local conditions and linked, through air, water, minerals, histories and systems, to all other beings on earth. For Baldwin, concentrated on the US polity, racial innocence was precisely the mechanism by which US whites denied these material bonds and refused to acknowledge, let alone redress, the histories that had created their deadly current configuration. At a planetary level, too, such disavowal permits the massive everyday predation, theft, and hoarding that underpin the "cult of true babyhood" today—the system of sacrifice demanded, as M Murphy describes it, by "rich, white, settler colonial, heteronormative reproduction . . . babymaking with expensive strollers assembled in supply chain capitalist webs . . . fossil-fuel guzzling SUVs fed through pipelines . . . oil turned into piles of plastic toys destined for landfills and then microplastic gyres . . . white property relations with empty rooms . . . all the many forms of white possession and enablement."[103] Within this context the stories that infant mortality statistics tell are not self-evident. Under US colonial racial capitalism, they have been used time and again to tell a self-aggrandizing story of white biological and moral supremacy and Black maternal, family, and community pathology, and as an apologia for colonial and racial-capitalist violence that robs from and poisons the ecology of Black infant life. They have deflected official attention from the lifegiving elements of that ecology gathered by

Black maternity, paternity, kinship, midwifery, care, and collective life around Black infant life and survival.

When Black infant mortality entered public view in the late nineteenth century, it did so as part of a broader "condemnation of Blackness"—to use Khalil Gibran Muhammad's phrasing—as white health statisticians like Frederick Hoffman proclaimed that the much higher rates of Black infant mortality, far from cause for alarm or intervention, signaled the evolutionary inferiority of a dying race.[104] Though challenged at the time by Black leaders including W.E.B. Du Bois and Mary Church Terrell, this sadistic rationalization, which remained influential for many years, effaced both the conditions that threatened Black infants' life chances and the lived experiences of Black maternal, parental, and community grief and loss. By the second decade of the twentieth century, health authorities belatedly enfolded Black infants into their biopolitical accounting. Yet like the timespan of biopolitical concern, its scope was racially bifurcated. These official incitements to life—as we see from Dr. Thompson's account that opened the introduction—were largely characterized by a studied inattention to the structures of violence that imperiled Black infant life. In other words health authorities' biopolitical concern for Black infant mortality left intact the necropolitical conditions at the root of Black infants' vulnerability to premature death. The "Healthy Baby Begins with You" campaign serves as yet another cautionary tale, demonstrating the persistence of that dynamic, even in the face of scientific consensus to the contrary.

At the same time, infant mortality statistics can tell another story. The stories and sense that we make of infant mortality statistics, the uses to which we—however we define that "we"—put them, remain political questions. Insofar as, as Nash suggests, the crisis frame risks pairing urgent rhetoric with political inaction, perhaps the current deemphasis of Black infant survival offers an important pause for acknowledging and acting on what we already know. Global infant mortality statistics tell us that it is not only possible but actual that 998 or 999 babies per 1,000 can live to see their first birthday, when basic supports can be counted on: paid parental leave, universal health care, clean water, midwives. They also show us that, even encased in the toxic and temporary protections of SUVs and strollers, the white settler babies supposedly protected by the cult of true babyhood are not doing so well. Even in the relatively good numbers for white infants, we see the lethality of our racial-capitalist medical system, as they die at four times the rate of so-called "peer countries." Globally, nationally, and at smaller scales, numbers track along colonial, racist, class, gender, and ability hierarchies and also reflect local particularities of care—and broader social, institutional, and political supports for that care—that can amplify or mitigate those structural factors.

Leith Mullings's observations from two decades ago remain relevant: the measures actually needed to transform the conditions that threaten Black infant survival in the United States are deep, redistributive, transformative, and ultimately beneficial for all babies, birthing people, and those who care for and about them. The birth justice movement's emphasis on the content and power of care that truly sees and supports birthing people in their wholeness and in their connections with community life and on shifting institutional protocols signals important potentials for such broad and deep transformation. It is crucial to push state entities and institutions away from innocence and toward accountability to this leadership, this collective work that is already midwifing a world where Black infants, maternity, gestation, and communities thrive.

Notes

Preface

1. Amani Nuru-Jeter et al., "'It's the Skin You're In': African-American Women Talk about Their Experiences of Racism. An Exploratory Study to Develop Measures of Racism for Birth Outcome Studies," *Maternal and Child Health Journal* 1, no. 13 (2009): 29–39, https://doi.org/10.1007/s10995-008-0357-x; Leith Mullings, "Resistance and Resilience: The Sojourner Syndrome and the Social Context of Reproduction in Central Harlem," *Transforming Anthropology* 13, no. 2 (2005): 79–91; Leith Mullings and Alaka Wali, *Stress and Resilience: The Social Context of Reproduction in Central Harlem* (New York: Kluwer Academic / Plenum Publishers, 2001); Michael C. Lu and Neal Halfon, "Racial and Ethnic Disparities in Birth Outcomes: A Life-Course Perspective," *Maternal and Child Health Journal* 7, no. 1 (2003): 13–30; Camara Phyllis Jones, "Levels of Racism: A Theoretic Framework and a Gardener's Tale," *American Journal of Public Health* 90, no. 8 (August 2000): 1212–15; and F. M. Jackson et al., "Examining the Burdens of Gendered Racism: Implications for Pregnancy Outcomes among College-Educated African American Women," *Maternal and Child Health Journal*, no. 5 (2001): 95–107.

2. "Underground Railroad for New Life," Birthing Project USA, August 24, 2021, www.birthingprojectusa.org; and Haile Eshe Cole, Paula X. Rojas, and Jennie Joseph, "Building a Movement to Birth a More Just and Loving World," National Perinatal Task Force, March 2018.

3. Erica Nelson, "Race to Equity: A Baseline Report on the State of Racial Disparities in Dane County," Race to Equity, Madison, WI, 2014.

4. Dána-Ain Davis, "Obstetric Racism: The Racial Politics of Pregnancy, Labor, and Birthing," *Medical Anthropology* 38, no. 7 (October 2019): 560–73, https://doi.org/10.1080/01459740.2018.1549389.

5. Keisha La'Nesha Goode, "Birthing, Blackness, and the Body: Black Midwives and Experiential Continuities of Institutional Racism," City University of New York, 2014, https://academicworks.cuny.edu/gc_etds/423, 31–32, 182–85.

6. Audre Lorde, *Sister Outsider* (New York: Crossing Press, 1984); Dorothy Roberts, *Killing the Black Body: Race, Reproduction, and the Meaning of Liberty* (New York: Penguin Random House, 1998); and Angela Davis, "The Legacy of Slavery: Standards for a New Womanhood," in *Women, Race, and Class* (New York: Penguin Random House, 1981), 3–29.

7. "Letter of Support for Midwives of Color Chair and Inner Council Resignation," *AROMidwifery* (blog), May 27, 2012, https://aromidwifery.wordpress.com/letter-of-support-for-midwives-of-color-chair-and-inner-council-resignation/.

8. Eve Tuck, "Suspending Damage: A Letter to Communities," *Harvard Educational Review* 73, no. 3 (2009): 409–28.

9. Richard A. Meckel, *Save the Babies: American Public Health Reform and the Prevention of Infant Mortality, 1850–1929* (Baltimore, MD: Johns Hopkins University Press, 1990). Sociologist David Armstrong argues that the "invention of infant mortality" proper occurred in in the 1870s, meaning that infants took form as a discrete form and phase of life, from birth to the first year or two, distinct from both late-term fetuses and older children. David Armstrong, "The Invention of Infant Mortality," *Sociology of Health & Illness* 8, no. 3 (1986): 211–32.

10. Nick Estes, *Our History Is the Future: Standing Rock versus the Dakota Access Pipeline, and the Long Tradition of Indigenous Resistance* (New York: Verso, 2019).

11. Wangui Muigai, "An Awful Gladness: African American Experiences of Infant Death from Slavery to the Great Migration," PhD dissertation, Princeton University, 2017, 177. See also Monica Casper, *Babylost: Racism, Survival, and the Quiet Politics of Infant Mortality, from A to Z* (New Brunswick, NJ: Rutgers University Press, 2022).

12. Claudia Jones, "An End to the Neglect of the Problems of the Negro Woman!," *Political Affairs,* June 1949, 51–67, esp. 53.

13. Loretta Ross, "Conceptualizing Reproductive Justice Theory," in *Radical Reproductive Justice,* ed. Loretta Ross et al. (New York: The Feminist Press at CUNY, 2017).

14. Loretta Ross and Rickie Solinger, *Reproductive Justice: An Introduction* (Oakland: University of California Press, 2017), 71; "Visioning New Futures for Reproductive Justice Declaration 2023," SisterSong Women of Color Reproduc-

tive Justice Collective, January 2023, www.sistersong.net/visioningnewfutures-forrj; and M Murphy, "Against Population, Towards Alterlife," in *Making Kin Not Population*, ed. Adele Clarke and Donna Haraway, 101–24 (Chicago: Prickly Paradigm Press, 2018). On abolition and reproductive justice, see Dorothy Roberts, *Torn Apart: How the Child Welfare System Destroys Black Families—and How Abolition Can Build a Safer World* (New York: Basic Books, 2022). As Jasmine Syedullah writes, "abolition is always already present in black feminist communities of care" (see Jasmine Syedullah, "'Becoming More Ourselves': Four Emergent Strategies of Black Feminist Congregational Abolition" *Palimpsest* 11, no. 1 [2022]: 110).

15. Julia Oparah and Alicia Bonaparte, eds., *Birthing Justice: Black Women, Pregnancy, and Childbirth* (New York: Routledge, 2015); "Birth Justice—Black Women Birthing Justice," July 28, 2020, www.blackwomenbirthingjustice.com/birth-justice; "Birth Justice," accessed June 1, 2023; https://southernbirthjustice.org/birth-justice; "Our Work," Black Mamas Matter Alliance, accessed August 13, 2023, https://blackmamasmatter.org/our-work/; and "Respectful Maternity Care," *National Birth Equity Collaborative* (blog), accessed August 13, 2023, https://birthequity.org/rm.

16. Michele Goodwin, *Policing the Womb: Invisible Women and the Criminalization of Motherhood* (Cambridge, UK: Cambridge University Press, 2020); and Roberts, *Killing the Black Body*.

17. "Visioning New Futures for Reproductive Justice Declaration 2023," SisterSong Women of Color Reproductive Justice Collective.

Introduction

1. Frederick Hoffman, *Race Traits and Tendencies of the American Negro* (American Economic Association, 1896), 2.

2. Hoffman, *Race Traits*, 37.

3. Khalil Gibran Muhammad, *The Condemnation of Blackness: Race, Crime, and the Making of Modern Urban America, with a New Preface* (Cambridge, MA: Harvard University Press, 2019), 40.

4. "Infant mortality," or sometimes "infantile mortality," had a fairly loose meaning until it was codified, in the United States, in the Children's Bureau reports of the later 1910s, as mortality during the first year of life. Before that time, the term was often used to signify death up to the age of five years. For a Foucauldian analysis of the term's emergence as a sign of the problematization of the phenomenon in the UK, see Armstrong, "Invention of Infant Mortality."

5. Hoffman, *Race Traits*, 42. In New York, 87.42 per thousand for Blacks under 15, versus 47.06 for whites; in Washington, 159.93 for Blacks under 5, versus 65.04 for whites. The oldest category ranges from an anomalous slightly higher rate for whites over 65 in New York City to Brooklyn's 96 per thousand for whites to 144 per thousand for Blacks, with most cities showing Black death rates about 25 percent higher than the white rate for that age group. Mortality tables from New Orleans, Charleston, and Richmond provide even more striking evidence, offering detailed data on both infant and early child mortality. Infant mortality in New Orleans, according to the 1890 census, was 269.4 per thousand for whites, compared to 430.2 per thousand for Blacks. An even more pronouncedly disparate rate of survival was in evidence in Charleston, where the rate was 200.4 per thousand for whites, compared to 461.7 per thousand among Blacks. In Richmond, 529.6 of every thousand Black infants—more than half of all babies born—died before their first birthday, compared to 186.9 of their white counterparts: "a mortality so great," according to Hoffman (*Race Traits*, 45), "that no greater fecundity could balance the loss."

6. Hoffman, *Race Traits*, 45. Earlier in the chapter, Hoffman sounds an initial note of caution about his statistical representations of infant life and death. Regarding "a comparative statement of the birth rates of both races," he writes, "it must be admitted that information on this point is almost entirely wanting, and that no trustworthy conclusion as to the comparative fecundity can be arrived at" (*Race Traits*, 33). But after acknowledging the lack of this essential factor—the birth rate is the denominator of the infant mortality rate calculation—he evinces no further hesitation in drawing unequivocal conclusions.

7. Muhammad, *Condemnation of Blackness*, 35.

8. Hoffman, *Race Traits*, 44–45; 42.

9. Hoffman, *Race Traits*, 56

10. Hoffman, *Race Traits*, 55

11. Hoffman, *Race Traits*, 57

12. Hoffman, *Race Traits*, 34

13. Stewart Thompson, "Factors That Influence Infant Mortality," *American Journal of Public Health* 11, no. 5 (1920): 415–20.

14. Thompson, "Factors That Influence Infant Mortality," 416.

15. Robin Bernstein, *Racial Innocence: Performing American Childhood from Slavery to Civil Rights* (New York: NYU Press, 2011).

16. Florida's brutally coercive racialized agricultural labor regimes persisted through the twentieth century and into the twenty-first. Sean Sellers, Greg Asbed, and the Coalition of Imokalee Workers, "The History and Evolution of Forced La-

bor in Florida Agriculture," *Race/Ethnicity: Multidisciplinary Global Contexts* 5, no. 1 (2011): 29–49.

17. Thompson, "Factors That Influence Infant Mortality," 418.

18. Gertrude Jacinta Fraser, *African American Midwifery in the South* (Cambridge, MA: Harvard University Press, 1998); Muigai, "An Awful Gladness"; Alicia D. Bonaparte, "'The Satisfactory Midwife Bag': Midwifery Regulation in South Carolina, Past and Present Considerations," *Social Science History* 38, no. 1–2 (2014): 155–82, https://doi.org/10.1017/ssh.2015.14; and Annie Menzel, "The Midwife's Bag, or, the Objects of Black Infant Mortality Prevention," *Signs: Journal of Women in Culture and Society* 46, no. 2 (January 1, 2021): 283–309, https://doi.org/10.1086/710806.

19. Thompson, "Factors That Influence Infant Mortality," 419.

20. Thompson, "Factors That Influence Infant Mortality," 419.

21. On the malignant midwife as a key framing, see Wangui Muigai, "Framing Black Infant and Maternal Mortality," *Journal of Law, Medicine & Ethics* 50, no. 1 (2022): 85–91.

22. "A Healthy Baby Begins with You," Office of Minority Health, US Department of Health and Human Services, 2008, https://minorityhealth.hhs.gov/Assets/pdf/checked/brochure.pdf.

23. Natali Valdez describes a strikingly parallel disjunction between research and interventions in maternal obesity during pregnancy, in *Weighing the Future: Race, Science, and Pregnancy Trials in the Postgenomic Era* (Berkeley: University of California Press, 2022).

24. Naomi Murakawa, "Racial Innocence: Law, Social Science, and the Unknowing of Racism in the US Carceral State," *Annual Review of Law and Social Science* 15 (2019): 474.

25. James Baldwin, "My Dungeon Shook: Letter to My Nephew on the One Hundredth Anniversary of the Emancipation," *Baldwin: Collected Essays* (New York: Library of America, 1998), 292.

26. Ruth Wilson Gilmore, "Abolition Geography and the Problem of Innocence," in *Abolition Geography: Essays toward Liberation* (New York: Verso, 2022).

27. Muhammad, *Condemnation of Blackness*, 62–64; Kelly Miller, "A Review of Hoffman's Race Traits and Tendencies of the American Negro," American Negro Academy, Occasional Papers No. 1, 1897; and W.E.B. Du Bois, "Race Traits and Tendencies of the American Negro by Frederick L. Hoffman, F.S.S. [Review]," *Annals of the American Academy of Political and Social Science* 9 (January 1897): 127–33.

28. Du Bois, "Race Traits and Tendencies of the American Negro."

29. W.E.B. Du Bois, *The Philadelphia Negro: A Social Study.* Philadelphia: University of Pennsylvania Press, 1996 [1899]; and W.E.B. Du Bois, *Mortality among Negroes in Cities,* Proceedings of the Conference for Investigations of City Problems, held at Atlanta University, May 26–27, 1896, Atlanta University Publications, No. 1.

30. Alison Parker, *Unceasing Militant: The Life of Mary Church Terrell.* Chapel Hill: University of North Carolina Press, 2020.

31. Fraser, *African American Midwifery in the South,* 260; Valerie Lee, *Granny Midwives and Black Women Writers: Double-Dutched Readings* (New York: Routledge, 1996); Onnie Lee Logan, as told to Katherine Clark, *Motherwit: An Alabama Midwife's Story* (New York: Dutton, 1989); and Margaret Charles Smith and Linda Janet Holmes, *Listen to Me Good: The Life Story of an Alabama Midwife* (Columbus: Ohio State University Press, 1996).

32. "What is Birth Justice?"; Julia Chinyere Oparah with Black Women Birthing Justice, "Introduction: Beyond Coercion and Malign Neglect," in *Birthing Justice: Black Women, Pregnancy, and Childbirth,* ed. Julia Chinyere Oparah and Alicia D. Bonaparte (New York: Routledge, 2015): 1–18; and "Birth Justice Network," Southern Birth Justice Network, accessed August 13, 2023, https://southernbirthjustice .org/birth-justice.

33. The formulation of white settler reproductive futurity builds on Black feminist theorizations of reproduction, mothering, and motherhood within the matrix of enslavement and ownership, including those of Angela Davis, Hortense Spillers, Alexis Pauline Gumbs, Joy James, Jennifer Morgan, and Alys Weinbaum; queer-of-color critique, especially Jafari Allen's engagement with Lee Edelman's argument against "reproductive futurism"; and Indigenous feminist and decolonial scholarship on settler futurity including that of Eve Tuck and Rubén A Gaztambide-Fernández, Tuck and K. Wayne Yang, M Murphy, and Alexis Shotwell. Key sources include Angela Davis, "Reflections on the Black Woman's Role in the Community of Slaves," *The Black Scholar* 3, no. 4 (December 1971): 2–15; Joy James, "The Womb of Western Theory: Trauma, Time Theft, and the Captive Maternal," *Challenging the Punitive Society: Carceral Notebooks* 12 (2016): 253–96; Saidiya Hartman, "The Belly of the World: A Note on Black Women's Labors," *Souls* 18, no. 1 (March 14, 2016): 166–73; Alexis Pauline Gumbs, "M/other Ourselves: A Black Queer Feminist Genealogy for Radical Mothering," in *Revolutionary Mothering: Love on the Front Lines,* ed. Alexis Pauline Gumbs, China Martens and Mai'a Williams (Oakland, CA: PM Press, 2016), 19–31; Jasmine Syedullah, "The Hearts We Beat: Black Feminist Freedom in the Hold of Slavery," lecture presented at Gender Talks, Women's and Gender Studies Department, Berea

College, February 10, 2021, www.youtube.com/watch?v = rh9XfeKva8c; Jennifer L. Morgan, *Reckoning with Slavery: Gender, Kinship, and Capitalism in the Early Black Atlantic* (Durham, NC: Duke University Press, 2021); Alys Eve Weinbaum, *The Afterlife of Reproductive Slavery: Biocapitalism and Black Feminism's Philosophy of History* (Durham, NC: Duke University Press, 2019); Jafari Sinclaire Allen, "For 'the Children' Dancing the Beloved Community," *Souls* 11, no. 3 (2009): 311–26, doi:10.1080/10999940903088945; Eve Tuck and Rubén A. Gaztambide-Fernández, "Curriculum, Replacement, and Settler Futurity," *Journal of Curriculum Theorizing* 29, no. 1 (2013): 72–89; Eve Tuck and K. Wayne Yang, "Decolonization Is Not a Metaphor," *Decolonization: Indigeneity, Education & Society* 1, no. 1 (2012): 1–40; M Murphy, "Against Population, Towards Alterlife," in *Making Kin Not Population*, ed. Adele Clarke and Donna Haraway, 101–24 (Chicago: Prickly Paradigm Press); and Alexis Shotwell, *Against Purity: Living Ethically in Compromised Times* (Minneapolis: University of Minnesota Press, 2016).

34. Baldwin, "My Dungeon Shook," 292.

35. On resonances between Baldwin's contestations of white devaluation and Black Lives Matter, see Eddie S. Glaude Jr., "James Baldwin and Black Lives Matter," in Susan J. McWilliams, ed., *A Political Companion to James Baldwin*, 361–72 (Lexington: University Press of Kentucky, 2017).

36. Baldwin, "My Dungeon Shook," 293.

37. Baldwin, "My Dungeon Shook," 292.

38. Kirstine Taylor, "Racial Capitalism and the Production of Racial Innocence," *Theory & Event* 24, no. 3 (2021): 702–29.

39. Cedric J. Robinson, *Black Marxism: The Making of the Black Radical Tradition*, 2nd ed. (Chapel Hill: University of North Carolina Press, 2000).

40. Jodi Melamed, "Racial Capitalism," *Critical Ethnic Studies* 1, no. 1 (2015): 76–85. In essence, Taylor is arguing that Baldwin's analytic converges with what Susan Koshy, Lisa Marie Cacho, Jodi A. Byrd, and Brian Jordan Jefferson term "colonial racial capitalism." See Brian Jordan Jefferson et al., introduction to *Colonial Racial Capitalism* (Durham, NC: Duke University Press, 2022).

41. Taylor, "Racial Capitalism and the Production of Racial Innocence," 712.

42. Baldwin, "White Problem," 75–76. As Kevin Bruyneel shows, Baldwin's relationship with the US's founding reality and disavowal of Indigenous genocide is complex. As in this passage, Baldwin's rhetoric often depicts genocide as a fait accompli, erasing ongoing Indigenous presence and politics; and his "we" aligns him uneasily with the same America whose innocence he indicts with eloquent fire. At the same time, the positioning of genocide as materially constitutive of the polity itself also militates against the innocence that inheres in what Bruyneel

calls "settler memory." Kevin Bruyneel, *Settler Memory: The Disavowal of Indigeneity and the Politics of Race in the United States* (Chapel Hill: University of North Carolina Press, 2021), 97–98.

43. Baldwin, "Talk to Teachers," 681–82.

44. See also Roberto Sirvent and Danny Haiphong, *American Exceptionalism and American Innocence: A People's History of Fake News—From the Revolutionary War to the War on Terror* (New York: Simon and Schuster, 2019).

45. This masculinist tendency in Baldwin's rhetoric of slavery is marked, even as his use of the term "flesh" resonates with Hortense Spillers's use of the term to signify European enslavers' disqualification of African peoples from normative Eurocentric gender categories, manifesting in their undiscriminating patterns of torture and brutalizing labor demands. Hortense Spillers, *Black, White, and in Color: Essays on American Literature and Culture* (Chicago: University of Chicago Press, 2003), 203–29.

46. Joy James, "The Womb of Western Theory: Trauma, Time Theft, and the Captive Maternal," *Carceral Notebooks* 12, no. 1 (2016): 255.

47. These predatory dynamics—as well as Black women's ongoing insurgency against them—persist into the present in what Alys Eve Weinbaum, drawing on Saidiya Hartman, names "the afterlife of reproductive slavery." Weinbaum, *Afterlife of Reproductive Slavery*.

48. Morgan, *Reckoning with Slavery*, 247.

49. Morgan, *Reckoning with Slavery*, 226.

50. Morgan, *Reckoning with Slavery*, 226.

51. Roberts, *Killing the Black Body*, 172–87.

52. Karen Scott, Laura Britton, and Monica McLemore, "The Ethics of Perinatal Care for Black Women: Dismantling the Structural Racism in 'Mother Blame' Narratives," *Journal of Perinatal and Neonatal Nursing* 33, no. 2 (2019): 108–15.

53. Juliet Hooker, *White Grievance/Black Grief* (Princeton, NJ: Princeton University Press, 2023), 37.

54. Hakima Tafunzi Payne, "Anti-Racism and Anti-Oppression Work in Midwifery," Facebook Group, October 7, 2015; also see Dána-Ain Davis, *Reproductive Injustice: Racism, Pregnancy, and Premature Birth* (New York: NYU Press, 2019), 182.

55. Tiffany L. Green et al., "Rethinking Bias to Achieve Maternal Health Equity: Changing Organizations, Not Just Individuals," *Obstetrics & Gynecology* 137, no. 5 (May 2021): 935–40.

56. Jennifer C. Nash, *Birthing Black Mothers* (Durham, NC: Duke University Press, 2021), and "Birthing Black Mothers: Birth Work and the Making of Black

Maternal Political Subjects. *WSQ: Women's Studies Quarterly* 47, no. 3–4 (Fall/ Winter 2019): 30.

57. Michel Foucault, *The History of Sexuality*, vol. 1 (New York: Pantheon Books, 1978), and Foucault, *"Society Must Be Defended": Lectures at the Collège de France, 1975–76* (1997; reprint, New York: Picador, 2003), 245.

58. Foucault, *History of Sexuality*, 139.

59. Ian Hacking, *The Taming of Chance* (New York: Cambridge University Press, 1990), 21–22.

60. Foucault, *"Society Must Be Defended,"* 243–44.

61. Foucault, *"Society Must Be Defended,"* 254–55.

62. Foucault, *"Society Must Be Defended,"* 256.

63. Paul Apostolidis, *Breaks in the Chain: What Immigrant Workers Can Teach America about Democracy* (Minneapolis: University of Minnesota Press, 2010), 97–98.

64. M Murphy, *Seizing the Means of Reproduction: Entanglements of Feminism, Health, and Technoscience* (Durham, NC: Duke University Press, 2012), 44.

65. Morgan, *Reckoning with Slavery*, 42. See also Stephanie Smallwood, *Saltwater Slavery: A Middle Passage from Africa to American Diaspora* (Cambridge, MA: Harvard University Press, 2007). Scott Lauria Morgensen makes a similar argument with regard to the naturalization of settler-colonial states and erasure of Indigenous genocide and ongoing presence within theorizations of biopolitics. Scott Lauria Morgensen, "The Biopolitics of Settler Colonialism: Right Here, Right Now," *Settler Colonial Studies* 1, no. 1 (2011): 52–76.

66. Smallwood, *Saltwater Slavery*; and Morgan, *Reckoning with Slavery*, 89–109.

67. Murphy, *Seizing the Means of Reproduction*, 37; Achille Mbembe, "Necropolitics," *Public Culture* 15, no. 1 (2003): 11–40; and Didier Fassin, "Another Politics of Life Is Possible," *Theory, Culture, & Society* 26, no. 5 (2009): 4–60, 53.

68. Ann Laura Stoler, *Race and the Education of Desire: Foucault's "History of Sexuality" and the Colonial Order of Things* (Durham, NC: Duke University Press, 1995); and Alexander G. Weheliye, *Habeas Viscus: Racializing Assemblages, Biopolitics, and Black Feminist Theories of the Human* (Durham, NC: Duke University Press, 2014).

69. James, "Womb of Western Theory," 267–68.

70. While part of a long note on both biopolitics and neoliberal governmentality, the quote here specifically refers to Foucault on neoliberal economics. M Murphy, *The Economization of Life* (Durham, NC: Duke University Press, 2017), 149n17.

71. In Kyla Schuller's terms, by the mid-nineteenth century, white infant mortality became a key site of "sentimental biopower" for the white polity. Kyla Schuller, *The Biopolitics of Feeling: Race, Sex, and Science in the 19th Century* (Durham, NC: Duke University Press, 2019), 3–4.

72. Murphy, *Economization of Life*, 24.

73. Richard Meckel, "Racialism and Infant Death," in *Migrants, Minorities, and Health: Historical and Contemporary Studies,* ed. Laura Marks and Michael Worboys, 70–92 (1997; reprint, New York: Routledge, 2003).

74. Meckel, *Save the Babies*, 200–11.

75. A. K. Driscoll and D. M. Ely, "Infant Mortality in the United States, 2020," *National Vital Statistics Reports* 71, no. 5 (2022). Linda Villarosa, "Why America's Black Mothers and Babies Are in a Life-or-Death Crisis," *New York Times Magazine*, April 2018, www.nytimes.com/2018/04/11/magazine/black-mothers-babies-death-maternal-mortality.html. Douglas Almond, Kenneth Y. Chay, and Michael Greenstone (in "Civil Rights, the War on Poverty, and Black-White Convergence in Infant Mortality in the Rural South and Mississippi," Working Paper No. 07-04, MIT Department of Economics, 2006), note that the disparity diminished, though it did not close, during the 1960–1980 period, which they link with civil rights agitation, community-based activism, and antipoverty programs. The widening disparity after 1980 corresponds with the increasing neoliberalization of the state, including drastic cuts under Reagan and the "end of welfare as we [knew] it" under Clinton. See also Rongal D. Nikola, "The Political Determinants of Health: The Impact of Political Factors on Black and White Infant Mortality Rates in the United States," PhD dissertation, University of New Mexico, 2013, 13.

76. LaKisha Michelle Simmons, "Black Feminist Theories of Motherhood and Generation: Histories of Black Infant and Child Loss in the United States," *Signs: Journal of Women in Culture and Society* 46, no. 2 (January 1, 2021): 331–35.

77. Casper, *Babylost*.

78. Karl Marx, *Capital: A Critique of Political Economy, Volume* 1, translated by Ben Fowkes. (New York: Penguin Classics, 1990), 163. As C. Riley Snorton writes, "The recurrent practice of enumerating the dead . . . seems to conform to the logics of accumulation that structure racial capitalism." C. Riley Snorton, *Black on Both Sides: A Racial History of Trans Identity* (Minneapolis: University of Minnesota Press, 2017), viii.

79. Emma Kowal, *Trapped in the Gap: Doing Good in Indigenous Australia* (New York: Berghahn Books, 2015).

80. As Zakiyyah Iman Jackson writes, "Although antiblackness relationally distributes differential material effects across the color line, in the making of the

color line, the experience of 'race' confounds comparative study." See Zakiyyah Iman Jackson, *Becoming Human: Matter and Meaning in an Antiblack World* (New York: NYU Press, 2020), 212.

81. Ruha Benjamin, "Black AfterLives Matter: Cultivating Kindness as Reproductive Justice," in *Making Kin Not Population*, ed. Adele E. Clarke and Donna Haraway, 41–65 (Chicago: Prickly Paradigm Press, 2018).

82. Data from the National Center for Health Statistics for the period linked birth/infant death file in Driscoll and Ely, "Infant Mortality in the United States, 2020."

83. "Infant Mortality by Country 2023," *World Population Review*, February 4, 2023, https://worldpopulationreview.com/country-rankings/infant-mortality-rate-by-country.

84. Alexandra M. Stern, *Eugenic Nation: Faults and Frontiers of Better Breeding in Modern America* (Oakland: University of California Press, 2016); Laura Briggs, *Somebody's Children: The Politics of Transracial and Transnational Adoption* (Durham, NC: Duke University Press, 2012); and Laura Briggs, *How All Politics Became Reproductive Politics: From Welfare Reform to Foreclosure to Trump* (Oakland: University of California Press, 2017).

85. Robyn Powell, "Disability Reproductive Justice," *University of Pennsylvania Law Review* 170 (October 7, 2022); Claudia Malacrida, "Mothering and Disability: From Eugenics to Newgenics," in *Routledge Handbook of Disability Studies*, 2nd edition, ed. Nick Watson and Simo Vehmas (New York: Routledge University Press, 2020); and Robyn Powell, "From Carrie Buck to Britney Spears: Strategies for Disrupting the Ongoing Reproductive Oppression of Disabled People," *Virginia Law Review Online* 246 (August 10, 2021).

86. Farah Diaz-Tello, "Invisible Wounds: Obstetric Violence in the United States," *Reproductive Health Matters* 24, no. 47 (May 2016): 56–64, https://doi.org/10.1016/j.rhm.2016.04.004; and March of Dimes and PeriStats, "Total Cesarean Deliveries by Maternal Race/Ethnicity: United States, 2019–2021 Average," www.marchofdimes.org/peristats/data?reg=99&top=8&stop=356&lev=1&slev=1&obj=1.

87. Hazel Carby, *Reconstructing Womanhood : The Emergence of the Afro-American Woman Novelist* (New York: Oxford University Press, 1987); and Bernstein, *Racial Innocence*.

88. M Murphy, "Alterlife and Decolonial Chemical Relations," *Cultural Anthropology* 32, no. 4 (2017): 494–503; and Tuck, "Suspending Damage."

89. Roberts's classic analysis of the "crack baby epidemic" offers one of the most horrific recent examples of this dynamic. Roberts, *Killing the Black Body*, 157.

90. Mbembe, "Necropolitics," 27.

91. Christen A. Smith, "Facing the Dragon: Black Mothering, Sequalae, and Gendered Necropolitics in the Americas," *Transforming Anthropology* 24, no. 1 (2016): 38. Smith builds on Dani McClain's argument that anti-Black state violence is a primary reproductive justice concern, as incidents of police killings result in "feelings of trauma and fear of loss related to maternity" for many Black women. Dani McClain, "The Murder of Black Youth Is a Reproductive Justice Issue," *The Nation*, August 13, 2014, www.thenation.com/article/archive/murder-black-youth-reproductive-justice-issue/.

92. Smith, "Facing the Dragon," 32.

93. Smith, "Facing the Dragon," 42.

94. Erica S. Lawson, "Bereaved Black Mothers and Maternal Activism in the Racial State," *Feminist Studies* 44, no. 3 (2018): 713–35.

95. Kwate and Threadcraft, "Dying Fast."

96. Eve Jablonka and Marion J. Lamb, *Evolution in Four Dimensions: Genetic, Epigenetic, Behavioral, and Symbolic Variation in the History of Life* (Cambridge, MA: MIT Press, 2005).

97. Jackson, *Becoming Human*, 205.

98. Valdez, *Weighing the Future*.

99. Naa Oyo A. Kwate and Shatema Threadcraft, "Dying Fast and Dying Slow in Black Space," *Du Bois Review: Social Science Research on Race* 14, no. 2 (2018): 535–56, 538.

100. Bernstein, *Racial Innocence*, 43; Bernstein argues that this polarization eclipsed children who were neither white nor Black from the dominant public imagination.

101. George Shulman, *American Prophecy: Race and Redemption in American Political Culture* (Minneapolis: University of Minnesota Press, 2008), 134.

102. Bernstein, *Racial Innocence*, 33.

103. Collier Meyerson, "Adults Think Black Girls Are Older Than They Are—and It Matters," *The Nation*, July 6, 2017, www.thenation.com/article/archive/adults-thinks-black-girls-are-older-than-they-are-and-it-matters/.

104. Salimah H. Meghani et al., "Time to Take Stock: A Meta-Analysis and Systematic Review of Analgesic Treatment Disparities for Pain in the United States," *Pain Medicine* 13, no. 2 (2012): 150–74; and Kelly M. Hoffman et al., "Racial Bias in Pain Assessment and Treatment Recommendations, and False Beliefs about Biological Differences between Blacks and Whites," *Proceedings of the National Academy of Sciences USA* 113, no. 16 (2016): 4296–301.

105. Bernstein, *Racial Innocence*, 221.

106. Ebony Elizabeth Thomas, *The Dark Fantastic: Race and the Imagination from Harry Potter to the Hunger Games* (New York: NYU Press, 2019), 55–56; and Christina Sharpe, *In the Wake: On Blackness and Being* (Durham, NC: Duke University Press, 2016), 80. On refusing "the Child" as the avatar of heteronormative "reproductive futurism," see Lee Edelman, *No Future: Queer Theory and the Death Drive* (Durham, NC: Duke University Press, 2004).

107. Hoffman, *Race Traits*, 115; and Robert J. Karp and Bobby Gearing, "The Death of Burghardt Du Bois, 1899: Implications for Today," *Journal of the National Medical Association* 107, no. 1 (February 1, 2015): 68–74.

108. Roberts, *Killing the Black Body*, 157.

109. Davis, *Reproductive Injustice*, 101–102.

110. Davis, *Reproductive Injustice*, 101–105

111. W.E.B. Du Bois, *Black Reconstruction in America, 1860–1880* (1935; New York: The Free Press, 1998), 700. This concept has been taken up by labor historian David Roediger as well as, more recently, political theorist Ella Myers. David Roediger, *The Wages of Whiteness: Race and the Making of the American Working Class* (New York: Verso, 1991); and Ella Myers, *The Gratifications of Whiteness: W. E. B. Du Bois and the Enduring Rewards of Anti-Blackness* (New York: Oxford University Press, 2022).

112. Du Bois, *Black Reconstruction in America*, 700.

113. Morgan, *Reckoning with Slavery*, 210–11.

114. Heidi Kiiwetinepinesiik Stark, "Criminal Empire: The Making of the Savage in a Lawless Land," *Theory & Event* 19, no. 4 (2016), muse.jhu.edu/article/633282.

115. Weinbaum casts *Black Reconstruction* as "opening up of the question of the sexual and reproductive politics of slavery and of slave women's insurgency against the system of slavery." While Du Bois's paradigm-shifting account of enslaved people's insurgency and, ultimately, their decisive refusal of the slave system as a *general strike* figures the slaves-cum-revolutionary workers as male, the book's opening chapters nevertheless explicitly bring into view the reproductive and sexual violence and exploitation at the heart of that slave system and in its aftermath. It thus "clears space" for Black feminist accounts, beginning with Davis's 1971 "Black Woman's Role in the Community of Slaves," that centers enslaved Black women's structural vulnerability to *and* insurgent refusals of this reproductive and sexual violence. Weinbaum, *Afterlife of Reproductive Slavery*, 67.

116. Stephanie Jones-Rogers, *They Were Her Property: White Women as Slaveowners in the American South* (New Haven, CT: Yale University Press, 2019).

117. Margaret McCrae, *Mothers of Massive Resistance: White Women and the Politics of White Supremacy* (New York: Oxford University Press, 2018).

118. Stephanie R. M. Bray and Monica R. McLemore, "Demolishing the Myth of the Default Human That Is Killing Black Mothers," *Frontiers in Public Health* 9, article no. 675788 (May 24, 2021), doi:10.3389/fpubh.2021.675788.

119. Lisa Beard, *If We Were Kin: Race, Identification, and Intimate Political Appeals* (New York: Oxford University Press, 2023).

120. Gilmore, "Race and Globalization," 261.

121. Miriam Ticktin, "A World without Innocence," *American Ethnologist* 44, no. 4 (2017): 577–90.

122. Gayatri C. Spivak, "Can the Subaltern Speak?," in *Marxism and the Interpretation of Culture*, ed. Lawrence Grossberg and Cary Nelson, 271–313 (Chicago: University of Illinois Press, 1988).

123. Gloria Wekker, *White Innocence: Paradoxes of Colonialism and Race* (Durham, NC: Duke University Press, 2016).

124. Roxane Dunbar-Ortiz draws on Sherene Razack's work on innocence to articulate a deliberate refusal of accountability for the ways that the past manifestly shapes the present—the ways that violent settler-colonial aggression lives on in US militarism and imperialism, as well as the ways that the settler-colonial state's political map actively effaces Indigenous sovereignty, resistance, and relations with lands and waters through borders, place names, and the property regime. Roxanne Dunbar-Ortiz, *An Indigenous Peoples' History of the United States* (Boston: Beacon Press, 2014), 229–30. Mary Louise Fellows and Sherene Razack, "The Race to Innocence: Hierarchical Relations among Women," *Gender, Race & Justice* 1 (1995): 335; and Sherene Razack, *Dark Threats and White Knights: The Somalia Affair, Peacekeeping, and the New Imperialism* (Toronto: University of Toronto Press, 2004).

125. Kevin Bruyneel, "'Happy Days' (of the White Settler Imaginary) Are Here Again," *Theory & Event* 20, no. 1 (2017): 44–54.

126. These include "the assumption that we and our work are fundamentally benevolent"; the assumption of neutrality or transcendence of the power relationships that we critique and describe; the location of the "worst" colonialism in the past, thus denying the "ongoingness" of racial and colonial violence in the present day, and self-presentation as agents of progressive futurity and not also of colonial institutions and racial power. Alissa Macoun, "Colonising White Innocence: Complicity and Critical Encounters," in *The Limits of Settler Colonial Reconciliation*, ed. Sarah Maddison, Tom Clark, and Ravi de Costa, 85–102 (Singapore: Springer, 2016), 86–94.

127. Tuck and Yang, "Decolonization Is Not a Metaphor," 10; see Corey Snelgrove, Rita Dhamoon, and Jeff Corntassel, "Unsettling Settler Colonialism: The

Discourse and Politics of Settlers, and Solidarity with Indigenous Nations," *Decolonization: Indigeneity, Education & Society* 3, no. 2 (2014): 1–32, for a genealogy of the term "settler" as well as of settler colonial studies.

128. Tuck and Yang, "Decolonization Is Not a Metaphor," 4.

129. Hoffman, *Race Traits*, 323–26. As Paul Lawrie notes, by the 1920s Hoffman had revised his positions on Blacks and Indigenous peoples alike, deeming them "stagnant" rather than doomed. Paul Lawrie, *Forging a Laboring Race: The African American Worker in the Progressive Imagination* (New York University Press: New York, 2016), 37.

130. Cato Sells, *Indian Babies—How to Keep them Well* (Washington, DC: Government Printing Office, 1916).

131. Sells, *Indian Babies*; and Bonnie McElhinny, "'Kissing a Baby Is Not at All Good for Him': Infant Mortality, Medicine, and Colonial Modernity in the U.S.-Occupied Philippines," *American Anthropologist* 107, no. 2 (2005): 183–94.

132. Manu Karuka (Vimalassery), Juliana Hu Pegues, and Alyosha Goldstein, "Introduction: On Colonial Unknowing," *Theory & Event* 19, no. 4 (2016), muse.jhu.edu/article/633283.

133. Kim TallBear, "Caretaking Relations, Not American Dreaming," *Kalfou: A Journal of Comparative and Relational Ethnic Studies* 6, no. 1 (2019); Kim Anderson, *A Recognition of Being: Reconstructing Native Womanhood* (Toronto: Women's Press, 2016); and Dorothy E. Roberts, "Prison, Foster Care, and the Systemic Punishment of Black Mothers," *UCLA Law Review* 59, no. 6 (2012): 1474–1501.

134. Dorothy Roberts, *Torn Apart: How the Child Welfare System Destroys Black Families—and How Abolition Can Build a Safer World* (New York: Basic Books, 2022), 24.

135. Tanya Katerí Hernández, *Racial Innocence: Unmasking Latino Anti-Black Bias and the Struggle for Equality* (Boston: Beacon Press, 2022).

136. Schuller, *Biopolitics of Feeling*, 16.

137. Simone Browne, *Dark Matter: On the Surveillance of Blackness* (Durham, NC: Duke University Press, 2015).

138. Alondra Nelson, *Body and Soul: The Black Panther Party and the Fight against Medical Discrimination* (Minneapolis: University of Minnesota Press, 2011), xii.

139. Brianna Theobald, *Reproduction on the Reservation: Pregnancy, Childbirth, and Colonialism in the Long Twentieth Century* (Chapel Hill: University of North Carolina Press, 2019), 48.

140. Joia Crear-Petty et al., "Moving Towards Anti-Racist Praxis in Medicine," *Lancet* 396, no. 10249 (2020): 451–53.

Chapter 1. The Cult of True Babyhood

1. Richard C. Cabot and Edith K. Richie, "The Influence of Race on the Infant Mortality of Boston in 1909," *Boston Medical and Surgical Journal* 162, no. 7J (1910): 199–202; and Meckel, "Racialism and Infant Death," 81.

2. AASPIM, 1911.

3. Alisa Klaus, *Every Child a Lion: The Origins of Maternal and Infant Health Policy in the US and France* (Ithaca, NY: Cornell University Press, 2019); and Meckel, *Save the Babies*, 116–18.

4. Meckel, *Save the Babies*, 117.

5. Khiara Bridges notes the nearly exclusive focus of early eugenic sterilization programs on "undesirable" poor whites, especially women— most famously Carrie Buck. Khiara Bridges, "White Privilege and White Disadvantage," *Virginia Law Review*, April 10, 2019, https://virginialawreview.org /articles/white-privilege-and-white-disadvantage/. Meckel, "Racialism and Infant Death."

6. Rana Hogarth, "Enslavement and Eugenics," presented at Dismantling Eugenics: A Convening, September 28, 2021, https://vimeo.com/642322721; and "The Shadow of Slavery in the Era of Eugenics," presented at the MacLean Center 2021-2022 Lecture Series "History of Medical Ethics," MacLean Center for Clinical Medical Ethics, University of Chicago, March 17, 2022, www.youtube.com /watch?v=doW44TmfWI8.

7. Carby, *Reconstructing Womanhood*.

8. Carby, *Reconstructing Womanhood*, 20.

9. Carby, *Reconstructing Womanhood*, 24.

10. Carby, *Reconstructing Womanhood*, 20.

11. Carby, *Reconstructing Womanhood*.

12. Carby, *Reconstructing Womanhood*.

13. Carby, *Reconstructing Womanhood*, 22.

14. Carby, *Reconstructing Womanhood*.

15. Carby, *Reconstructing Womanhood*, 23.

16. Carby, *Reconstructing Womanhood*, 23.

17. Spillers, *Black, White, and in Color*, 255.

18. Carby, *Reconstructing Womanhood*, 37.

19. Carby, *Reconstructing Womanhood*, 20.

20. Harriet Ann Jacobs, *Incidents in the Life of a Slave Girl: Written by Herself, with "A True Tale of Slavery" by John S. Jacobs* (1861; Cambridge, MA: Harvard University Press, 1969), 200; see also Davis, *Reproductive Injustice*, 45.

21. Morgan, *Reckoning with Slavery*, 211.

22. Dorothy Roberts, "Spiritual and Menial Housework," *Faculty Scholarship at Penn Carey Law* 1282 (1997): 71.

23. Morgan, *Reckoning with Slavery*, 210-12.

24. Roberts, "Spiritual and Menial Housework," 69-70.

25. Nancy Schrom Dye and Daniel Blake Smith, "Mother Love and Infant Death, 1750-1920," *Journal of American History* 73, no. 2 (1986): 329-53, 330.

26. Barbara Welter, "The Cult of True Womanhood: 1820-1860," *American Quarterly* 18, no. 2 part 1 (1966): 151-74.

27. Viviana A. Zelizer, *Pricing the Priceless Child: The Changing Social Value of Children* (New York: Basic Books, 1985), 8-9.

28. Carl N. Degler, *At Odds: Women and the Family in America from the Revolution to the Present* (New York: Oxford University Press, 1980), 73-74.

29. Dye and Smith, "Mother Love and Infant Death," 338-40.

30. V. Lynn Kennedy, *Born Southern: Childbirth, Motherhood, and Social Networks in the Old South* (Baltimore, MD: Johns Hopkins University Press, 2010), 80-81.

31. Zelizer, *Pricing the Priceless Child*, 25.

32. Dye and Smith, "Mother Love and Infant Death," 340.

33. Dye and Smith, "Mother Love and Infant Death," 340.

34. Dye and Smith, "Mother Love and Infant Death," 340.

35. Fanny Appleton Longfellow, *Mrs. Longfellow: Selected Journals and Letters*, ed. Edward Wageknecht (1848; New York: Longmans, Green, 1956), 129.

36. Dye and Smith, "Mother Love and Infant Death," 339.

37. Dye and Smith, "Mother Love and Infant Death," 340.

38. Dye and Smith, "Mother Love and Infant Death," 340.

39. Ann Douglas, "Heaven Our Home: Consolation Literature in the Northern United States, 1830-1880," *American Quarterly* 26, no. 5 (1974): 496-515.

40. Ann Cvetkovich, "Depression Is Ordinary: Public Feelings and Saidiya Hartman's 'Lose Your Mother,'" *Feminist Theory* 13, no. 2 (2012): 131-46. The "Public Feelings Project" from which this term arises is characterized by a critical queer and queer of color theoretical orientation, and the investigations that it has grounded have been focused on the generativity of negative affects—depression, exhaustion, despair—among marginalized potential counterpublics. See Ann Cvetkovich, "Public Feelings," *South Atlantic Quarterly* 106, no. 3 (2007): 459. While the focus here is on white and economically advantaged women, the key questions that these analysts pose—like "how does capitalism feel?"—perhaps get at the complex collective emotions of homebound, if relatively privileged, antebellum mothers.

41. Douglas, "Heaven Our Home," 496fn2.

42. Douglas, "Heaven Our Home," 496; and S. J. Kleinberg, *Women in the United States, 1830-1945* (New Brunswick, NJ: Rutgers University Press, 1999), 38.

43. Douglas, "Heaven Our Home," 508.

44. Douglas, "Heaven Our Home," 509.

45. Degler, *At Odds*, 74.

46. Zelizer, *Pricing the Priceless Child*, 3.

47. Zelizer, *Pricing the Priceless Child*, 11.

48. Zelizer, *Pricing the Priceless Child*, 11. .

49. Zelizer, *Pricing the Priceless Child*, 5.

50. Zelizer, *Pricing the Priceless Child*, 25.

51. Dye and Smith, "Mother Love and Infant Death," 339-40.

52. Dye and Smith, "Mother Love and Infant Death," 339.

53. Dye and Smith, "Mother Love and Infant Death," 339.

54. Dye and Smith, "Mother Love and Infant Death," 339.

55. Dye and Smith, "Mother Love and Infant Death," 340.

56. Carby, *Reconstructing Womanhood*, 27.

57. Dye and Smith, "Mother Love and Infant Death," 340.

58. Dye and Smith, "Mother Love and Infant Death," 340.

59. Welter, "Cult of True Womanhood," 171.

60. Catherine Clinton, *The Plantation Mistress: Woman's World in the Old South* (New York: Pantheon, 1982), 8; and Carby, *Reconstructing Womanhood*, 20.

61. Philippe Ariès, *Western Attitudes toward Death* (Baltimore, MD: Johns Hopkins University Press, 1974), 68, quoted in Zelizer, *Pricing the Priceless Child*, 26.

62. Dye and Smith, "Mother Love and Infant Death," 342.

63. Dye and Smith, "Mother Love and Infant Death," 342.

64. David Stannard, *The Puritan Way of Death: A Study in Religion, Culture, and Social Change* (New York: Oxford University Press, 1977), 465.

65. Dye and Smith, "Mother Love and Infant Death," 343.

66. Dye and Smith, "Mother Love and Infant Death," 340.

67. Much of the historiography of midwifery and childbirth reviewed in chapter 3, especially from the 1970s and 1980s, stresses this aspect of the rise of male medical authority; see also Barbara Ehrenreich and Deirdre English, *Witches, Midwives, and Nurses: A History of Woman Healers* (1973; reprint, New York: The Feminist Press, 2010).

68. Jacques Donzelot, *The Policing of the Family* (New York: Pantheon Books, 1979), 18.

69. Judith Leavitt, *Brought to Bed: Childbearing in America, 1750–1950* (New York: Oxford University Press, 1986).

70. Dye and Smith, "Mother Love and Infant Death," 344.

71. Dye and Smith, "Mother Love and Infant Death," 343.

72. Dye and Smith, "Mother Love and Infant Death," 342.

73. Dye and Smith, "Mother Love and Infant Death," 343.

74. Dye and Smith, "Mother Love and Infant Death," 343.

75. Jennifer L. Morgan, *Laboring Women: Reproduction and Gender in New World Slavery* (Philadelphia: University of Pennsylvania Press, 2004); and Sasha Turner, "The Nameless and the Forgotten: Maternal Grief, Sacred Protection, and the Archive of Slavery," *Slavery & Abolition: A Journal of Slave and Post-Slave Studies* 38, no. 2 (2017): 232–50.

76. Turner, "The Nameless," 232–33.

77. Turner, "The Nameless," 234.

78. Turner, "The Nameless," 234.

79. Jacobs, *Incidents in the Life of a Slave Girl: Written by Herself, with "A True Tale of Slavery" by John S. Jacobs.*

80. Shatema Threadcraft, *Intimate Justice: The Black Female Body and the Body Politic* (Oxford: Oxford University Press, 2016); Morgan, *Laboring Women*; and Toni Morrison, *Beloved* (New York: Knopf, 1988).

81. Turner, "The Nameless," 233.

82. Schuller, *Biopolitics of Feeling.*

83. Muigai, "An Awful Gladness," 37.

84. Turner, "The Nameless"; Deborah Gray White, *Ar'n't I a Woman? Female Slaves in the Plantation South*, 2nd edition (New York: Norton, 1999).

85. Muigai, "An Awful Gladness," 41, 48.

86. Saidiya Hartman, *Scenes of Subjection: Terror, Slavery, and Self-Making in Nineteenth-Century America* (New York: Oxford University Press, 1997), 98.

87. Zelizer, *Pricing the Priceless Child*, 11.

88. Frederick Douglass, *Narrative of the Life of Frederick Douglass* (1845; New York: Bedford/St. Martins, 2003), 41.

89. Turner, "The Nameless," 245.

90. Chris Dixon, *Perfecting the Family: Antislavery Marriages in Nineteenth-Century America* (Amherst: University of Massachusetts Press, 1997), 31.

91. In Dixon, *Perfecting the Family*, 32.

92. Dixon, *Perfecting the Family*, 31–32.

93. Hartman, *Scenes of Subjection*, 19.

94. Hartman, *Scenes of Subjection*, 20.

95. Hartman, *Scenes of Subjection*, 20.

96. Hartman, *Scenes of Subjection*, 21.

97. Khalil Gibran Muhammad, *The Condemnation of Blackness: Race, Crime, and the Making of Modern Urban America, with a New Preface* (Cambridge, MA: Harvard University Press, 2019).

98. Jim Downs, *Sick from Freedom: African-American Illness and Suffering during the Civil War and Reconstruction* (Oxford: Oxford University Press, 2012).

99. Joseph Camp Kennedy, *Preliminary Report on the 1860 Census* (Washington, DC: Government Printing office, 1862), 145–46; and John Haller, *Outcasts from Evolution: Scientific Attitudes of Racial Inferiority 1859–1900* (Urbana: University of Illinois Press, 1971), 40.

100. Downs, *Sick from Freedom*, 211fn43.

101. Downs, *Sick from Freedom*, 211fn43.

102. Michael W. Byrd and Linda Clayton, *An American Health Dilemma: Race, Medicine, and Health Care in the United States 1900–2000* (Cambridge, UK: Psychology Press, 2000), 387.

103. Haller, *Outcasts from Evolution*, 44–48.

104. Evelynn M. Hammonds and Susan M. Reverby, "Toward a Historically Informed Analysis of Racial Health Disparities since 1619," *American Journal of Public Health* 109, no. 10 (October 1, 2019): 1348–49.

105. Meckel, *Save the Babies*, 11.

106. Meckel, *Save the Babies*, 21.

107. Meckel, *Save the Babies*, 25.

108. Cybelle Fox, *Three Worlds of Relief: Race, Immigration, and the American Welfare State from the Progressive Era to the New Deal* (Princeton, NJ: Princeton University Press, 2012).

109. Meckel, *Save the Babies*, 25.

110. Meckel, "Racialism and Infant Death."

111. Richard H. Steckel, "A Peculiar Population: The Nutrition, Health, and Mortality of American Slaves from Childhood to Maturity," *Journal of Economic History* 46 (1986): 721–741, 733; and Downs, *Sick from Freedom*.

112. Edward Beardsley, *A History of Neglect: Health Care for Blacks and Mill Workers in the Twentieth-Century South* (Knoxville: University of Tennessee Press, 1990), 25.

113. Meckel, "Racialism and Infant Death," 71.

114. Meckel, "Racialism and Infant Death," 72.

115. Omar Ricks, "# (or, Counted without Counting)," *The Feminist Wire* (blog), August 20, 2015, https://thefeministwire.com/2015/08/or-counted-without-counting/.

116. See H. M. Folkes, "The Negro as a Health Problem," *Journal of the American Medical Association* (1910); Thomas Murrell, "Syphilis and the American Negro: A Medico-Sociologic Study," *JAMA* 14, no. 11 (1910): 46–49; and David McBride, *From TB to AIDS: Epidemics among Urban Blacks since* 1900 (Albany: SUNY University Press, 1991), 18–19.

117. Muigai, "An Awful Gladness," 63–64; see also Laura Briggs, "The Race of Hysteria: 'Overcivilization' and the 'Savage' Woman in Late Nineteenth-Century Obstetrics and Gynecology," *American Quarterly* 52, no. 2 (2000): 246–73.

118. Briggs, "Race of Hysteria."

119. Briggs, "Race of Hysteria," 254–55.

120. Briggs, "Race of Hysteria," 262–64.

121. Muigai, "An Awful Gladness," 183.

122. Hammonds and Reverby, "Toward a Historically Informed Analysis," 1349.

123. Hoffman, *Race Traits*, v.

124. Muhammad, *Condemnation of Blackness*, 51–52.

125. Hoffman, *Race Traits*, v; this same logic underpinned, four decades later, the Carnegie Foundation's choice of the Swedish Myrdal to survey race relations in the United States. See Ralph Ellison, "An American Dilemma," in *Shadow & Act* (New York: First Vintage International Edition, 1994).

126. Muhammad, *Condemnation of Blackness*, 53.

127. Muhammad, *Condemnation of Blackness*, 176.

128. Muhammad, *Condemnation of Blackness*, 48.

129. Hoffman, *Race Traits*, 37.

130. Muhammad, *Condemnation of Blackness*, 48.

131. Nancy Stepan, *The Idea of Race in Science: Great Britain* 1800–1960 (London: MacMillan Press, 1982), xvi.

132. Mary L. Heen, "Ending Jim Crow Life Insurance Rates," *Northwestern Journal of Law and Social Policy* 4, no. 2 (2009): 360–99, 375; and Megan J. Wolff, "The Myth of the Actuary: Life Insurance and Frederick L. Hoffman's 'Race Traits and Tendencies of the American Negro,'" *Public Health Reports* 121, no. 1 (2006): 84–91, 89.

133. Hoffman, *Race Traits*, 534–35.

134. Hoffman, *Race Traits*, 541.

135. Wolff, "Myth of the Actuary," 89; and Muhammad, *Condemnation of Blackness*, 42.

136. François Ewald, "Insurance and Risk," in *The Foucault Effect: Studies in Governmentality*, ed. Graham Burchell, Colin Gordon, and Peter Miller (Chicago: University of Chicago Press, 1991), 198.

137. Jonathan Levy, *Freaks of Fortune: The Emerging World of Capitalism and Risk in America* (Cambridge, MA: Harvard University Press, 2012).

138. Ewald, "Insurance and Risk," 199.

139. Ladelle McWhorter, *Racism and Sexual Oppression in Anglo-America: A Genealogy* (Bloomington: Indiana University Press, 2009), 201.

140. Hoffman, *Race Traits*, 37.

141. Hoffman, *Race Traits*.

142. As W.E.B. Du Bois notes in his critical review of Hoffman's *Race Traits*, most Blacks were still living in rural areas at the time of Hoffman's study, and yet Hoffman uses almost exclusively urban statistics to draw broad conclusions about African American existence. See Du Bois's "Race Traits and Tendencies of the American Negro by Frederick L. Hoffman, F.S.S. [Review]," *Annals of the American Academy of Political and Social Science* 9 (January 1897): 127–33. In chapter 1 of his treatise, however, Hoffman notes the enormous demographic shift of African Americans from the countryside to the cities. He writes that the "phenomenal increase in the colored population of southern cities during the past thirty years is perhaps the most convincing evidence of the changed conditions at the South, as affecting the future of the colored population" (Hoffman, *Race Traits*, 11). He writes: "It is true that most of the collected statistics have reference only to the large cities; but in view of the tendency of the colored population to migrate from the country to the cities in ever increasing numbers, and at the age period most favorable for a low general death rate, the proof of an excessive mortality rate is of the greatest economic and social significance" (Hoffman, *Race Traits*, 38). Despite his lack of data on rural areas, Hoffman's emphasis on this "migratory tendency" thus casts his analysis not only as a diagnosis of present pathologies but as the shape of things ineluctably to come.

143. Hoffman, *Race Traits*, 42. In New York, 87.42 per thousand for Blacks under 15, versus 47.06 for whites; in Washington, 159.93 for Blacks under 5, versus 65.04 for whites. The oldest category ranges from an anomalous slightly higher rate for whites over 65 in New York City to Brooklyn's 96 per thousand for whites to 144 per thousand for Blacks, with most cities showing Black death rates about 25 percent higher than the white rate for that age group. Mortality tables from New Orleans, Charleston, and Richmond provide even more striking evidence,

offering detailed data on both infant and early child mortality. Infant mortality in New Orleans, according to the 1890 census, was 269.4 per thousand for whites, compared to 430.2 per thousand for Blacks. An even more pronouncedly disparate rate of survival was in evidence in Charleston, where the rate was 200.4 per thousand for whites, compared to 461.7 per thousand among Blacks. In Richmond, 529.6 out of every thousand Black infants—over half of all babies born—died before their first birthday, compared to 186.9 of their white counterparts: "a mortality so great," according to Hoffman, "that no greater fecundity could balance the loss" (Hoffman, *Race Traits*, 43–45).

144. "Infant mortality," or sometimes "infantile mortality," had a fairly loose meaning until it was codified, in the United States, in the Children's Bureau reports of the later 1910s, as mortality during the first year of life. Before that time, the term was often used to signify death up to the age of five years. For a Foucauldian analysis of the term's emergence as a sign of the problematization of the phenomenon in the UK, see Armstrong, "Invention of Infant Mortality," 211–32.

145. Hoffman, *Race Traits*, 45. Earlier in the chapter, Hoffman had sounded an initial note of caution about his statistical representations of infant life and death. Regarding "a comparative statement of the birth rates of both races," he writes, "it must be admitted that information on this point is almost entirely wanting, and that no trustworthy conclusion as to the comparative fecundity can be arrived at" (Hoffman, *Race Traits*, 33). But after acknowledging the lack of this essential factor—the birth rate is the denominator of the infant mortality rate calculation—he evinces no further hesitation in drawing unequivocal conclusions.

146. Hoffman, *Race Traits*, 44–45; 42.

147. Hoffman, *Race Traits*, 56.

148. Hoffman, *Race Traits*, 55.

149. Hoffman, *Race Traits*, 57.

150. Hoffman, *Race Traits*, 84.

151. Hartman, *Scenes of Subjection*, 21.

152. Hoffman, *Race Traits*, 51. He admits that "the mortality from diarrhoeal disease is largely subject to sanitary conditions, which no doubt have some influence in producing [the much higher] negro mortality rate." But overall, in Hoffman's view, the impact of sanitary conditions is minimal. Hoffman, *Race Traits*, 66.

153. Hoffman, *Race Traits*, 84.

154. Hoffman, *Race Traits*, 178.

155. Hoffman, *Race Traits*, 181.

156. Hoffman, *Race Traits*, 16.

157. Hoffman, *Race Traits*, 182.

158. Hoffman, *Race Traits*, 229–34.

159. Hoffman (*Race Traits*, 178) writes: "No considerable crossing of negroes with white females has ever taken place . . . the few cases that occur cannot possibly have affected the traits and tendencies of the race."

160. Hoffman, *Race Traits*, 236.

161. Hoffman, *Race Traits*, 197–98.

162. Jared Sexton, *Amalgamation Schemes: Antiblackness and the Critique of Multiracialism* (Minneapolis: University of Minnesota Press, 2008) 32; and compare with Haller, *Outcasts from Evolution*, 51.

163. Hoffman, *Race Traits*, 311.

164. Hoffman (*Race Traits*, 197) writes that there is "abundant proof that there is a natural aversion between some races and that attempts to cross this natural barrier, determined by the 'law of similarity' have invariably lead to the most disastrous consequences." Similarly: "That races of similar culture and physical and psychical development can intermarry to mutual advantage is too patent a fact to need instances in its support . . . children of mixed parentage of Indo-German stock, irrespective of nationality, are superior to the parents. . . . It is an entirely different matter when Germans and Italians, English and Spaniards, Swedes and Turks intermarry and have children. And it may be said, only with emphasis, that the cross-breed of white men and colored women is, as a rule, a product inferior to both parents, physically and morally" (Hoffman, *Race Traits*, 179–80). Hoffman, *Race Traits*, 181.

165. Hoffman, *Race Traits*, 181, italics in the original. Josiah Nott (1804–1873), surgeon and physician, influential proponent of polygenism and apologist for US slavery, argued on that basis. With George Gliddon, Nott carried forward his teacher Samuel Morton's project of tracing the polygenetic origins of humanity through skull measurements, *Crania Americana* (1839), in the 1854 treatise *Types of Mankind*. See Haller, *Outcasts from Evolution*, 79–85.

166. Hoffman, *Race Traits*, 174.

167. Hoffman, *Race Traits*, 175.

168. Hoffman, *Race Traits*, 189.

169. Hoffman, *Race Traits*, 197–98.

170. Hoffman, *Race Traits*, 184.

171. Hoffman, *Race Traits*, 185.

172. Hoffman, *Race Traits*, 206–207.

173. Hoffman, *Race Traits*, 311.

174. Hoffman, *Race Traits*, 208.

175. Hoffman, *Race Traits*, 67.

176. Downs, *Sick from Freedom*.

177. Haller, *Outcasts from Evolution*, 49–50.

178. Briggs, "Race of Hysteria," 262.

179. Hoffman, *Race Traits*, 95.

180. Hoffman, *Race Traits*, 238. This particular illegitimacy statistic becomes something of a refrain—e.g., "the low state of sexual morality among the colored population . . . [demonstrated by the increasing] illegitimate births in Washington . . . show more emphatically the tendency of the race towards a low level of sexual immorality and vice" (Hoffman, *Race Traits*, 235). See also a more extended discussion of the unfavorable comparison with white illegitimacy (Hoffman, *Race Traits*, 238).

181. Carby, *Reconstructing Womanhood*.

182. Carby, *Reconstructing Womanhood*, 23.

183. Carby, *Reconstructing Womanhood*, 24.

184. Hartman, *Scenes of Subjection*, 21; compare with Frank B. Wilderson, *Red, White & Black: Cinema and the Structure of U.S. Antagonisms* (Durham, NC: Duke University Press, 2010), and Stephen H. Marshall, "The Political Life of Fungibility," *Theory & Event* 15, no. 3 (2012).

185. Welter, "Cult of True Womanhood," 154; quoted in Carby, *Reconstructing Womanhood*, 25.

186. Carby, *Reconstructing Womanhood*, 27.

187. Carby, *Reconstructing Womanhood*, 30.

188. Hoffman, *Race Traits*, 327. While McWhorter does not treat the 1896 *Race Traits* in her analysis, she similarly points out that Hoffman had previously blamed African Americans' "inferior womanhood" for race decline in his 1892 article, "Vital Statistics of the Negro." McWhorter, *Racism and Sexual Oppression*.

189. Hoffman, *Race Traits*, 236, emphasis added.

190. Hoffman, *Race Traits*, 208.

191. Hoffman, *Race Traits*, 62.

192. Hoffman, *Race Traits*.

193. Hoffman, *Race Traits*, 62–63. As Harriet Washington notes: "Historically, African Americans have been subjected to exploitative, abusive involuntary experimentations at a rate far higher than other ethnic groups. Thus, although the heightened African American wariness of medical research and institutions reflects a situational hypervigilance, it is [not] a *baseless* fear of harm. . . . That is why I refer to African Americans fears of medical professionals and institutions as iatrophobia . . . the fear of medicine." See Harriet Washington, *Medical*

Apartheid: The Dark History of Medical Experimentation on Black Americans from Colonial Times to the Present (New York: Doubleday, 2008), 21.

194. Hoffman, *Race Traits*, 63.

195. Hoffman, *Race Traits*, 69.

196. Hoffman, *Race Traits*, 311.

197. Carby, *Reconstructing Womanhood*, 30.

198. Berg as quoted in Carby, *Reconstructing Womanhood*, 26.

199. Carby, *Reconstructing Womanhood*, 28.

200. Hartman, *Scenes of Subjection*, 17–19. Hartman also writes about the sadomasochistic pleasures that attach to white empathic representations of the slave coffle, as not only the wounds of the lash but the wielding of the whip are imaginatively experienced (Hartman, *Scenes of Subjection*, 19). I do not enter into a psychoanalytic interpretation of Hoffman's text, but it is not a stretch to read a grim sadistic pleasure in his exhaustive enumerations of Black wretchedness, as well as his emphasis on "helping" the Black race—though chances of survival are remote—by depriving them utterly of any assistance, and a masochistic triumph—as well as a neat encapsulation of the biopolitical death function's evolutionary logic—in his characterization of Anglo-Saxons as having attained their current purity through long ages of suffering and death. Hoffman, *Race Traits*, 310–18.

201. Carby, *Reconstructing Womanhood*, 28.

202. Hoffman, *Race Traits*, 45.

203. Hoffman, *Race Traits*, 95. He employs the formulation "waste of life" several times in discussions of African American mortality more generally. Hoffman, *Race Traits*, 38, 45, 61.

204. Hoffman, *Race Traits*, 246–47.

205. Lauren Berlant, "The Subject of True Feeling," in *Cultural Pluralism, Identity Politics, and the Law,* ed. Austin Sarat and Thomas Kearns (Ann Arbor: University of Michigan Press, 1999). Berlant's account of "the subject of true feeling" is a critique of the notion that the "image of the traumatized worker," in our own era the victim of sweatshop atrocities, "produces *feeling* and with it something akin to *consciousness* that can lead to *action*" (Berlant, "Subject of True Feeling," 49). Berlant argues that the righteous display of the suffering of racial, national, geographical others as a transparent call to action risks figuring the suffering subject as pre-political, as well as reinscribing US/Global North citizenship as a natural state of security in which the traumatized worker fundamentally has no place. While Berlant, tracing the history of this subject position, highlights the child laborer, not the enslaved person, as the nineteenth-century figure

around which this dynamic condensed, Carby's argument prefigures this argument to a significant extent.

206. Sells, *Indian Babies*.

207. Hoffman, *Race Traits*, 241.

208. Hoffman, *Race Traits*, 241–42.

209. Hoffman, *Race Traits*, 241.

210. In Levy, *Freaks of Fortune*, 109.

211. Hoffman, *Race Traits*, 209–11; and Wolff, "Myth of the Actuary."

212. Ewald, "Insurance and Risk," 198.

213. Ewald, "Insurance and Risk," 202–203.

214. Anthony P. Damico, "Health Coverage by Race and Ethnicity, 2010–2021," *Kaiser Family Foundation* (blog), December 20, 2022, www.kff.org/racial-equity-and-health-policy/issue-brief/health-coverage-by-race-and-ethnicity/.

215. Muhammad, *Condemnation of Blackness*, 91.

216. Heen, "Ending Jim Crow."

217. Robert Lieberman, *Shifting the Color-Line: Race and the American Welfare State* (Cambridge, MA: Harvard University Press, 1999); and Fox, *Three Worlds of Relief*.

218. Hammonds and Reverby, "Toward a Historically Informed Analysis," 1348–49.

219. Du Bois, "Race Traits," 127.

220. Du Bois, "Race Traits," 133.

221. Du Bois, "Race Traits," 128.

222. Turner, "The Nameless," 232–33.

223. Du Bois, "Race Traits," 129.

224. Du Bois, "Race Traits," 129.

225. Du Bois, "Race Traits," 129.

226. Du Bois, "Race Traits," 130.

227. Du Bois, "Race Traits," 130.

228. Du Bois, "Race Traits," 130.

229. Du Bois, "Race Traits," 131.

230. Du Bois, "Race Traits," 132.

231. Du Bois, "Race Traits," 132.

232. Du Bois, "Race Traits," 132.

233. Du Bois, "Race Traits," 133.

234. Du Bois, "Race Traits," 133.

235. For example, Du Bois, *Atlanta University Study* No. 3: "Some Efforts of American Negroes for Their Own Social Betterment. Report of an Investigation

under the Direction of Atlanta University; Together with the Proceedings of the Third Conference for the Study of the Negro Problems," held at Atlanta University, Atlanta, Georgia, May 25-26, 1898. Although the tone of the review is restrained, Du Bois's engagement with Hoffman's treatise left a mark. In the 1940 essay "Race: Autobiography of a Concept," Du Bois mentions his gladness at seeing all of Hoffman's ideas debunked. See W.E.B. Du Bois, *Dusk of Dawn: The Autobiography of a Race Concept* (1940; New York: Schocken Books, 1984), 99.

236. Du Bois, *Philadelphia Negro*, 117; and Kevin Gaines, *Uplifting the Race: Black Leadership, Politics, and Culture in the Twentieth Century* (Chapel Hill: University of North Carolina Press, 1996), 194.

237. Gaines, *Uplifting the Race*, 166; also see Evelyn Brooks Higginbotham, *Righteous Discontent: The Women's Movement in the Black Baptist Church*, 1880-1920 (Cambridge, MA: Harvard University Press, 1993), 187-96.

238. Du Bois, *Philadelphia Negro*, 49; and Gaines, *Uplifting the Race*, 166. Cathy Cohen argues that *The Philadelphia Negro* initiated a scholarly "tradition of pathologizing the behaviors of the African American poor and working class, especially women" in "Deviance as Resistance: A New Agenda for the Study of Black Politics," *The Du Bois Review* 1, no. 1 (2004): 27-45, 33-34.

239. Muhammad, *Condemnation of Blackness*, 58.

240. Treva Lindsey, *Colored No More: Reinventing Black Womanhood in Washington, D.C.* (Urbana: University of Illinois Press, 2017), 10.

241. Joy James, "The Profeminist Politics of W. E. B. Du Bois with Respects to Anna Julia Cooper and Ida B. Wells Barnett," in *W. E. B. Du Bois on Race and Culture*, ed. Bernard W. Bell, Emily R. Grosholz, and James B. Stewart (New York: Routledge, 1996), 152.

242. Ida B. Wells-Barnett, *Southern Horrors and Other Writings; The Anti-Lynching Campaign of Ida B. Wells*, 1892-1900, ed. Jaqueline Jones Royster (Boston: Bedford/St. Martin, 1996).

243. Jacqueline Goldsby, *A Spectacular Secret: Lynching in American Life and Literature* (Chicago: University of Chicago Press, 2006), 49.

244. Muhammad, *Condemnation of Blackness*, 61.

245. Vivian May, *Anna Julia Cooper, Visionary Black Feminist: A Critical Introduction* (New York: Routledge, 2007), 149.

246. Anna Julie Cooper, "What Are We Worth?" in *The Voice of Anna Julia Cooper, including "A Voice from the South" and Other Important Essays, Papers, and Letters*, ed. Charles Lemert and Esme Bhan (Lanham, MD: Rowman & Littlefield, 1998), 170-71.

247. Carol Wayne White, "Anna Julia Cooper: Radical Relationality and the Ethics of Interdependence," in *African American Political Thought*, ed. Melvin Rogers and Jack Turner (Chicago: University of Chicago Press, 2021), 196.

248. James, "Profeminist Politics of W. E. B. Du Bois," 142. See also Erica Richardson, "Beyond the Negro Problem: The Engagement between Literature and Sociology in the Age of the New Negro," PhD dissertation, Columbia University, 2018.

249. Du Bois, *Dusk of Dawn*, 32.

250. Du Bois, *Dusk of Dawn*, 221-22; and David Levering-Lewis, *W.E.B. Du Bois, 1868-1919: Biography of a Race* (New York: Henry Holt & Co, 1993), 276.

251. Cornel West, "Black Strivings in a Twilight Civilization," in *The Cornel West Reader* (New York: Basic Civitas Books, 1999), 87-118, 92-93.

252. Levering-Lewis, *W.E.B. Du Bois*, 275.

253. Levering-Lewis, *W.E.B. Du Bois*, 276-77.

Chapter 2. Three Forms of Innocence in W.E.B.
Du Bois's "Of the Passing of the First-Born"

1. Levering-Lewis, *W.E.B. Du Bois*.

2. Freeden Blume Oeur, "Fever Dreams: WEB Du Bois and the Racial Trauma of COVID-19 and Lynching," *Ethnic and Racial Studies* 44, no. 5 (2021): 735-45. Blume Oeur argues that diphtheria, in which inflamed mucous membranes prevent breathing and make the patient's throat feel as if it is on fire, mirrors and extends the horror of lynching. Also look at the *Journal of the National Medical Association* article from 2015 on the contemporary meanings of Burghardt's death: Karp and Gearing, "Death of Burghardt Du Bois, 1899."

3. W.E.B. Du Bois, *The Autobiography of W.E.B. DuBois: a soliloquy on viewing my life from the last decade of its first century*. New York: International Publishers, 1968.

4. Muigai, "An Awful Gladness," 191-93.

5. W.E.B. Du Bois, *The Souls of Black Folk* (New York: Oxford University Press, 2007), 140. Levering-Lewis, *W.E.B. Du Bois*, 226-27; Shamoon Zamir, *Dark Voices: W.E.B. Du Bois and American Thought, 1888-1903* (Chicago: University of Chicago Press, 1995), 193; "Unto us a child is born" (Isaiah 9:6, King James Version); "and For unto you is born this day in the city of David a savior, which is Christ the Lord" (Luke 2:11, King James Version).

6. Du Bois, *Souls of Black Folk*, 140.

7. Du Bois, *Souls of Black Folk*, 140-41.

8. Du Bois, *Souls of Black Folk*, 141.

9. Du Bois, *Souls of Black Folk*, 141.

10. Du Bois, *Souls of Black Folk*, 141.

11. Du Bois, *Souls of Black Folk*, 143.

12. Levering-Lewis, *W.E.B. Du Bois*, 226; and Blume Oeur, "Fever Dreams," 737.

13. Du Bois, *Autobiography of W.E.B. DuBois*.

14. Du Bois, *Souls of Black Folk*, 142–43. The image (and legal constitution) of the house as man's refuge from external dominion comes from English common law: Sir Edward Coke's *The Institutes of the Laws of England* (1628) holds that "For a man's house is his castle, *et domus sua cuique est tutissimum refugium* [and each man's home is his safest refuge]." But as Welter makes clear, the gendered separation of spheres in the nineteenth century entrenched and elaborated this image, figuring the outside world as profane and dangerous, and home and hearth as the singular and sacred refuge of the storm-tossed public man—a figure clearly employed in this passage. Welter, "Cult of True Womanhood." Levering-Lewis (*W.E.B. Du Bois*, 227) rightly points out that Du Bois here effectively eclipses Nina's bereavement with his own.

15. Du Bois, *Souls of Black Folk*, 144.

16. Du Bois, *Souls of Black Folk*, 143.

17. Du Bois, *Souls of Black Folk*, 143.

18. Du Bois, *Souls of Black Folk*, 143.

19. Nahum Dimitri Chandler, *X—The Problem of the Negro as a Problem for Thought* (New York: Fordham University Press, 2014), 125.

20. Chandler, *X—The Problem of the Negro*, 144.

21. Chandler, *X—The Problem of the Negro*, 140.

22. I suggest an alternative reading of this ambivalence below following Paul Gilroy, *The Black Atlantic: Modernity and Consciousness* (Cambridge, MA: Harvard University Press, 1993).

23. Spenser as quoted in Hoffman: "Inferior forms of marriage . . . cannot develop to any great extent that powerful combination of feelings . . . affection, admiration, sympathy . . . which in so marvelous a manner has grown out of the sexual instinct. And in the absence of this complex passion . . . the supreme interest in life (the raising up of members of a new generation) disappears . . . a prevalent unchastity severs the higher from the lower components of the sexual relation: the root may produce a few leaves, but no true flower" (in Hoffman, *Race Traits*, 208).

24. The final uses of Love recede back into gendered respectability politics, with Gomer Du Bois cast as Love and Du Bois himself as Wisdom.

25. Du Bois, *Souls of Black Folk*, 144.

26. *Pace v. Alabama*, 106 U.S. 583 (1883) (106 U.S. 583).

27. Juliet Hooker, *Theorizing Race in the Americas: Douglass, Sarmiento, Du Bois, and Vasconcelos* (New York: Oxford University Press, 2017), 114.

28. Galia Ofek, *Representations of Hair in Victorian Literature and Culture* (Burlington, VT: Ashgate Publishing, 2009), 113.

29. Du Bois, *Souls of Black Folk*, 141.

30. Hoffman, *Race Traits*, 181.

31. Evelyn Hammonds, "New Technologies of Race," in *Processed Lives: Gender and Technology in Everyday Life*, ed. Jennifer Terry and Melodie Calvert (New York: Routledge, 1997), 110.

32. Mark M. Smith, *How Race Is Made: Slavery, Segregation, and the Senses* (Chapel Hill: University of North Carolina Press, 2006).

33. Du Bois, *Souls of Black Folks*, 176.

34. Melvin Rogers, "The People, Rhetoric, and Affect: On the Political Force of Du Bois' *The Souls of Black Folk.*" *American Political Science Review,* 106, no. 1 (2012): 192.

35. Hooker includes some nonfiction writings within the rubric of "mulatto fictions," including the 1897 "The Conservation of Races," 114, 118.

36. Claudia Tate, *Psychoanalysis and Black Novels: Desire and the Protocols of Race* (New York: Oxford University Press, 1998), 63.

37. Hooker, *Theorizing Race in the Americas*, 118.

38. Hooker, *Theorizing Race in the Americas*, 124.

39. Alys Eve Weinbaum, "Interracial Romance and Black Internationalism," in *Next to the Color Line: Gender, Sexuality, and W.E.B. Du Bois*, ed. Susan Gillman and Alys Eve Weinbaum (Minneapolis: University of Minnesota Press, 2007), 96–123.

40. Tate, *Psychoanalysis and Black Novels*, 70.

41. Farah Jasmine Griffin, "Black Feminists and Du Bois: Respectability, Protection, and Beyond," *Annals of the American Academy of Political and Social Science* 568, no. 1 (2000): 130–32.

42. "The Constructive View of Reparations with Olúfẹ́mi O. Táíwò," *Millennials Are Killing Capitalism* podcast, March 7, 2022.

43. A "glance" at statistics about Black migration in chapter 2 and a teacher's "glance" at the doomed student John in chapter 8.

44. Du Bois, *Souls of Black Folks*, 8.

45. Du Bois, *Souls of Black Folks*, 143.

46. Du Bois, *Souls of Black Folks*, 23.

47. Du Bois, *Souls of Black Folks*, 141.

48. Du Bois, *Souls of Black Folks*, 141.

49. Thomas Dumm, "Political Theory for Losers," in *Vocations of Political Theory*, ed. Jason A. Frank and John Tambornino (Minneapolis: University of Minnesota Press, 2000), 157.

50. Du Bois, *Souls of Black Folks*, 143.

51. From the *OED*: 1803 in Sir Walter Scott *Minstrelsy of the Scottish Border* (2nd edition) III. 391: "There, wan from her maternal throes, His Margaret, beautiful and mild, Sate in her bower, a pallid rose." From 1867, Mary Elizabeth Braddon, *Rupert Godwin* i: "Clara Westford's noble face is pale and wan this sunny morning." And in noun form: 1847 Tennyson *The Princess* iii. 9: "Melissa, tinged with wan from lack of sleep." Interestingly, the Anglo-Saxon etymological root of this word signifies a dark rather than a pale aspect.

52. Shawn Michelle Smith, "Second-Sight: Du Bois and the Black Masculine Gaze," in *Next to the Color Line: Gender, Sexuality, and W.E.B. Du Bois*, ed. Susan Gillman and Alys Eve Weinbaum (Minneapolis: University of Minnesota Press, 2007), 361.

53. Du Bois, *Souls of Black Folks*, 141.

54. Du Bois, *Souls of Black Folks*, 142.

55. Du Bois, *Souls of Black Folks*, 143.

56. Du Bois, *Souls of Black Folks*, 144.

57. Hazel V. Carby, *Race Men* (Cambridge, MA: Harvard University Press, 1998), 10.

58. Rogers, "People, Rhetoric, and Affect," 189.

59. Rogers, "People, Rhetoric, and Affect," 194.

60. Rogers, "People, Rhetoric, and Affect," 195.

61. Carby, *Race Men*, 12; and Raymond Williams, *Marxism and Literature* (New York: Oxford University Press, 1977), 133–34.

62. Rogers, "People, Rhetoric, and Affect," 200.

63. Du Bois, *Souls of Black Folks*, 144.

64. Du Bois, *Souls of Black Folks*, 143.

65. Du Bois, *Souls of Black Folks*, 143.

66. Morgan, *Laboring Women*, 114.

67. Morgan, *Laboring Women*, 114–15; and Londa Schiebinger, "Exotic Abortifacients and Lost Knowledge," *The Lancet* 371, no. 9614 (2008): 718.

68. Toni Morrison, *Beloved* (New York: Knopf, 1987); and Threadcraft, *Intimate Justice*; and Weinbaum, *Afterlife of Reproductive Slavery*.

69. White, *Ar'n't I a Woman?*.

70. Muigai, "An Awful Gladness," 182–98.

71. Mary Church Terrell, "Greetings from the National Association of Colored Women," *National Association Notes* 2 (March 1899).

72. Cornel West, *The Cornel West Reader* (New York: Basic Civitas Books, 1999), 106.

73. Harriet Jacobs, *Incidents in the Life of a Slave Girl* (1861; Cambridge, MA: Harvard University Press, 2009), 60.

74. Hartman, *Scenes of Subjection*, 107.

75. Fred Moten, "Uplift and Criminality," in *Next to the Color Line: Gender, Sexuality, and W.E.B. Du Bois*, ed. Susan Gillman and Alys Eve Weinbaum (Minneapolis: University of Minnesota Press, 2007), 337.

76. Moten, "Uplift and Criminality," 323.

77. It is noteworthy that, in *Souls of Black Folks*, the third mention of the Housatonic refers to Du Bois's stolen great-great grandmother, as the river that ran through the foreign land in which she found herself; this perhaps injects a shadow even into the sunny summer "before the veil" link to the sexual violence that Burghardt's hybridity brings to light. And/or, does it hearken back to a way of seeing that this ancestor brought to bear, torn away from yet still rooted in the "ontological totality" of her natal African community?

78. Du Bois, *Souls of Black Folks*, 99.

79. Lawrie Balfour, *Democracy's Reconstruction: Thinking Politically with W.E.B. Du Bois* (New York: Oxford University Press, 2011), 106; Molly Ladd-Taylor, *Mother-Work: Women, Child Welfare, and the State*, 1890–1930 (Champaign: University of Illinois Press, 1994); and Eileen Boris, "The Power of Motherhood: Black and White Activist Women Redefine the 'Political,'" *Yale Journal of Law and Feminism* 2 (1989): 25–49.

80. W.E.B. Du Bois, *Darkwater: Voices from within the Veil* (New York: Oxford University Press, 2007), 88.

81. Balfour, *Democracy's Reconstruction*, 100.

82. Hortense Spillers, "Mama's Baby, Papa's Maybe: An American Grammar Book," *Diacritics* 17, no. 2 (1987): 64–81; Spillers, *Black, White, and in Color*; and Alexis Pauline Gumbs, *Spill: Scenes of Black feminist fugitivity* (Durham, NC: Duke University Press, 2016).

83. Roberts, *Torn Apart*.

84. Joy James, *Transcending the Talented Tenth* (New York: Routledge, 1997), 44; Carby, *Race Men*; and Balfour, *Democracy's Reconstruction*, 100–102.

85. Ralph Waldo Emerson, "Experience," in *Essays: Second Series*, ed. Alfred Riggs Ferguson, Joseph Slater, and Jean Ferguson Carr, *The Collected Works of*

Ralph Waldo Emerson (Cambridge, MA: Belknap Press of Harvard University Press, 1971), 29; and Shannon Mariotti, "On the Passing of the First-Born Son: Emerson's 'Focal Distancing,' Du Bois' 'Second Sight,' and Disruptive Particularity," *Political Theory* 37 (2009): 351–74, 359.

86. Emerson, "Experience," 29.

Chapter 3. Innocence and Inheritance

1. Mary Church Terrell, *A Colored Woman in a White World* (1940; New York: G.K. Hall & Co, 1996), 151; and Lindsey, *Colored No More*, 47.

2. Terrell, *Colored Woman in a White World*, 106–107. See also Parker, *Unceasing Militant*, 52.

3. Terrell, *Colored Woman in a White World*, 107.

4. Davis, *Reproductive Injustice*.

5. Terrell, *Colored Woman in a White World*, 105; and Parker, *Unceasing Militant*, 46–47.

6. Judith Leavitt, *Brought to Bed* (New York: Oxford University Press, 2016).

7. Terrell, *Colored Woman in a White World*, 97.

8. Terrell, *Colored Woman in a White World*, 99.

9. Terrell, *Colored Woman in a White World*, 16.

10. Terrell, *Colored Woman in a White World*, 295.

11. Terrell, *Colored Woman in a White World*, 297.

12. Terrell, *Colored Woman in a White World*, 298.

13. The systematic failures of what Jina B. Kim calls "infrastructure" to support maternal and intergenerational Black life in particular resonates with Kim and Sami Schalk's theorization of crip-of-color critique. Sami Schalk and Jina B. Kim, "Integrating Race, Transforming Feminist Disability Studies," *Signs: Journal of Women in Culture and Society* 46, no. 1 (2020): 31–55.

14. Terrell, *Colored Woman in a White World*, 229.

15. Elizabeth McHenry, *To Make Negro Literature: Writing, Literary Practice, and African American Authorship* (Durham, NC: Duke University Press, 2021). As McHenry shows, however, Terrell translated these experiences into fictional form in her short story, "Betsy's Borrowed Baby." In that story a young Black college student traveling home to the South from her midwestern campus—like the sixteen-year-old Terrell herself—faces the assaults of white men, as well as being banned from the sleeping and dining cars. She adopts the strategy of "borrowing" a white neighbor's visiting granddaughter, a white toddler who needed accompaniment back north to her father. Passing as the child's nanny, she is able to travel

safely and comfortably within the whites-only accommodations of the train. Significantly, although Terrell submitted the story to many mainstream white journals, none would publish this story; the "whole truth," even in fictional form, could not appear in print.

16. Brittney Cooper, *Beyond Respectability*, 75.

17. Terrell, *Colored Woman in a White World*, 105.

18. Lindsey, *Colored No More*.

19. Pablo Neruda, *Odes to Common Things* (Boston: Bullfinch, 1994), 11–17.

20. Terrell, *Colored Woman in a White World*, 105.

21. Muigai, "An Awful Gladness," 177.

22. Jenny Edkins, *Trauma and the Memory of Politics* (Cambridge, UK: Cambridge University Press, 2003), xiv.

23. Parker, *Unceasing Militant*, 66, 92–93.

24. Muhammad, *Condemnation of Blackness*.

25. Pauli Murray, *The Autobiography of a Black Activist, Feminist, Lawyer, Priest, and Poet* (Knoxville: University of Tennessee Press, 1989), 232, in Brittney Cooper, *Beyond Respectability: The Intellectual Thought of Race Women* (Urbana: University of Illinois Press, 2017), 86.

26. Robert Gooding-Williams, *In the Shadow of Du Bois* (Cambridge, MA: Harvard University Press, 2009), 62; Cornel West, *Race Matters* (Boston: Beacon Press, 1993); Carby, *Race Men*; and Claudia Tate, *Domestic Allegories of Political Desire: The Black Heroine's Text at the Turn of the Century* (New York: Oxford University Press, 1992).

27. Terrell, "Greetings from the National Association of Colored Women to the National Council of Women" speech, 1900.

28. Du Bois, *Souls of Black Folks*, 144.

29. Muigai, "An Awful Gladness," 192.

30. Nella Larsen, *Quicksand* (New York: A.A. Knopf, 1928), 164, in Muigai, "An Awful Gladness," 196–97.

31. Koritha Mitchell, *Living with Lynching: African American Lynching Plays, Performance, and Citizenship*, 1890–1930 (Champaign: University of Illinois Press, 2011), 10.

32. Thank you to Sasha Turner for first bringing Grimké's play to my attention.

33. McKay, introduction to *Colored Woman in a White World*, xxxi.

34. Mitchell, *Living with Lynching*, 10.

35. Mitchell, *Living with Lynching*, 56.

36. Megan Ming Francis, "Ida B. Wells and the Economics of Racial Violence," *Items: Insights from the Social Sciences, Social Science Research Council,*

January 24, 2017, https://items.ssrc.org/reading-racial-conflict/ida-b-wells-and-the-economics-of-racial-violence/#:~:text = According%20to%20Wells%2C%20the%20logic,a%20captive%20black%20labor%20force.

37. Ida B. Wells-Barnett, *Crusade for Justice: The Autobiography of Ida B. Wells*, 2nd edition, ed. Alfreda M. Duster with a new foreword by Eve L. Ewing and a new afterword by Michelle Duster (Urbana, IL: University of Chicago Press, 2020), 56.

38. McHenry, *To Make Negro Literature*, 208.

39. Mary Church Terrell, "Lynching from a Negro's Point of View," *North American Review* (1904); and Wells-Barnett, *Southern Horrors and Other Writings*.

40. McHenry, *To Make Negro Literature*, 208, quoting Terrell, "Lynching from a Negro's Point of View."

41. H. G. Wells, preface to *Colored Woman in a White World*, i.

42. Cooper, *Beyond Respectability*, 69.

43. Muigai, "An Awful Gladness," 194.

44. Cooper, *Beyond Respectability*, 69.

45. Cooper, *Beyond Respectability*, 73–74.

46. Schuller, *Biopolitics of Feeling*, 37.

47. Mel Chen, *Animacies: Biopolitics, Mattering, Affect* (Durham, NC: Duke University Press, 2012).

48. Schuller, *Biopolitics of Feeling*, 13.

49. Schuller, *Biopolitics of Feeling*, 8.

50. Susan Lanzoni, "Sympathy in Mind (1876–1900)," *Journal of the History of Ideas* 70, no. 2 (2009): 285, quoted in Schuller, *Biopolitics of Feeling*, 56.

51. Schuller, *Biopolitics of Feeling*, 70.

52. Anna Julia Cooper, *A Voice from the South* (New York: Oxford University Press, 1892), iii.

53. Cooper, *Voice from the South*, 145.

54. Muigai, "An Awful Gladness," 201, also quoted in Schuller, *Biopolitics of Feeling*, 86.

55. Briggs, "Race of Hysteria."

56. Parker, *Unceasing Militant*, 46.

57. Schuller, *Biopolitics of Feeling*, 210.

58. Schuller, *Biopolitics of Feeling*.

59. Deva Woodly, "Black Feminist Visions and the Politics of Healing in the Movement for Black Lives," in *Women Mobilizing Memory*, ed. Ayşe Gül Altınay et al. (New York: Columbia University Press, 2019); Shatema Threadcraft, "North American Necropolitics and Gender: On #BlackLivesMatter and Black Femicide," *South Atlantic Quarterly* 116, no. 3 (2017): 553–79; and Naa Oyo A. Kwate and

Shatema Threadcraft, "Dying Fast and Dying Slow in Black Space," *Du Bois Review: Social Science Research on Race* 14, no. 2 (2018): 535-56.

60. Smith, "Facing the Dragon."

61. Schuller, *Biopolitics of Feeling*, 89; Davis, *Reproductive Injustice*; and Deirdre Cooper Owens, *Medical Bondage: Race, Gender, and the Origins of American Gynecology* (Athens: University of Georgia Press, 2017).

62. Terrell, *Colored Woman in a White World*, 41-42.

63. Terrell, *Colored Woman in a White World*, 161-62.

64. Terrell, *Colored Woman in a White World*, 451.

65. Terrell, "Lynching from a Negro's Point of View," 861-62.

66. Bromell, 153: Even a naturally kind and generous person could be corrupted by this power. In the *Narrative*, Douglass writes that when he had first met Mrs. Hugh Auld, she was kind and even maternal toward him: "But, alas! . . . The fatal poison of irresponsible power was already in her hands, and soon commenced its infernal work" (37). "Slavery," he concludes, "proved as injurious to her as to me" (40).

67. Harriet Jacobs sounds a similar note, though she reserves the term "brutalized" for enslaved people; see Jacobs, *Incidents in the Life of a Slave Girl*, 80.

68. March Church Terrell, "Purity and the Negro" speech, 1905.

69. Parker, *Unceasing Militant*, 142.

70. Douglass's public deeds, including his championing of women's rights, loom large in Terrell's writings. Notably, she writes in great detail in her autobiography about attending the World's Fair with Douglass and Paul Lawrence Dunbar in 1893, explicitly situating this event as taking place the year after her first pregnancy and loss in chapter 12, the chapter following "I Return to America." Indeed, Terrell successfully led the campaign for Douglass Day in Washington, DC—the first such officially recognized day for an African American. She and her husband were instrumental in the creation of the Frederick Douglass Memorial and Historical Organization, an effort led by his widow, Helen Pitts Douglass.

71. Terrell writes proudly of playing the role of Douglass in 1906, in a sixtieth anniversary reenactment of the Seneca Falls convention. See Terrell, *Colored Woman in a White World*, 169-71; and Mary Church Terrell, "I Remember Frederick Douglass," *Ebony* 8, no. 12 (October 1953): 72-76, 78-80.

72. Terrell, "Purity and the Negro."

73. Parker, *Unceasing Militant*, 133.

74. Parker, *Unceasing Militant*, 291

75. Terrell, "Lynching from a Negro's Point of View"; and Jones-Rogers, *They Were Her Property*.

76. Wells-Barnett, *Crusade for Justice*, 74. Dainty-Pelham was a white social reformer and former actress with long-standing roles at Chicago's Hull House, including founding the Hull House Players. On Dainty-Pelham's observations, see also Terry Anne Scott, *Lynching and Leisure: Race and the Transformation of Mob Violence in Texas* (Lafayette: University of Arkansas Press, 2022), 180.

77. Elizabeth G. McRae, *Mothers of Massive Resistance* (New York: Oxford University Press, 2018), 4.

78. Hazel Carby, "We Must Burn Them," *London Review of Books* 44, no. 10 (2022), www.lrb.co.uk/the-paper/v44/n10/hazel-v.-carby/we-must-burn-them, accessed February 1, 2023.

79. Carby, "We Must Burn Them."

80. Terrell, *Colored Woman in a White World*. Noaquia Callahan, "Heat of the Day: Mary Church Terrell and African American feminist transnational activism," PhD dissertation, University of Iowa, 2018.

81. Jones, "End to the Neglect of the Problems of the Negro Woman!," 16.

82. Dayo F. Gore, *Radicalism at the Crossroads: African American Women Activists in the Cold War* (New York: NYU Press, 2011), 74.

83. Gore, *Radicalism at the Crossroads*, 75; and Parker, *Unceasing Militant*, 282–83.

84. Gore, *Radicalism at the Crossroads*, 75.

85. Gore, *Radicalism at the Crossroads*, 83–84; and Parker, *Unceasing Militant*, 284–85.

86. W.E.B. Du Bois, "A Petition to the Human Rights Commission of the Social and Economic Council of the United Nations, and to the Several Delegations of the Member States of the United Nations," September 19, 1949, in Mary Church Terrell, Mary Church Terrell Papers: Speeches and Writings, 1866 to 1953; and "Petition to the U.N. Protesting Discrimination in the U.S. and the Rosa Ingram Case," 1949, Manuscript/Mixed Material, www.loc.gov/item/mss425490520/, Image 4.

87. "Petition to the U.N. Protesting Discrimination in the U.S. and the Rosa Ingram Case," www.loc.gov/item/mss425490520/ Image 5.

88. Parker, *Unceasing Militant*, 282–83. Gore, *Radicalism at the Crossroads*, 92.

89. Valdez, *Weighing the Future*, 4.

Chapter 4. The Midwife's Bag

1. McBride, *From TB to AIDS*, 10, 15. As Tera Hunter shows, Black women domestic workers in particular were singled out as vectors of TB and other illnesses

in the 1910s: "the black female servant was a metaphor for disease" (*To 'Joy My Freedom: Southern Black Women's Lives and Labors after the Civil War* [Cambridge, MA: Harvard University Press, 1997], 202; see more generally 187–218).

2. Shaka McGlotten, "Black Data," in *No Tea, No Shade: New Writings in Queer Black Studies*, ed. E. Patrick Johnson, 262–86 (Durham, NC: Duke University Press).

3. Most prominent was a municipal effort in Manhattan's Columbus Hill neighborhood. As Tanya Hart shows, however, the efficacy of this effort was hampered by the conviction that the Black population was "syphilis-soaked"; prenatal care was restricted to those who submitted to syphilis testing, and the mercury therapy used prenatally for positive diagnoses may well have done more harm than good. This had the effect of leaving the skyrocketing syphilis rates in Italian and other non-Black communities almost entirely unaddressed. See Tanya Hart, *Health in the City: Race, Poverty, and the Negotiation of Women's Health in New York City, 1915-1930* (New York: NYU Press, 2015).

4. Molly Ladd-Taylor, "'Grannies' and 'Spinsters': Midwife Education under the Sheppard-Towner Act," *Journal of Social History* 22, no. 2 (Winter 1988): 258.

5. Fraser, *African American Midwifery*; Ladd-Taylor, "'Grannies' and 'Spinsters'"; and Susan Smith, *Sick and Tired of Being Sick and Tired: Black Women's Health Activism in America, 1890-1950* (Philadelphia: University of Pennsylvania Press, 1995).

6. Fraser, *African American Midwifery in the South*; and Sharla M. Fett, "Consciousness and Calling: African American Midwives at Work in the Antebellum South," in *New Studies in the History of American Slavery*, ed. Edward Baptist and Stephanie Camp (Athens: University of Georgia Press, 2006).

7. Fraser, *African American Midwifery in the South*, 34; Ladd-Taylor, "'Grannies' and 'Spinsters,'" 258–60; Smith, *Sick and Tired of Being Sick and Tired*; and Judy Litoff, *The American Midwife Debate: A Sourcebook on Its Modern Origins* (Westport, CT: Greenwood Press, 1986), 113–14. In a study of infant mortality in rural Mississippi released the same year as the act was passed (1921), the Children's Bureau expressed concern about midwives' care—in particular, the near-universal nonuse of antibiotic ophthalmic drops to prevent blindness in newborns—and included "midwife control" among its recommendations. Nevertheless, in diagnosing the causes of infant mortality, it stressed the conditions of grinding poverty among the families in the study over these concerns. Moreover, it avoided ascribing a specifically racial pathology to Black midwives or mothers, portraying white midwives as more or less equally deficient and also noting that few Black families could afford the services of doctors.

8. Bonaparte, "'Satisfactory Midwife Bag.'"

9. Fraser, *African American Midwifery in the South*, 36.

10. Muigai, "An Awful Gladness," 145.

11. Muigai, "An Awful Gladness," 230.

12. Muigai, "An Awful Gladness," 145–54.

13. Logan as told to Clark, *Motherwit*, 53. Logan's autobiography, *Motherwit: An Alabama Midwife's Story*, was related orally to Katherine Clark. *Motherwit* is part of a small but significant genre of Black midwives' oral histories "as told to" a younger woman from outside the community, often a white woman (women's historian Linda Janet Holmes, coauthor of *Listen to Me Good* with Alabama midwife Margaret Charles Smith, is an exception; unlike other interlocutor/coauthors, she also spent several years with Alabama midwives in the course of graduate research and later public history projects), and often written in a style representing the midwife's vernacular speech patterns as interpreted by the interviewer. Fraser (*African American Midwifery in the South*, 3, 13) cautions her readers against taking these narratives as merely transparent accounts. Like any narration, midwives' narrations are shaped by a variety of factors, inter alia the power relationship between narrator and interviewer/transcriber, expectations of the interviewer, the agendas of either party, self-stylization on the part of the interviewee, or self- or community-protective framings by the narrator, particularly given that midwifery became illegal in many Southern states in the 1970s. See Christa Craven and Mara Glatzel, "Downplaying Difference: Historical Accounts of African American Midwives and Contemporary Struggles for Midwifery," *Feminist Studies* 36, no. 2 (2010): 330–58.

14. Smith, *Sick and Tired of Being Sick and Tired*, 122.

15. Fraser, *African American Midwifery in the South*, 114.

16. Smith and Holmes, *Listen to Me Good*, 100. The bag inspection was, in Beatrice Mongeau's assessment, "the official agency's first mechanism of control and the means through which the changes in the midwife's practice [were] to be brought about." Beatrice Bell Mongeau, "The 'Granny' Midwives: A Study of a Folk Institution in the Process of Social Disintegration," PhD dissertation, University of North Carolina at Chapel Hill, 1973, 83

17. Fraser, *African American Midwifery in the South*, 77.

18. Michel Foucault, *Discipline and Punish: The Birth of the Prison*, translated by Alan Sheridan (New York: Random House, 1977), 187–91.

19. Foucault, *Discipline and Punish*, 184–85.

20. James Ferguson, "Mississippi Midwives," *Journal of the History of Medicine and Allied Sciences* 5, no. 1 (1950): 85–95.

21. Fraser, *African American Midwifery in the South*, 77.

22. Hartman, *Scenes of Subjection*, 138.

23. Browne, *Dark Matters*, 9.

24. Kelena Reid Maxwell, "Birth behind the Veil: African American Midwives and Mothers in the Rural South, 1921–1962," PhD dissertation, Rutgers University, 2009.

25. Maxwell, "Birth behind the Veil."

26. Edna Roberts and Rene Reeb, "Mississippi Public Health Nurses: A Partnership that Worked," *Public Health Nursing* 11, no. 1 (1994): 57–63, cited in Fraser, *African American Midwifery in the South*, 109, my emphasis.

27. Susan Smith, Sick and Tired, 130.

28. Maxwell, "Birth behind the Veil."

29. Marie Campbell, *Folks Do Get Born* (New York: Garland Publishing, 1942).

30. Hartman, *Scenes of Subjection*, 160. Intrusions into Black private space were not limited to these nominally benign visits. Rather, home visits can be thought of as situated on the less violent end of a spectrum of white intrusions that precluded the stabilization of a private sphere for African Americans. Elsa Barkley Brown notes that during Reconstruction in Richmond, Virginia, as Black citizens began to occupy the city's public spaces, "raids on black homes, which made all space public and subject to the interests of the state, obliterated any possible distinctions between public and private spheres" (Elsa Barkley Brown, "Negotiating and Transforming the Public Sphere," 115). On the very constitution of "the private" as predicated on the exclusion of Black women's reproductive lives and Black kinship at the very outset of racial capitalism, see Morgan, *Reckoning with Slavery*, 49, 210–11.

31. Jill Quadagno, *The Color of Welfare: How Racism Undermined the War on Poverty* (New York: Oxford University Press, 1996), 119–20.

32. Evelyn Brooks Higginbotham, "African-American Women's History and the Metalanguage of Race," *Signs* 17, no. 2 (1992): 265.

33. Browne, *Dark Matters*, 10.

34. Richard W. Wertz and Dorothy C. Wertz, *Lying-In: A History of Childbirth in America* (New Haven, CT: Yale University Press, 1989), 214, Bureau of Child Hygiene, Texas State Board of Health, 1925, in Litoff, *American Midwife Debate*, 70–76; and Lee, *Granny Midwives and Black Women Writers*, 39, 44.

35. Fraser, *African American Midwifery in the South*, 68.

36. Fraser, *African American Midwifery in the South*, 74.

37. Ladd-Taylor, "'Grannies' and 'Spinsters,'" 264.

38. Toni Morrison, *Song of Solomon* (New York: Knopf, 1977).

39. Fraser, *African American Midwifery in the South*, 103, 131; and Diane Vecchio, *Merchants, Midwives, and Laboring Women: Italian Migrants in Urban America* (Champaign: University of Illinois Press, 2006).

40. Ladd-Taylor, "'Grannies' and 'Spinsters'", 275fn71; and Carolyn Moehling and Melissa Thomasson, "Saving Babies: The Contribution of Sheppard-Towner to the Decline in Infant Mortality in the 1920s," National Bureau of Economic Research Working Paper, April 2012, www.nber.org/papers/w17996. In their working paper, Moehling and Thomasson in fact find that visiting nurse programs under Sheppard-Towner specifically were effective in attaining the significant reductions of around 8 per 1,000 in Black infant mortality. These programs, however, were implemented very unevenly, and as such the overall reduction was much less. Moehling and Thomasson conclude that the reduction for whites was in fact part of a preexisting trend, and that Sheppard-Towner programs in themselves did not significantly contribute to this decline.

41. Logan as told to Clark, *Motherwit*; and Smith and Holmes, *Listen to Me Good*; and Debra Ann Susie, *In the Way of Our Grandmothers: A Cultural View of Twentieth-Century Midwifery in Florida* (Athens: University of Georgia Press, 1988).

42. Browne, *Dark Matters*, 16.

43. Ferguson, "Mississippi Midwives."

44. Fraser discusses the pervasive "symbolism of the color white" in official descriptions of midwives' garments (*African American Midwifery in the South*, 115).

45. Carolyn Conant Van Blarcom, "Rat Pie: Among the Black Midwives of the South," *Harper's* 60 (February 1930): 331.

46. Sara Ahmed, *Queer Phenomenology: Orientations, Objects, Others* (Durham, NC: Duke University Press, 2006), 111.

47. Smith and Holmes, *Listen to Me Good*, 75. Midwife Smith links this blinkered perception of training with the unrealistic standards that the state attempted to impose on mothers, whose preparedness for birth (with new linens and baby clothes) midwives were instructed to police. Looking back to a time and place where "people lived in newspaper houses . . . with flour holding it together," she comments on the disconnection of the prescriptions from the realities of the context: "can't nobody prepare what they don't have" (Smith and Holmes, *Listen to Me Good*, 75). Like Lea's health administrators' fetishized policy documents in contemporary Australia, the enunciation of these imperatives for improving infant health was itself attributed transformative power, regardless of their irrelevance to the context that they were meant to transform.

48. Smith and Holmes, *Listen to Me Good*, 64.

49. Ahmed, *Queer Phenomenology*, 164.

50. Fraser, *African American Midwifery in the South*, 109.

51. Smith and Holmes, *Listen to Me Good*, 286; Fraser, *African American Midwifery in the South*, 187-188; and Fett, "Consciousness and Calling."

52. Smith and Holmes, *Listen to Me Good*, 100.

53. Fraser, *African American Midwifery in the South*, 113.

54. Ahmed, *Queer Phenomenology*, 111.

55. Smith and Holmes, *Listen to Me Good*, 100.

56. Beginning in the early twentieth century, a common accusation against immigrant and Black midwives was that they spread filth and disease through internally examining their patients with unclean hands. In fact, physicians were responsible for the deaths of many more women from puerperal fever, as they transmitted virulent microbes on their hands. This remained the case even after the necessity of antisepsis was proven by the work of Oliver Wendell Holmes, Ignaz Semmelweiss, Joseph Lister, and Louis Pasteur—conclusions that many physicians resisted (obstetrician Charles Meigs asserted that "doctors were gentlemen and gentlemen's hands were clean" (in Wertz and Wertz, *Lying-In*, 122). A 1930 study by the New York Academy of Medicine showed that cases attended (mostly immigrant) midwives resulted in significantly fewer maternal mortalities than physician-attended births (Wertz and Wertz, *Lying-In*, 215).

57. Carby, *Reconstructing Womanhood*, 39.

58. Schiebinger, "Exotic Abortifacients and Lost Knowledge"; and compare with Vimalassery, Pegues, and Goldstein, "Introduction: On Colonial Unknowing."

59. Fraser, *African American Midwifery in the South*, 119.

60. Hartman, *Scenes of Subjection*; and Lisa Nakamura and Peter Chow-White, eds., *Race after the Internet* (New York: Routledge, 2012).

61. Ahmed, *Queer Phenomenology*, 112.

62. George Stoney, "*All My Babies*" in *Film: Book 1: The Audience and the Filmmaker*, ed. Robert Hughes (New York: Grove Press, 1959), 77.

63. Though the demonstrations and sit-ins did not yield any immediate concessions, its setbacks served to sharpen Dr. King's future strategies and to broaden criteria of success; he writes: "When we planned our strategy for Birmingham months later, we spent many hours assessing Albany and trying to learn from its errors. Our appraisals not only helped to make our subsequent tactics more effective, but revealed that Albany was far from an unqualified failure. Though lunch counters remained segregated, thousands of Negroes were added to the voting

registration roll." Martin Luther King Jr., *The Autobiography of Martin Luther King, Jr.* (New York: Grand Central Publishing, 2001).

64. Lynne Jackson, "The Production of George Stoney's Film *All My Babies: A Midwife's Own Story*," *Film History* 1 (1987): 376.

65. Jackson, "Production of George Stoney's Film," 369.

66. Jackson, "Production of George Stoney's Film," 371.

67. Wangui Muigai, "'Something Wasn't Clean': Black Midwifery, Birth, and Postwar Medical Education in *All My Babies*," *Bulletin of the History of Medicine* 93, no. 1 (2019): 83.

68. Stoney, "*All My Babies*."

69. Muigai, "'Something Wasn't Clean,'" 108.

70. "Maternal Health Committee. Selected Case Report of Maternal Death," *Virginia Medical Monthly* 61 (1942): 35-37; in Fraser *African American Midwifery in the South*, 133.

71. Muigai, "'Something Wasn't Clean,'" 108-109.

72. Browne, *Dark Matters*, 21.

73. Stoney, "*All My Babies*," 83.

74. Smith and Holmes, *Listen to Me Good*.

75. Lee, *Granny Midwives and Black Women Writers*, 45.

76. Fraser, *African American Midwifery in the South*, 114.

77. Smith and Holmes, *Listen to Me Good*, 99.

78. Smith and Holmes, *Listen to Me Good*, 101.

79. Smith and Holmes, *Listen to Me Good*, 100.

80. Stoney, "All My Babies," 83.

81. Browne, *Dark Matters*, 21.

82. Ahmed, *Queer Phenomenology*, 147.

83. Fraser, *African American Midwifery in the South*, 96.

84. Smith and Holmes, *Listen to Me Good*, 84-85; Logan as told to Clark, *Motherwit*, 89, 142; and Susie, *In the Way of Our Grandmothers*, 166.

85. Fraser, *African American Midwifery in the South*, 163; and Smith and Holmes, *Listen to Me Good*, 76.

86. Fraser, *African American Midwifery in the South*, 163; and Logan as told to Clark, *Motherwit*, 95.

87. "Midwives in Texas," Bureau of Child Hygiene, Texas State Board of Health, Austin, 1925.

88. Ahmed, *Queer Phenomenology*, 165.

89. Robbie Davis-Floyd, "The Technocratic Body: American Childbirth As Cultural Expression," *Social Science & Medicine* 38, no. 8 (1994): 1125-40.

90. Fraser, *African American Midwifery in the South*, 260.

91. Fraser, *African American Midwifery in the South*, 95–96.

92. Gertrude Fraser, "Modern Bodies, Modern Minds: Midwifery and Reproductive Change in an African American Community," in *Conceiving the New World Order*, ed. Faye Ginsburg and Rayna Rapp, 42–58 (Berkeley: University of California Press, 1995).

93. Fraser, *African American Midwifery in the South*, 260.

94. Saraswathi Vedam et al., "The Giving Voice to Mothers Study: Inequity and Mistreatment during Pregnancy and Childbirth in the United States," *Reproductive Health* 16, no. 1 (2019): 1–18.

95. Ahmed, *Queer Phenomenology*, 129.

96. "White House Blueprint for Addressing the Maternal Health Crisis," June 2022. For a cautionary take on this turn, see Nash, "Birthing Black Mothers," 30.

Chapter 5. From Infants in Crisis to Maternal Health Crisis

1. "White House Blueprint for Addressing the Maternal Health Crisis," June 2022, 7.

2. Goode, "Birthing, Blackness, and the Body," 29–32; Appendix A.

3. Caleb J. Jang and Henry C. Lee, "A Review of Racial Disparities in Infant Mortality in the US," *Children* (Basel, Switzerland) 9, no. 2 (February 14, 2022): 257, doi:10.3390/children9020257.

4. Davis, "Obstetric Racism."

5. The campaign appears to be no longer active; although still hosted on the OMH website, and is the first result via search engines if searched by name, this brochure is no longer available if searched by name through that website's search function. However, it is still linked to other public service provider sites. Head Start, the national program of the US Department of Health and Human Services Administration for Children and Families, still offers an introduction and a link to the brochure. See https://eclkc.ohs.acf.hhs.gov/family-support-well-being /article/healthy-baby-begins-you. The Texas Department of Health and Human Services also lists the program among its "Resources for Providers," www.dshs .texas.gov/maternal-child-health/healthy-texas-mothers-babies/providers /resources-providers.

6. Garth Graham, MD MPH, deputy assistant secretary for minority health, "A Healthy Baby Begins with You: Update from the Office of Minority Health," August 2, 2011, US Department of Health and Human Services.

7. Fleda Mask Jackson et al., "Examining the Burdens of Gendered Racism"; Fleda Mask Jackson, "Race, Stress & Social Support: Addressing the Crisis in Black Infant Mortality," Joint Center for Political and Economic Studies, Health Policy Institute, Washington, DC, 2007, www.jointcenter.org; Fleda Mask Jackson, Diane L. Rowley, and Tracy Curry Owens, "Contextualized Stress, Global Stress, and Depression in Well-Educated, Pregnant, African-American Women," *Women's Health Issues* 22, no. 3 (May 2012): E329–E336; and Arline T. Geronimus et al., "Do US Black Women Experience Stress-Related Accelerated Biological Aging? A Novel Theory and First Population-based Test of Black-White Differences in Telomere Length," *Human Nature* 21 (2010): 19–38.

8. Mullings and Wali, *Stress and Resilience.*

9. L. Mullings et al., "Qualitative Methodologies and Community Participation in Examining Reproductive Experiences: The Harlem Birth Right Project," *Maternal and Child Health Journal* 5, no. 2 (2001): 85–93.

10. Mullings et al., "Qualitative Methodologies and Community Participation," 92.

11. Mullings, "Resistance and Resilience."

12. Mullings, "Resistance and Resilience," 87.

13. Mullings, "Resistance and Resilience," 88.

14. "During the data analysis phase of the research, physiological evidence that women who experience more prenatal stress and anxiety have significantly higher rates of adverse birth outcomes became available." Mullings, "Resistance and Resilience," 81.

15. Arline T. Geronimus et al., "'Weathering' and Age Patterns of Allostatic Load Scores among Blacks and Whites in the United States," *American Journal of Public Health* 96, no. 5 (2006): 826–33.

16. Geronimus et al., "'Weathering' and Age Patterns."

17. Geronimus et al., "'Weathering' and Age Patterns"; N. L. Jones et al., "Life Course Approaches to the Causes of Health Disparities," *American Journal of Public Health* 109 (2019): S48–S55; Tyan Parker Dominguez et al., "Racial Differences in Birth Outcomes: the Role of General, Pregnancy, and Racism Stress," *Health Psychology* 27, no. 2 (2008): 194–203; and Sarah Mustillo et al., "Self-Reported Experiences of Racial Discrimination and Black-White Differences in Preterm and Low-Birthweight Deliveries: The CARDIA Study," *American Journal of Public Health* 94, no. 12 (2004): 2125–31. For a critical race feminist synthesis of research on these intergenerational impacts of racism, see Shannon Sullivan, *The Physiology of Sexist and Racist Oppression* (New York: Oxford University Press, 2015), 99–127.

18. Jablonka and Lamb, *Evolution in Four Dimensions*.

19. Fatima L.C. Jackson, Mihai D. Niculescu, and Robert T. Jackson, "Conceptual Shifts Needed to Understand the Dynamic Interactions of Genes, Environment, Epigenetics, Social Processes, and Behavioral Choices," *American Journal of Public Health* 103, no. 1 (2013): S33-S42; and Richard C. Francis, *Epigenetics: How Environment Shapes Our Genes* (New York: W. W. Norton, 2011), 43-44.

20. Zaneta M. Thayer and Christopher W. Kuzawa, "Biological Memories of Past Environments: Epigenetic Pathways to Health Disparities," *Epigenetics* 6, no. 7 (2011):798-803, 800.

21. Sullivan, *Physiology of Sexist and Racist Oppression*, 113; and Francis, *Epigenetics*, 38-44.

22. Sullivan, *Physiology of Sexist and Racist Oppression*, 117.

23. Dorothy Roberts, *Fatal Invention: How Science, Politics, and Big Business Re-create Race in the Twenty-first Century* (New York: The New Press, 2012).

24. Valdez, *Weighing the Future*, 10.

25. Scott, Britton, and McLemore, "Ethics of Perinatal Care for Black Women."

26. Valdez, *Weighing the Future*, 197.

27. Tuck, "Suspending Damage."

28. Valdez, *Weighing the Future*, 201.

29. Lu and Halfon, "Racial and Ethnic Disparities in Birth Outcomes."

30. Lu and Halfon, "Racial and Ethnic Disparities in Birth Outcomes," 22.

31. Lu and Halfon, "Racial and Ethnic Disparities in Birth Outcomes."

32. "Unnatural Causes: When the Bough Breaks," episode, *Unnatural Causes: Is Inequality Making Us Sick?* PBS, California Newsreel, 2008.

33. Mullings, "Resistance and Resilience," 87-88.

34. Mullings, "Resistance and Resilience," 87.

35. Valdez , *Weighing the Future*, 47; Loretta Ross and Rickie Solinger, *Reproductive Justice: An Introduction* (Oakland: University of California Press, 2017), 100; and Ross, "Conceptualizing Reproductive Justice Theory," 190-91; and Wendy Brown, "American Nightmare: Neoliberalism, Neoconservatism, and De-Democratization," *Political Theory* 34 (2006): 690-715.

36. Miranda Waggoner, *The Zero Trimester: Pre-Pregnancy Care and the Politics of Reproductive Risk* (Berkeley: University of California Press, 2017), 13.

37. Waggoner, *Zero Trimester*, 19.

38. "Program History (PPE)," Office of Minority Health, Department of Health and Human Services, accessed March 6, 2023, www.minorityhealth.hhs.gov/omh/content.aspx?ID = 10240&lvl = 3&lvlID = 9.

39. "College Peer Educators Fighting the Infant Mortality Battle," *Minority Nurse*, March 20, 2013.

40. Valdez, *Weighing the Future*, 19.

41. For just a few examples: "Recent Steps By the State of Ohio to End Infant Mortality by Senator Shannon Jones," Cradle Cincinnati, July 21, 2014, www.cradlecincinnati.org/blog/2014/07/21/recent-steps-by-the-state-of-ohio-to-end-infant-mortality-by-senator-shannon-jones; Fault Lines, "America's Infant Mortality Crisis," *Al-Jazeera*, September 26, 2013, www.aljazeera.com/program/fault-lines/2013/9/26/americas-infant-mortality-crisis; and Crocker Stephenson, "City Vows To Fight Infant Mortality," *Milwaukee Journal Sentinel*, January 24, 2011.

42. Nash, *Birthing Black Mothers*, 12.

43. Kristin Sziarto, "Whose Reproductive Futures? Race-Biopolitics and Resistance in the Black Infant Mortality Reduction Campaigns in Milwaukee," *Environment and Planning D: Society and Space* 35, no. 2 (2017): 299–318, https://doi.org/10.1177/0263775816655803.

44. Khiara Bridges, *Reproducing Race: An Ethnography of Pregnancy as a Site of Racialization* (Berkeley: University of California Press, 2012); and Khiara Bridges, "Pregnancy, Medicaid, State Regulation, and the Production of Unruly Bodies," *Northwestern Journal of Law & Social Policy* 3, no. 1 (2008): 62–102.

45. Davis, *Reproductive Injustice*.

46. Davis, *Reproductive Injustice*, 203–204.

47. Davis, *Reproductive Injustice*, 86–87.

48. Davis, *Reproductive Injustice*, 87.

49. White House Blueprint, 7.

50. White House Blueprint, 38

51. White House Blueprint, 18.

52. Along with issuing its own declaration, the American Public Health Association has created an interactive map of declarations that racism is a public health crisis by health/public health bodies, states, localities, and other entities: see "Our Analysis: Declarations of Racism as a Public Health Crisis," accessed August 13, 2023, www.apha.org/topics-and-issues/health-equity/racism-and-health/racism-declarations.

53. See "Joint Statement: Collective Action Addressing Racism," www.acog.org/news/news-articles/2020/08/joint-statement-obstetrics-and-gynecology-collective-action-addressing-racism; "Apology to People of Color for APA's Role in Promoting, Perpetuating, and Failing to Challenge Racism, Racial Discrimination, and Human Hierarchy in U.S.," www.apa.org/about/policy/racism-apology;

"AMA Board of Trustees Pledges Action against Racism, Police Brutality," www
.ama-assn.org/press-center/press-releases/ama-board-trustees-pledges-action-
against-racism-police-brutality; "Our Analysis: Declarations of Racism as a Public Health Crisis," www.apha.org/policies-and-advocacy/public-health-policy-
statements/policy-database/2021/01/13/structural-racism-is-a-public-health-
crisis; and "Ending Structural Racism," www.nih.gov/ending-structural-racism.

54. Linda Villarosa, "Why America's Black Mothers and Babies Are in a Life-
or-Death Crisis," *New York Times Magazine*, April 11, 2018, www.nytimes.com
/2018/04/11/magazine/black-mothers-babies-death-maternal-mortality
.html. See also Linda Villarosa, *Under the Skin: The Hidden Toll of Racism on American Lives* (New York: Doubleday, 2022).

55. Nash, *Birthing Black Mothers*, 3.

56. Jonathan Capeheart, "Capeheart: Tonya Lewis Lee on the Black Maternal
Mortality Crisis and the New Film *Aftershock*," *Washington Post Live*, July 6, 2022,
www.washingtonpost.com/podcasts/capehart/tonya-lewis-lee-on-aftershock-
and-americas-black-maternal-mortality-crisis/; Beandra July, "'*Aftershock*' Review: A Moving Ode to the Black Family," *New York Times*, July 19, 2022; and "'*Aftershock*': Film Explores Disproportionate Black Maternal Mortality in U.S., Could
Worsen after *Roe*," *Democracy Now*, July 25, 2022. www.democracynow.org/2022
/7/25/aftershock_film_black_maternal_mortality_crisis.

57. Tonya Jackson Lee and Paula Eiselt, directors, *Aftershock*, ABC News Studios, Onyx Collective, Hulu, 2022.

58. Abigail Abrams, "Women of the Year: Jennie Joseph Wants to Fix the Black
Maternal Mortality Crisis One Midwife at a Time," *TIME Magazine*, March 2, 2022,
https://time.com/collection/women-of-the-year/6150545/jennie-joseph/.

59. Rojas's Texas practice, Mama Sana, offers a similar model of care that she
terms the *maternal justice* model, offering high-quality care to a largely Latine patient base regardless of documentation status. Cole, Rojas, and Joseph, "Building
a Movement to Birth a More Just and Loving World."

60. Bridges, *Reproducing Race*.

61. Davis, *Reproductive Injustice*, 179.

62. "Birthing Project—Madison, WI," www.facebook.com/BirthingProject-
MadisonWI/.

63. "Underground Railroad for New Life," Birthing Project USA, www.birth-
ingprojectusa.org.

64. Lillian Maddox-Whitehead, "Birthing Project Nashville," Metro
Davidson County Nashville Public Health Department, in Davis, *Reproductive Injustice*, 181.

65. Davis, *Reproductive Injustice*, 180–81. In 2018, Madison, Wisconsin, became a Birthing Project site. Tia Murray and Annie Menzel, "Black Infant Mortality: Continuities, Contestations and Care," in *The Edinburgh Companion to the Politics of American Health*, ed. Martin Halliwell and Sophie A. Jones (Edinburgh: Edinburgh University Press, 2022), 245.

66. Davis, *Reproductive Injustice*, 94–98. Serena Williams's highly publicized postpartum brush with death from a blood clot was a prime example of diagnostic lapse. Serena Williams, "How Serena Williams Saved Her Own Life," *Elle*, April 2022.

67. Davis, *Reproductive Injustice,* 98–109

68. Cooper Owens, *Medical Bondage*, 112.

69. Davis, "Obstetric Racism"; Dána-Ain Davis, "Reproducing while Black: The Crisis of Black Maternal Health, Obstetric Racism and Assisted Reproductive Technology," *Reproductive and Biomedical Society Online* 11 (November 1, 2020): 56–64, www.ncbi.nlm.nih.gov/pmc/articles/PMC7710503/; Karen Scott and Dána-Ain Davis, "Obstetric Racism: Naming and Identifying a Way Out of Black Women's Adverse Medical Experiences," *American Anthropologist* 123 (2021): 681–84, https://doi.org/10.1111/aman.13559; and Karen A. Scott and Indra Lusero, "The First Tool to Name Obstetric Racism Might Finally Push Policymakers Into Action," *Ms.*, October 4, 2023.

70. See, e.g., Scott, Britton, and McLemore, "Ethics of Perinatal Care for Black Women"; Stephanie Bray and Monica McLemore, "Demolishing the Myth of the Default Human That Is Killing Black Mothers," *Frontiers in Public Health* 9 (2021): 675788; and Julia Chinyere Oparah et al., *Battling over Birth: Black Women and the Maternal Health Care Crisis in California* (Oakland, CA: Black Women Birthing Justice, 2016); and Alicia D. Bonaparte and Julia Chinyere Oparah, eds., *Birthing Justice: Black Women, Pregnancy, and Childbirth*, 2nd edition (New York: Routledge, 2023).

71. Bray and McLemore, "Demolishing the Myth of the Default Human."

72. Toni M. Bond Leonard, "Laying the Foundations for a Reproductive Justice Movement," in *Radical Reproductive Justice*, ed. Loretta Ross et al. (New York: The Feminist Press, 2017).

73. Ross, "Conceptualizing Reproductive Justice Theory," 175.

74. Ross and Solinger, *Reproductive Justice*, 9.

75. Ross, "Conceptualizing Reproductive Justice Theory."

76. Ross, "Conceptualizing Reproductive Justice Theory," 323; Ross and Solinger, *Reproductive Justice*, 96–106; and Zakiya Luna, *Reproductive Rights as Human Rights: Women of Color and the Fight for Reproductive Justice* (New York: NYU Press, 2020).

77. Bailey, Moya, and Whitney Peoples. "Towards a Black Feminist Health Science Studies." *Catalyst: Feminism, Theory, Technoscience*, vol. 3, no. 2, fall 2017, 14.

78. SisterSong Women of Color Reproductive Justice Collective and coauthors, "Visioning New Futures for Reproductive Justice Declaration 2023," January 2023, www.sistersong.net/visioningnewfuturesforrj.

79. Roberts, *Torn Apart*, 301

80. "What Is Birth Justice?" www.blackwomenbirthingjustice.com/birth-justice. Also see Ross, "Conceptualizing Reproductive Justice," 189; Biany Pérez, "Birthing Sexual Freedom and Healing: A Survivor Mother's Birth Story," in *Birthing Justice: Black Women, Pregnancy, and Childbirth*, ed. Julia Chinyere Oparah and Alicia D. Bonaparte (New York: Routledge, 2015): 106–11; and Oparah with Black Women Birthing Justice, "Introduction: Beyond Coercion and Malign Neglect," 1–18.

81. "Birth Justice," Southern Birth Justice Network, https://southernbirthjustice.org/birth-justice.

82. Cole, Rojas, and Joseph, "Building a Movement to Birth a More Just and Loving World," 19.

83. "Perinatal Safe Spots," National Perinatal Task Force, https://perinataltaskforce.com/safe-spots/.

84. Cole, Rojas, and Joseph, "Building a Movement to Birth a More Just and Loving World," 25–26.

85. Cole, Rojas, and Joseph, "Building a Movement to Birth a More Just and Loving World," 23.

86. Kenneth J. Gruber, Susan H. Cupito, and Christina F. Dobson, "Impact of Doulas on Healthy Birth Outcomes," *Journal of Perinatal Education* 22, no. 1 (2013): 49–58, https://doi.org/10.1891/1058-1243.22.1.49; and Mariel Rivera, "Transitions in Black and Latinx Community-Based Doula Work in the US During COVID-19," *Frontiers in Sociology* 6 (March 11, 2021): 611350, https://doi.org/10.3389/fsoc.2021.611350. Black newborns' simply being cared for by a Black physician after birth—whether pediatrician, neonatologist, or family practice doctor—lessened the inequity between Black and white infant mortality by half. Brad N. Greenwood, Rachel R. Hardeman, and Aaron Sojourner, "Physician-patient Racial Concordance and Disparities in Birthing Mortality for Newborns," *Proceedings of the National Academy of Sciences* 117, no. 35 (August 17, 2020): 21194–200.

87. White House Blueprint, 44.

88. White House Blueprint, 48

89. "Black Mamas Matter Toolkit," Black Mamas Matter, June 2016, https://blackmamasmatter.org/our-work/toolkits/.

90. Jennie Joseph, "We cannot save Black women in America if we don't start telling the truth." https://blackmaternalhealthcaucus-underwood.house.gov/sites/evo-subsites/blackmaternalhealthcaucus-underwood.house.gov/files/wysiwyg_uploaded/Jennie%27s%20OP-ED.%2010%2019%202019%20final_JD%20format.pdf. Accessed May 2, 2023.

91. Third World Women's Alliance, Bay Area Chapter records, Sophia Smith Collection, SSC-MS-00697, Smith College Special Collections, Northampton, Massachusetts, accessed July 12, 2021, https://findingaids.smith.edu/repositories/2/archival_objects/139167.

92. Birthing While Black: Examining America's Black Maternal Health Crisis," Hearing before the Committee on Oversight and Reform," US House of Representatives, 117th Congress, first session, May 6, 2021.

93. Nash, "Birthing Black Mothers," 30.

94. Goode, "Birthing, Blackness, and the Body"; P. Mimi Niles and Michelle Drew, "Constructing the Modern American Midwife: White Supremacy and White Feminism Collide," *Nursing Clio* (October 22, 2020), https://nursingclio.org/2020/10/22/constructing-the-modern-american-midwife-white-supremacy-and-white-feminism-collide/. See also Christa Craven, *Pushing for Midwives: Homebirth Mothers and the Reproductive Rights Movement* (Philadelphia: Temple University Press, 2010).

95. Porchia-Albert, "Public Hearing."

96. Murray and Menzel, "Black Infant Mortality: Continuities, Contestations and Care."

97. Oparah et al., "Creativity, Resilience and Resistance: Black Birthworkers' Responses to the COVID19 Pandemic," *Frontiers in Sociology* 6 (2021): 63629.

98. Cherene Sherrard-Johnson, introduction to Christina Sharpe, "BLACK. STILL. LIFE.," Nellie Y. McKay Lecture, UW-Madison Institute for the Humanities, October 19, 2017.

99. Abrams, "Jennie Joseph Wants to Fix the Black Maternal Mortality Crisis One Midwife at a Time"; SisterSong, "Birth Justice Care Fund," www.sistersong.net/bjcarefund.

100. Murakawa, "Racial Innocence," 486.

101. Green et al., "Rethinking Bias to Achieve Maternal Health Equity," 936.

102. Green et al., "Rethinking Bias to Achieve Maternal Health Equity," 937.

103. Murphy, "Against Population, Towards Alterlife."

104. Muhammad, *Condemnation of Blackness*.

Bibliography

Abrams, Abigail. "Women of the Year: Jennie Joseph Wants to Fix the Black Maternal Mortality Crisis One Midwife at a Time." *TIME Magazine*, March 2, 2022. https://time.com/collection/women-of-the-year/6150545/jennie-joseph/.

Aftershock. ABC News Studios, Onyx Collective, Hulu, 2022.

"Aftershock: Film Explores Disproportionate Black Maternal Mortality in U.S., Could Worsen after *Roe*." *Democracy Now*, July 25, 2022. www.democracy-now.org/2022/7/25/aftershock_film_black_maternal_mortality_crisis.

Ahmed, Sara. *Queer Phenomenology: Orientations, Objects, Others*. Durham, NC: Duke University Press, 2006.

Allen, Jafari Sinclaire. "For 'the Children' Dancing the Beloved Community." *Souls: A Critical Journal of Black Politics, Culture, and Society* 11, no. 3 (2009): 311–26, doi:10.1080/10999940903088945.

Almond, Douglas, Kenneth Y. Chay, and Michael Greenstone. "Civil Rights, the War on Poverty, and Black-White Convergence in Infant Mortality in the Rural South and Mississippi." Working Paper No. 07-04. MIT Department of Economics, 2006.

"AMA Board of Trustees Pledges Action against Racism, Police Brutality." American Medical Association, June 7, 2020. www.ama-assn.org/press-center/press-releases/ama-board-trustees-pledges-action-against-racism-police-brutality.

American Association for Study and Prevention of Infant Mortality: Transactions of the Second Annual Meeting. Chicago, IL, Nov. 16–18, 1911.

Anderson, Kim. *A Recognition of Being: Reconstructing Native Womanhood*. Toronto: Women's Press, 2016.

"Apology to People of Color for APA's Role in Promoting, Perpetuating, and Failing to Challenge Racism, Racial Discrimination, and Human Hierarchy in U.S." American Psychological Association, October 29, 2021. www.apa.org/about/policy/racism-apology.

American Association for Study and Prevention of Infant Mortality: Transactions of the Second Annual Meeting. Chicago, IL, Nov. 16–18, 1911.

Apostolidis, Paul. *Breaks in the Chain: What Immigrant Workers Can Teach America about Democracy*. Minneapolis: University of Minnesota Press, 2010.

Ariès, Philippe. *Western Attitudes toward Death*. Baltimore, MD: Johns Hopkins University Press, 1974.

Armstrong, David. "The Invention of Infant Mortality." *Sociology of Health & Illness* 8, no. 3 (1986): 211–32.

Bailey, Moya, and Whitney Peoples. "Toward a Black Feminist Health Science Studies." *Catalyst: Feminism, Theory, Technoscience*, 3, no. 3 (Fall 2017): 14.

Baldwin, James. *The Fire Next Time*. New York: Dial Press, 1963.

———. "My Dungeon Shook: Letter to My Nephew on the One Hundredth Anniversary of the Emancipation." In *Baldwin: Collected Essays*. New York: Library of America, 1998.

———. "A Talk to Teachers." In *Baldwin: Collected Essays*. New York: Library of America, 1998.

———. "The White Problem." In *The Cross of Redemption: Uncollected Essays*. New York: Pantheon Books, 2010.

Balfour, Lawrie. *Democracy's Reconstruction: Thinking Politically with W.E.B. Du Bois*. New York: Oxford University Press, 2011.

Beard, Lisa. *If We Were Kin: Race, Identification, and Intimate Political Appeals*. New York: Oxford University Press, 2023.

Beardsley, Edward. *A History of Neglect: Health Care for Blacks and Mill Workers in the Twentieth-Century South*. Knoxville: University of Tennessee Press, 1990.

Benjamin, Ruha. "Black AfterLives Matter: Cultivating Kindness as Reproductive Justice." In *Making Kin Not Population*, edited by Adele Clarke and Donna Haraway, 41–65. Chicago: Prickly Paradigm Press, 2018.

Berlant, Lauren. "The Subject of True Feeling." In *Cultural Pluralism, Identity Politics, and the Law*, edited by Austin Sarat and Thomas Kearns, 49–84. Ann Arbor: University of Michigan Press, 1999.

Bernstein, Robin. *Racial Innocence: Performing American Childhood from Slavery to Civil Rights*. New York: NYU Press, 2011.

"Birth Justice." Southern Birth Justice Network. Accessed July 1, 2023. https://
southernbirthjustice.org/birth-justice.

"Birth Justice Care Fund." SisterSong. Accessed December 12, 2022. www
.sistersong.net/bjcarefund.

"Birthing Project-Madison, WI." Facebook. Accessed June 30, 2021. www
.facebook.com/BirthingProjectMadisonWI/.

"Birthing While Black: Examining America's Black Maternal Health Crisis."
Hearing before the Committee on Oversight and Reform, US House of
Representatives, 117th Congress, first session, May 6, 2021.

"Black Mamas Matter Toolkit." Black Mamas Matter, June 2016. https://
blackmamasmatter.org/our-work/toolkits/.

Blume Oeur, Freeden. "Fever Dreams: WEB Du Bois and the Racial Trauma of
COVID-19 and Lynching." *Ethnic and Racial Studies* 44, no. 5 (2021): 735–45.

Bonaparte, Alicia D. "'The Satisfactory Midwife Bag': Midwifery Regulation in
South Carolina, Past and Present Considerations." *Social Science History* 38,
no. 1–2 (2014): 155–82.

Boris, Eileen. "The Power of Motherhood: Black and White Activist Women
Redefine the 'Political.'" *Yale Journal of Law and Feminism* 2 (1989): 25–49.

Braddon, Mary Elizabeth. *Rupert Godwin*. 1867; London: Forgotten Books,
2018.

Bray, Stephanie R. M., and Monica R. McLemore. "Demolishing the Myth of the
Default Human That Is Killing Black Mothers." *Frontiers in Public Health* 9
(May 24, 2021): 675788. doi:10.3389/fpubh.2021.675788.

Bridges, Khiara. "Pregnancy, Medicaid, State Regulation, and the Production of
Unruly Bodies." *Northwestern Journal of Law & Social Policy* 3, no. 1 (2008):
62–102.

———. *Reproducing Race: An Ethnography of Pregnancy as a Site of Racialization.*
Berkeley: University of California Press, 2012.

———. "White Privilege and White Disadvantage." *Virginia Law Review*, April 10,
2019. https://virginialawreview.org/articles/white-privilege-and-white-
disadvantage/.

Briggs, Laura. *How All Politics Became Reproductive Politics: From Welfare Reform
to Foreclosure to Trump*. Oakland: University of California Press, 2017.

———. "The Race of Hysteria: 'Overcivilization' and the 'Savage' Woman in Late
Nineteenth-Century Obstetrics and Gynecology." *American Quarterly* 52, no.
2 (2000): 246–73.

———. *Somebody's Children: The Politics of Transracial and Transnational
Adoption*. Durham, NC: Duke University Press, 2012.

Brown, Elsa Barkley. "Negotiating and Transforming the Public Sphere: African American Political Life in the Transition from Slavery to Freedom." *Public Culture* 1, no. 7 (1994): 107–46.

Brown, Wendy. "American Nightmare: Neoliberalism, Neoconservatism, and De-Democratization." *Political Theory* 34 (2006): 690–715.

Browne, Simone. *Dark Matters: On the Surveillance of Blackness*. Durham, NC: Duke University Press, 2015.

Bruyneel, Kevin. "'Happy Days' (of the White Settler Imaginary) Are Here Again." *Theory & Event* 20, no. 1 (2017): 44–54.

———. *Settler Memory: The Disavowal of Indigeneity and the Politics of Race in the United States*. Chapel Hill: University of North Carolina Press, 2021.

Byrd, Michael W., and Linda Clayton. *An American Health Dilemma: Race, Medicine, and Health Care in the United States* 1900–2000. Cambridge, UK: Psychology Press, 2000.

Cabot, Richard C., and Edith K. Richie. "The Influence of Race on the Infant Mortality of Boston in 1909." *Boston Medical and Surgical Journal* 162, no. 7 (1910): 199–202.

Callahan, Noaquia. "Heat of the Day: Mary Church Terrell and African American Feminist Transnational Activism." PhD dissertation, University of Iowa, 2018.

Campbell, Marie. *Folks Do Get Born*. New York: Garland Publishing, 1942.

Capeheart, Jonathan. "Capeheart: Tonya Lewis Lee on the Black Maternal Mortality Crisis and the New Film *Aftershock*." *Washington Post Live*, July 6, 2022. www.washingtonpost.com/podcasts/capehart/tonya-lewis-lee-on-af-tershock-and-americas-black-maternal-mortality-crisis/.

Carby, Hazel. *Race Men*. Cambridge, MA: Harvard University Press, 1998.

———. *Reconstructing Womanhood: The Emergence of the Afro-American Woman Novelist*. New York: Oxford University Press, 1987.

———. "We Must Burn Them." *London Review of Books* 44, no. 10 (2022), www.lrb.co.uk/the-paper/v44/n10/hazel-v.-carby/we-must-burn-them.

Casper, Monica. *Babylost: Racism, Survival, and the Quiet Politics of Infant Mortality, from A to Z*. New Brunswick, NJ: Rutgers University Press, 2022.

Chandler, Nahum Dimitri. *X—The Problem of the Negro as a Problem for Thought*. New York: Fordham University Press, 2013.

Chen, Mel. *Animacies: Biopolitics, Mattering, Affect*. Durham, NC: Duke University Press, 2012.

Clinton, Catherine. *The Plantation Mistress: Woman's World in the Old South*. New York: Pantheon, 1982.

Cohen, Cathy. "Deviance as Resistance: A New Agenda for the Study of Black Politics." *The Du Bois Review* 1, no. 1 (2004): 27–45.

Cole, Haile Eshe, Paula X. Rojas, and Jennie Joseph. "Building a Movement to Birth a More Just and Loving World." National Perinatal Task Force, March 2018.

"College Peer Educators Fighting the Infant Mortality Battle." *Minority Nurse.* March 20, 2013.

"The Constructive View of Reparations with Olúfẹ́mi O. Táíwò." *Millennials Are Killing Capitalism* podcast, March 7, 2022. https://millennialsarekillingcapitalism.libsyn.com/the-constructive-view-of-reparations-with-olfmi-o-tw.

Cooper, Anna Julia. *A Voice from the South.* New York: Oxford University Press, 1892.

———. "What Are We Worth?" In *The Voice of Anna Julia Cooper, Including "A Voice from the South" and Other Important Essays, Papers, and Letters,* edited by Charles Lemert and Esme Bhan. Lanham, MD: Rowman & Littlefield, 1998.

Cooper, Brittney. *Beyond Respectability: The Intellectual Thought of Race Women.* Urbana: University of Illinois Press, 2017.

Cooper Owens, Deidre. *Medical Bondage: Race, Gender, and the Origins of American Gynecology.* Athens: University of Georgia Press, 2017.

Cradle Cincinnati. "Recent Steps by the State of Ohio To End Infant Mortality by Senator Shannon Jones." July 21, 2014. www.cradlecincinnati.org/blog /2014/07/21/recent-steps-by-the-state-of-ohio-to-end-infant-mortality-by-senator-shannon-jones.

Craven, Christa. *Pushing for Midwives: Homebirth Mothers and the Reproductive Rights Movement.* Philadelphia: Temple University Press, 2010.

Craven, Christa, and Mara Glatzel. "Downplaying Difference: Historical Accounts of African American Midwives and Contemporary Struggles for Midwifery." *Feminist Studies* 36, no. 2 (2010): 330–58.

Crear-Perry, Joia, Aletha Maybank, Mia Keeys, Nia Mitchell, and Dawn Godbolt. "Moving Towards Anti-Racist Praxis in Medicine." *Lancet* 396, no. 10249 (2020): 451–53.

Cvetkovich, Ann. "Depression Is Ordinary: Public Feelings and Saidiya Hartman's 'Lose Your Mother.'" *Feminist Theory* 13, no. 2 (2012): 131–46.

Damico, Anthony P. "Health Coverage by Race and Ethnicity, 2010–2021." *Kaiser Family Foundation* (blog), December 20, 2022. www.kff.org/racial-equity-and-health-policy/issue-brief/health-coverage-by-race-and-ethnicity/.

Davis, Angela. "Reflections on the Black Woman's Role in the Community of
Slaves." *The Black Scholar* 3, no. 4 (December 1971): 2–15.

———. *Women, Race, and Class.* New York: Penguin Random House, 1981.

Davis, Dána-Ain. "Obstetric Racism: The Racial Politics of Pregnancy, Labor,
and Birthing." *Medical Anthropology* 38, no. 7 (October 2019): 560–73.

———. "Reproducing while Black: The Crisis of Black Maternal Health,
Obstetric Racism and Assisted Reproductive Technology." *Reproductive
Biomedical Society Online* 11 (November 1, 2020): 56–64.

———. *Reproductive Injustice: Racism, Pregnancy, and Premature Birth.* New York:
NYU Press, 2019.

Davis-Floyd, Robbie. "The Technocratic Body: American Childbirth as Cultural
Expression." *Social Science & Medicine* 38, no. 8 (1994): 1125–40.

Degler, Carl N. *At Odds: Women and the Family in America from the Revolution to
the Present.* New York: Oxford University Press, 1980.

Diaz-Tello, Farah. "Invisible Wounds: Obstetric Violence in the United States."
Reproductive Health Matters 24, no. 47 (May 2016): 56–64.

Dixon, Chris. *Perfecting the Family: Antislavery Marriages in Nineteenth-Century
America.* Amherst: University of Massachusetts Press, 1997.

Dominguez, Tyan Parker, Christine Dunkel-Schetter, Laura M. Glynn, Calvin
Hobel, and Curt A. Sandman. "Racial Differences in Birth Outcomes: The
Role of General, Pregnancy, and Racism Stress." *Health Psychology* 27, no. 2
(2008): 194–203.

Donzelot, Jacques. *The Policing of the Family.* New York: Pantheon Books, 1979.

Douglas, Ann. "Heaven Our Home: Consolation Literature in the Northern
United States, 1830–1880." *American Quarterly* 26, no. 5 (1974): 496–515.

Douglass, Frederick. *Narrative of the Life of Frederick Douglass.* 1845; New York:
Bedford/St. Martins, 2003.

Downs, Jim. *Sick from Freedom: African-American Illness and Suffering during the
Civil War and Reconstruction.* Oxford, UK: Oxford University Press, 2012.

Driscoll, A. K., and D. M. Ely. "Infant Mortality in the United States, 2020."
National Vital Statistics Reports 71, no. 5 (2022).

W.E.B. Du Bois. *The Autobiography of W.E.B. DuBois: A soliloquy on viewing my life
from the last decade of its first century.* New York: International Publishers,
1968.

———. *Black Reconstruction in America, 1860–1880.* New York: The Free Press,
1998.

———. *Darkwater: Voices from within the Veil.* New York: Oxford University Press,
2007.

———. *Dusk of Dawn: The Autobiography of a Race Concept.* 1940; New York: Schocken Books, 1984.

———. *Mortality among Negroes in Cities,* Proceedings of the Conference for Investigations of City Problems, held at Atlanta University, May 26–27, 1896. Atlanta University Publications, No. 1.

———. *Petition to the U.N. Protesting Discrimination in the U.S. and the Rosa Ingram Case.* 1949. In *Mary Church Terrell Papers: Speeches and Writings, 1866 to 1953.* Manuscript/Mixed Material. www.loc.gov/item/mss425490520/, images 1–4.

———. *The Philadelphia Negro: A Social Study.* 1899; Philadelphia: University of Pennsylvania Press, 1996.

———. "Race Traits and Tendencies of the American Negro by Frederick L. Hoffman, F.S.S. [Review]." *Annals of the American Academy of Political and Social Science* 9 (January 1897): 127–33.

———. "Some Efforts of American Negroes for Their Own Social Betterment. Report of an Investigation under the Direction of Atlanta University; Together with the Proceedings of the Third Conference for the Study of the Negro Problems." Atlanta University, Atlanta, GA, May 25, 1898.

———. *The Souls of Black Folk.* New York: Oxford University Press, 2007.

Dumm, Thomas. "Political Theory for Losers." In *Vocations of Political Theory,* edited by Jason A. Frank and John Tambornino, 145–64. Minneapolis: University of Minnesota Press, 2000.

Dunbar-Ortiz, Roxanne. *An Indigenous Peoples' History of the United States.* Boston, MA: Beacon Press, 2014.

Dye, Nancy Schrom, and Daniel Blake Smith. "Mother Love and Infant Death, 1750–1920." *Journal of American History* 73, no. 2 (1986): 329–53.

Edelman, Lee. *No Future: Queer Theory and the Death Drive.* Durham, NC: Duke University Press, 2004.

Edkins, Jenny. *Trauma and the Memory of Politics.* Cambridge, UK: Cambridge University Press, 2003.

Ehrenreich, Barbara, and Deirdre English. *Witches, Midwives, and Nurses: A History of Woman Healers.* 1973; reprint, New York: The Feminist Press, 2010.

Ellison, Ralph. "An American Dilemma." In *Shadow & Act.* New York: First Vintage International Edition, 1994.

Emerson, Ralph Waldo. *The Collected Works of Ralph Waldo Emerson,* edited by Alfred Riggs Ferguson, Joseph Slater, and Jean Ferguson Carr. Cambridge, MA: The Belknap Press of Harvard University Press, 1971.

"Ending Structural Racism." National Institutes of Health. Accessed November 15, 2022. www.nih.gov/ending-structural-racism.

England, Pam, and Rob Horowitz. *Birthing from Within*. Albuquerque, NM: Partera Press, 1998.

Estes, Nick. *Our History Is the Future: Standing Rock versus the Dakota Access Pipeline, and the Long Tradition of Indigenous Resistance*. New York: Verso, 2019.

Ewald, François. "Insurance and Risk." In *The Foucault Effect: Studies in Governmentality*, edited by Graham Burchell, Colin Gordon, and Peter Miller, 197-210. Chicago: University of Chicago Press, 1991.

Fassin, Didier. "Another Politics of Life Is Possible." *Theory, Culture, & Society* 26, no. 5 (2009): 4-60.

Fault Lines. "America's Infant Mortality Crisis." *Al-Jazeera*. September 26, 2013. www.aljazeera.com/program/fault-lines/2013/9/26/americas-infant-mortality-crisis.

Fellows, Mary Louise, and Sherene Razack. "The Race to Innocence: Hierarchical Relations Among Women." *Gender, Race & Justice* 1 (1995): 335-52.

Ferguson, James. "Mississippi Midwives." *Journal of the History of Medicine and Allied Sciences* 5, no. 1 (1950): 85-95.

Fett, Sharla M. "Consciousness and Calling: African American Midwives at Work in the Antebellum South." In *New Studies in the History of American Slavery*, edited by Edward E. Baptist and Stephanie M. H. Camp, 64-86. Athens: University of Georgia Press, 2006.

Folkes, H. M. "The Negro as a Health Problem." *Journal of the American Medical Association* 55, no. 15 (1910): 1246-47.

Foucault, Michel. *Discipline and Punish: The Birth of the Prison*. Translated by Alan Sheridan. New York: Random House, 1977.

——. *The History of Sexuality*. Vol. 1. New York: Pantheon Books, 1978.

——. *"Society Must Be Defended": Lectures at the Collège de France, 1975-76*. 1997; reprint, New York: Picador, 2003.

Fox, Cybelle. *Three Worlds of Relief: Race, Immigration, and the American Welfare State from the Progressive Era to the New Deal*. Princeton, NJ: Princeton University Press, 2012.

Francis, Megan Ming. "Ida B. Wells and the Economics of Racial Violence." *Items: Insights from the Social Sciences, Social Science Research Council*, January 24, 2017. https://items.ssrc.org/reading-racial-conflict/ida b wells and the economics of racial violence/#:~:text=According%20to%20Wells%2C%20the%20logic,a%20captive%20black%20labor%20force.

Francis, Richard C. *Epigenetics: How Environment Shapes Our Genes.* New York: W. W. Norton, 2011.

Fraser, Gertrude Jacinta. *African American Midwifery in the South: Dialogues of Birth, Race, and Memory.* Cambridge, MA: Harvard University Press, 1998.

———. "Modern Bodies, Modern Minds: Midwifery and Reproductive Change in an African American Community." In *Conceiving the New World Order,* edited by Faye Ginsburg and Rayna Rapp, 42–58. Berkeley: University of California Press, 1995.

Gaines, Kevin. *Uplifting the Race: Black Leadership, Politics, and Culture in the Twentieth Century.* Chapel Hill: University of North Carolina Press, 1996.

Gaskin, Ina May. *Ina May's Guide to Childbirth.* New York: Bantam Books, 2003.

———. *Spiritual Midwifery.* Summertown, TN: Book Publishing Company, 2010.

Geronimus, Arline T., Margaret Hicken, Danya Keene, and John Bound. "'Weathering' and Age Patterns of Allostatic Load Scores among Blacks and Whites in the United States." *American Journal of Public Health* 96, no. 5 (2006): 826–33.

Geronimus, Arline T., Margaret T. Hicken, Jay A. Pearson, Sarah J. Seashols, Kelly L. Brown, and Tracey Dawson Cruz. "Do US Black Women Experience Stress-Related Accelerated Biological Aging? A Novel Theory and First Population-based Test of Black-White Differences in Telomere Length." *Human Nature* 21 (2010): 19–38.

Gilmore, Ruth Wilson. "Abolition Geography and the Problem of Innocence." In *Abolition Geography: Essays toward Liberation.* New York: Verso, 2022.

———. "Race and Globalization." In *Geographies of Global Change: Remapping the World,* edited by Ronald J. Johnston, Peter J. Taylor, and Michael J. Watts, 261–74. New York: Wiley-Blackwell, 2002.

Gilroy, Paul. *The Black Atlantic: Modernity and Double Consciousness.* Cambridge, MA: Harvard University Press, 1993.

Glaude Jr., Eddie S. "James Baldwin and Black Lives Matter." In *A Political Companion to James Baldwin,* edited by Susan J. McWilliams, 361–72. Lexington: University of Kentucky Press, 2017.

Goldsby, Jacqueline. *A Spectacular Secret: Lynching in American Life and Literature.* Chicago: University of Chicago Press, 2006.

Goode, Keisha. *Birthing, Blackness and the Body: Black Midwives and the Pursuit of Reproductive Justice.* New York: Columbia University Press, forthcoming.

Goode, Keisha La'Nesha. "Birthing, Blackness, and the Body: Black Midwives and Experiential Continuities of Institutional Racism." City University of New York, 2014. https://academicworks.cuny.edu/gc_etds/423.

Goode, Keisha, and Barbara Katz Rothman. "African-American Midwifery, a History and a Lament." *American Journal of Economics and Sociology* 76, no. 1 (2017): 65–94.

Gooding-Williams, Robert. *In the Shadow of Du Bois*. Cambridge, MA: Harvard University Press, 2009.

Goodwin, Michele. *Policing the Womb: Invisible Women and the Criminalization of Motherhood*. Cambridge, UK: Cambridge University Press, 2020.

Gore, Dayo F. *Radicalism at the Crossroads: African American Women Activists in the Cold War*. New York: NYU Press, 2011.

Graham, Garth. "A Healthy Baby Begins with You: Update from the Office of Minority Health." August 2, 2011. Deputy Assistant Secretary for Minority Health. Office of Minority Health of the US Department of Health and Human Services.

Green, Tiffany L., Jasmine Y. Zapata, Heidi W. Brown, and Nao Hagiwara. "Rethinking Bias to Achieve Maternal Health Equity: Changing Organizations, Not Just Individuals." *Obstetrics & Gynecology* 137, no. 5 (May 2021): 935–40.

Greenwood, Brad N., Rachel R. Hardeman, and Aaron Sojourner. "Physician-patient Racial Concordance and Disparities in Birthing Mortality for Newborns." *Proceedings of the National Academy of Sciences* 117, no. 35 (August 17, 2020): 21194–200.

Griffin, Farah Jasmine. "Black Feminists and Du Bois: Respectability, Protection, and Beyond." *The ANNALS of the American Academy of Political and Social Science* 568, no. 1 (March 1, 2000): 28–40.

Gruber, Kenneth J., Susan H. Cupito, and Christina F. Dobson. "Impact of Doulas on Healthy Birth Outcomes." *Journal of Perinatal Education* 22, no. 1 (2013): 49–58, https://doi.org/10.1891/1058-1243.22.1.49.

Gumbs, Alexis Pauline. "M/Other Ourselves: A Black Queer Feminist Genealogy for Radical Mothering." In *Revolutionary Mothering; Love on the Front Lines*, edited by Alexis Pauline Gumbs, China Martens, and Mai'a Williams, 19–31. Oakland, CA: PM Press, 2016.

———. *Spill: Scenes of Black Feminist Fugitivity*. Durham, NC: Duke University Press.

Hacking, Ian. *The Taming of Chance*. New York: Cambridge University Press, 1990.

Haller, John. *Outcasts from Evolution: Scientific Attitudes of Racial Inferiority 1859–1900*. Urbana: University of Illinois Press, 1971.

Hammonds, Evelyn. "New Technologies of Race." In *Processed Lives: Gender and Technology in Everyday Life*, edited by Jennifer Terry and Melodie Calvert, 107–22. New York: Routledge, 1997.

Hammonds, Evelynn M., and Susan M. Reverby. "Toward a Historically Informed Analysis of Racial Health Disparities since 1619." *American Journal of Public Health* 109, no. 10 (2019): 1348-49.

Hart, Tanya. *Health in the City: Race, Poverty, and the Negotiation of Women's Health in New York City, 1915-1930.* New York: NYU Press, 2015.

Hartman, Saidiya. "The Belly of the World: A Note on Black Women's Labors." *Souls* 18, no. 1 (March 14, 2016): 166-73.

———. *Scenes of Subjection: Terror, Slavery, and Self-Making in Nineteenth-century America.* New York: Oxford University Press, 1997.

"A Healthy Baby Begins with You." Office of Minority Health of the US Department of Health and Human Services. https://eclkc.ohs.acf.hhs.gov /family-support-well-being/article/healthy-baby-begins-you. Accessed June 15, 2023.

Heen, Mary L. "Ending Jim Crow Life Insurance Rates." *Northwestern Journal of Law and Social Policy* 4, no. 2 (2009): 360-99.

Hernández, Tanya Katerí. *Racial Innocence: Unmasking Latino Anti-Black Bias and the Struggle for Equality.* Boston, MA: Beacon Press, 2022.

Higginbotham, Evelyn Brooks. "African-American Women's History and the Metalanguage of Race." *Signs* 17, no. 2 (1992): 251-74.

———. *Righteous Discontent: The Women's Movement in the Black Baptist Church, 1880-1920.* Cambridge, MA: Harvard University Press, 1993.

Hoffman, Frederick Ludwig. *Race Traits and Tendencies of the American Negro.* American Economic Association, 1896.

Hoffman, Kelly M., Sophie Trawalter, Jordan R. Axt, and M. Norman Oliver. "Racial Bias in Pain Assessment and Treatment Recommendations, and False Beliefs about Biological Differences between Blacks and Whites." *Proceedings of the National Academy of Sciences USA* 113, no. 16 (2016): 4296-4301.

Hogarth, Rana. "Enslavement and Eugenics." Presented at Dismantling Eugenics: A Convening, September 28, 2021. https://vimeo.com /642322721.

———. "The Shadow of Slavery in the Era of Eugenics." Presented at the MacLean Center 2021-2022 Lecture Series: "History of Medical Ethics," MacLean Center for Clinical Medical Ethics, University of Chicago, March 17, 2022. www.youtube.com/watch?v=doW44TmfWI8.

Hooker, Juliet. "Black Protest / White Grievance: On the Problem of White Political Imaginations Not Shaped by Loss." *South Atlantic Quarterly* 116, no. 3 (2017): 483-504.

———. *Theorizing Race in the Americas: Douglass, Sarmiento, Du Bois, and Vasconcelos.* New York: Oxford University Press, 2017.

———. *White Grievance/Black Grief.* Princeton, NJ: Princeton University Press, 2023.

"Infant Mortality by Country 2023." *World Population Review*, February 4, 2023. https://worldpopulationreview.com/country-rankings/infant-mortality-rate-by-country.

Jablonka, Eve, and Marion J. Lamb. *Evolution in Four Dimensions: Genetic, Epigenetic, Behavioral, and Symbolic Variation in the History of Life.* Cambridge, MA: MIT Press, 2005.

Jackson, Fatima L. C., Mihai D. Niculescu, and Robert T. Jackson. "Conceptual Shifts Needed to Understand the Dynamic Interactions of Genes, Environment, Epigenetics, Social Processes, and Behavioral Choices." *American Journal of Public Health* 103, no. 1 (2013): S33–42.

Jackson, Fleda Mask. "Race, Stress and Social Support: Addressing the Crisis in Black Infant Mortality." Joint Center for Political and Economic Studies, Health Policy Institute, Washington, DC, 2007. www.jointcenter.org.

Jackson, Fleda Mask, Mona T. Phillips, and Carol J. R. Hogue. "Examining the Burdens of Gendered Racism: Implications for Pregnancy Outcomes among College-Educated African American Women." *Maternal and Child Health Journal*, no. 5 (2001): 95–107.

Jackson, Fleda Mask, Diane L. Rowley, and Tracy Curry Owens. "Contextualized Stress, Global Stress, and Depression in Well-Educated, Pregnant, African-American Women." *Women's Health Issues* 22, no. 3 (May 2012): E329–E336.

Jackson, Lynne. "The Production of George Stoney's Film All My Babies: A Midwife's Own Story." *Film History* 1 (1987): 367–92.Jackson, Zakiyyah Iman. *Becoming Human: Matter and Meaning in an Antiblack World.* New York: NYU Press, 2020.

Jacobs, Harriet. *Incidents in the Life of a Slave Girl.* 1861; Cambridge, MA: Harvard University Press, 2009.

Jacobs, Harriet Ann. *Harriet Ann Jacobs, Incidents in the Life of a Slave Girl: Written by Herself, with "A True Tale of Slavery" by John S. Jacobs.* Cambridge, MA: Harvard University Press, 1861.

James, Joy. "The Profeminist Politics of W. E. B. Du Bois with Respects to Anna Julia Cooper and Ida B. Wells Barnett." In *W. E. B. Du Bois on Race and Culture*, edited by Bernard W. Bell, Emily R. Grosholz, and James B. Stewart, 141–60. New York: Routledge, 1996.

——. *Transcending the Talented Tenth.* New York: Routledge, 1997.

——. "The Womb of Western Theory: Trauma, Time Theft, and the Captive Maternal." *Challenging the Punitive Society: Carceral Notebooks* 12, no. 1 (2016): 253–96.

Jang, Caleb J., and Henry C. Lee. "A Review of Racial Disparities in Infant Mortality in the US." *Children* (Basel, Switzerland) 9, no. 2 (February 14, 2022): 257, doi:10.3390/children9020257.

Jefferson, Brian Jordan, Jodi A. Byrd, Lisa Marie Cacho, and Susan Koshy. Introduction to *Colonial Racial Capitalism*, 1–30. Durham, NC: Duke University Press, 2022.

"Joint Statement: Collective Action Addressing Racism." American College of Obstetricians and Gynecologists, August 27, 2020. www.acog.org/news /news-articles/2020/08/joint-statement-obstetrics-and-gynecology-collective-action-addressing-racism.

Jones, Camara Phyllis. "Levels of Racism: A Theoretic Framework and a Gardener's Tale." *American Journal of Public Health* 90, no. 8 (August 2000): 1212–15.

Jones, Claudia. "An End to the Neglect of the Problems of the Negro Woman!" *Political Affairs* (June 1949): 51-67.

Jones, N. L., S. E. Gilman, T. L. Cheng, S. S. Drury, C. V. Hill, and A. T. Geronimus. "Life Course Approaches to the Causes of Health Disparities." *American Journal of Public Health* 109 (2019): S48–55.

Jones-Rogers, Stephanie. *They Were Her Property: White Women as Slave Owners in the American South.* New Haven, CT: Yale University Press, 2019.

Joseph, Jennie, "We cannot save Black women in America if we don't start telling the truth." Black Maternal Health Caucus website, https:// blackmaternalhealthcaucus-underwood.house.gov/sites/evo-subsites /blackmaternalhealthcaucus-underwood.house.gov/files/wysiwyg_up-loaded/Jennie%27s%20OP-ED.%2010%2019%202019%20final_JD%20 format.pdf. Accessed May 2, 2023.

July, Beandra. "'Aftershock' Review: A Moving Ode to the Black Family." *New York Times*, July 19, 2022.

Karp, Robert J., and Bobby Gearing. "The Death of Burghardt Du Bois, 1899; Implications for Today." *Journal of the National Medical Association* 107, no. 1 (February 1, 2015): 68–74.

Karuka (Vimalassery), Manu, Juliana Hu Pegues, and Alyosha Goldstein. "Introduction: On Colonial Unknowing." *Theory & Event* 19, no. 4 (2016). muse.jhu.edu/article/633283.

Kennedy, John Camp. *Preliminary Report on the 1860 Census.* Washington, DC: Government Printing Office, 1862.

Kennedy, V. Lynn. *Born Southern: Childbirth, Motherhood, and Social Networks in the Old South.* Baltimore, MD: Johns Hopkins University Press, 2010.

King Jr., Martin Luther. *The Autobiography of Martin Luther King, Jr.* New York: Grand Central Publishing, 2001.

Klaus, Alisa. *Every Child a Lion: The Origins of Maternal and Infant Health Policy in the US and France.* Ithaca, NY: Cornell University Press, 2019.

Kleinberg, S. J. *Women in the United States, 1830-1945.* New Brunswick, NJ: Rutgers University Press, 1999.

Kline, Wendy. *Coming Home: How Midwives Changed Birth.* New York: Oxford University Press, 2019.

Kowal, Emma. *Trapped in the Gap: Doing Good in Indigenous Australia.* New York: Berghahn Books, 2015.

Kwate, Naa Oyo A., and Shatema Theadcraft. "Dying Fast and Dying Slow in Black Space." *Du Bois Review: Social Science Research on Race* 14, no. 2 (2018): 535-56.

Ladd-Taylor, Molly. "'Grannies' and 'Spinsters': Midwife Education under the Sheppard-Towner Act." *Journal of Social History* 22, no. 2 (Winter 1988): 255-75.

———. *Mother-Work: Women, Child Welfare, and the State, 1890-1930.* Champaign: University of Illinois Press, 1994.

Lanzoni, Susan. "Sympathy in Mind (1876-1900)." *Journal of the History of Ideas* 70, no. 2 (2009): 265-87.

Larsen, Nella. *Quicksand.* New York: A. A. Knopf, 1928.

Lawrie, Paul. *Forging a Laboring Race: The African American Worker in the Progressive Imagination.* New York: NYU Press, 2016.

Lawson, Erica S. "Bereaved Black Mothers and Maternal Activism in the Racial State." *Feminist Studies* 44, no. 3 (2018): 713-35.

Leavitt, Judith. *Brought to Bed.* New York: Oxford University Press, 2016.

———. *Brought to Bed: Childbearing in America, 1750-1950.* New York: Oxford University Press, 1986.

Lee, Valerie. *Granny Midwives and Black Women Writers: Double-Dutched Readings.* New York: Routledge, 1996.

Leonard, Toni M. Bond. "Laying the Foundations for a Reproductive Justice Movement." In *Radical Reproductive Justice,* edited by Loretta Ross and et al., 39-49. New York: Feminist Press at CUNY, 2017.

"Letter of Support for Midwives of Color Chair and Inner Council Resignation." Aromidwifery (blog), May 27, 2012. https://aromidwifery.wordpress.com/letter-of-support-for-midwives-of-color-chair-and-inner-council-resignation/.

Levering-Lewis, David. *W.E.B. Du Bois, 1868–1919: Biography of a Race.* New York: Henry Holt & Co, 1993.

Levy, Jonathan. *Freaks of Fortune: The Emerging World of Capitalism and Risk in America.* Cambridge, MA: Harvard University Press, 2012.

Lieberman, Robert. *Shifting the Color-Line: Race and the American Welfare State.* Cambridge, MA: Harvard University Press, 1999.

Lindsey, Treva. *Colored No More: Reinventing Black Womanhood in Washington, D.C.* Champaign: University of Illinois Press, 2017.

Litoff, Judy. *The American Midwife Debate: A Sourcebook on Its Modern Origins.* Westport, CT: Greenwood Press, 1986.

Logan, Onnie Lee, as told to Katherine Clark. *Motherwit: An Alabama Midwife's Story.* New York: Dutton, 1989.

Longfellow, Fanny Appleton. *Mrs. Longfellow: Selected Journals and Letters,* edited by Edward Wagenknecht. 1848; New York: Longmans, Green, 1956.

Lorde, Audre. *Sister Outsider.* New York: Crossing Press, 1984.

Lu, Michael C., and Neal Halfon. "Racial and Ethnic Disparities in Birth Outcomes: A Life-Course Perspective." *Maternal and Child Health Journal 7,* no. 1 (2003): 13–30.

Luna, Zakiya. *Reproductive Rights as Human Rights: Women of Color and the Fight for Reproductive Justice.* New York: NYU Press, 2020.

Macoun, Alissa. "Colonising White Innocence: Complicity and Critical Encounter." In *The Limits of Settler Colonial Reconciliation,* edited by Sarah Maddison, Tom Clark, and Ravi de Costa, 85–102. Singapore: Springer, 2016.

Maddox-Whitehead, Lillian. "Birthing Project Nashville." Metro Davidson County, Nashville Public Health Department, 2008.

Malacrida, Claudia. "Mothering and Disability: From Eugenics to Newgenics." Chapter 33 in *Routledge Handbook of Disability Studies,* second edition, edited by Nick Watson and Simo Vehmas. New York: Routledge University Press, 2020.

McKay, Nellie Y. "Introduction." In *A Colored Woman in a White World,* ed. Mary Church Terrell. New York: G.K. Hall, 1996.

March of Dimes and PeriStats. "Total Cesarean Deliveries by Maternal Race/Ethnicity: United States, 2019–2021 Average." Accessed July 10, 2023. www.marchofdimes.org/peristats/data?reg=99&top=8&stop=356&lev=1&slev=1&obj=1.

Mariotti, Shannon. "On the Passing of the First-Born Son: Emerson's 'Focal Distancing,' Du Bois' 'Second Sight,' and Disruptive Particularity." *Political Theory* 37 (2009): 351–74.

Marshall, Stephen H. "The Political Life of Fungibility." *Theory & Event* 15, no. 3 (2012).

Marx, Karl. *Capital: A Critique of Political Economy, Volume 1.* Translated by Ben Fowkes. New York: Penguin Classics, 1990.

Maternal Health Committee. "Selected Case Report of Maternal Death." *Virginia Medical Monthly* 61 (1942): 35–37.

Maxwell, Kelena Reid. "Birth behind the Veil: African American Midwives and Mothers in the Rural South, 1921–1962." PhD dissertation, Rutgers University, 2009.

May, Vivian. *Anna Julia Cooper, Visionary Black Feminist: A Critical Introduction.* New York: Routledge, 2007.

Mbembe, Achille. "Necropolitics." *Public Culture* 5, no. 1 (2003): 11–40.

McBride, David. *From TB to AIDS: Epidemics among Urban Blacks since 1900.* Albany, NY: SUNY University Press, 1991.

McClain, Dani. "The Murder of Black Youth Is a Reproductive Justice Issue." *The Nation*, August 14, 2014. www.thenation.com/article/archive/murder-black-youth-reproductive-justice-issue/.

McCrae, Margaret. *Mothers of Massive Resistance: White Women and the Politics of White Supremacy.* New York: Oxford University Press, 2018.

McElhinny, Bonnie. "'Kissing a Baby Is Not at All Good for Him': Infant Mortality, Medicine, and Colonial Modernity in the U.S.-Occupied Philippines." *American Anthropologist* 102, no. 2 (2005): 183–94.

McGlotten, Shaka. "Black Data." In *No Tea, No Shade: New Writings in Queer Black Studies*, edited by E. Patrick Johnson, 262–86. Durham, NC: Duke University Press, 2016.

McHenry, Elizabeth. *To Make Negro Literature: Writing, Literary Practice, and African American Authorship.* Durham, NC: Duke University Press, 2021.

McRae, Elizabeth G. *Mothers of Massive Resistance.* New York: Oxford University Press, 2018.

McWhorter, Ladelle. *Racism and Sexual Oppression in Anglo-America: A Genealogy.* Bloomington: Indiana University Press, 2009.

Meckel, Richard. "Racialism and Infant Death." In *Migrants, Minorities, and Health: Historical and Contemporary Studies*, edited by Laura Marks and Michael Worboys, 70–92. 1997; reprint, New York: Routledge, 2003.

———. *Save the Babies: American Public Health Reform and the Prevention of Infant Mortality*, 1850-1929. Baltimore, MD: Johns Hopkins University Press, 1990.

Meghani, Salimah H., et al. "Time to Take Stock: A Meta-Analysis and Systematic Review of Analgesic Treatment Disparities for Pain in the United States." *Pain Medicine* 13, no. 2 (2012): 150-74.

Melamed, Jodi. "Racial Capitalism." *Critical Ethnic Studies* 1, no. 1 (2015): 76-85.

Menzel, Annie. "The Midwife's Bag, or, the Objects of Black Infant Mortality Prevention." *Signs: Journal of Women in Culture and Society* 46, no. 2 (January 1, 2021): 283-309, https://doi.org/10.1086/710806.

Meyerson, Collier. "Adults Think Black Girls Are Older Than They Are—and It Matters." *The Nation*, July 6, 2017. www.thenation.com/article/archive /adults-thinks-black-girls-are-older-than-they-are-and-it-matters/.

"Midwives in Texas." Bureau of Child Hygiene, Texas State Board of Health, Austin, 1925.

Miller, Kelly. "A Review of Hoffman's Race Traits and Tendencies of the American Negro." American Negro Academy, Occasional Papers No. 1, 1897

Mitchell, Koritha. *Living with Lynching: African American Lynching Plays, Performance, and Citizenship*, 1890-1930. Champaign: University of Illinois Press, 2011.

Moehling, Carolyn, and Melissa Thomasson. "Saving Babies: The Contribution of Sheppard-Towner to the Decline in Infant Mortality in the 1920s." National Bureau of Economic Research, April 2012.

Mongeau, Beatrice Bell. "The 'Granny' Midwives: A Study of a Folk Institution in the Process of Social Disintegration." PhD dissertation, University of North Carolina at Chapel Hill, 1973.

Morgan, Jennifer L. *Laboring Women: Reproduction and Gender in New World Slavery*. Philadelphia: University of Pennsylvania Press, 2004.

———. *Reckoning with Slavery: Gender, Kinship, and Capitalism in the Early Black Atlantic*. Durham, NC: Duke University Press, 2021.

Morgensen, Scott Lauria. "The Biopolitics of Settler Colonialism: Right Here, Right Now." *Settler Colonial Studies* 1, no. 1 (2011): 52-76.

Morrison, Toni. *Beloved*. New York: Knopf, 1988.

———. *Song of Solomon*. New York: Knopf, 1977.

Moten, Fred. "Uplift and Criminality." In *Next to the Color Line: Gender, Sexuality, and W.E.B. Du Bois*, edited by Susan Gillman and Alys Eve Weinbaum, 317-49. Minneapolis: University of Minnesota Press, 2007.

Muhammad, Khalil Gibran. *The Condemnation of Blackness: Race, Crime, and the Making of Modern Urban America, with a New Preface.* Cambridge, MA: Harvard University Press, 2019.

Muigai, Wangui. "An Awful Gladness: African American Experiences of Infant Death from Slavery to the Great Migration." PhD dissertation, Princeton University, 2017.

———. "Framing Black Infant and Maternal Mortality." *Journal of Law, Medicine & Ethics* 50, no. 1 (2022): 85–91.

———. "'Something Wasn't Clean': Black Midwifery, Birth, and Postwar Medical Education in All My Babies." *Bulletin of the History of Medicine* 93, no. 1 (2019): 82–113.

Mullings, Leith. "Resistance and Resilience: The Sojourner Syndrome and the Social Context of Reproduction in Central Harlem." *Transforming Anthropology* 13, no. 2 (2005): 79–91.

Mullings, Leith, et al. "Qualitative Methodologies and Community Participation in Examining Reproductive Experiences: The Harlem Birth Right Project." *Maternal and Child Health Journal* 5, no. 2 (2001): 85–93.

Mullings, Leith, and Alaka Wali. *Stress and Resilience: The Social Context of Reproduction in Central Harlem.* New York: Kluwer Academic / Plenum Publishers, 2001.

Murakawa, Naomi. "Racial Innocence: Law, Social Science, and the Unknowing of Racism in the US Carceral State." *Annual Review of Law and Social Science* 15 (2019): 473–93.

Murphy, M. "Against Population, Towards Alterlife." In *Making Kin Not Population*, edited by Adele Clarke and Donna Haraway, 101–24. Chicago: Prickly Paradigm Press, 2018.

———. "Alterlife and Decolonial Chemical Relations." *Cultural Anthropology* 32, no. 4 (2017): 494–503.

———. *The Economization of Life.* Durham, NC: Duke University Press, 2017.

———. *Seizing the Means of Reproduction: Entanglements of Feminism, Health, and Technoscience.* Durham, NC: Duke University Press, 2012.

Murray, Pauli. *The Autobiography of a Black Activist, Feminist, Lawyer, Priest, and Poet.* Knoxville: University of Tennessee Press, 1989.

Murray, Tia, and Annie Menzel. "Black Infant Mortality: Continuities, Contestations and Care." In *The Edinburgh Companion to the Politics of American Health*, edited by Martin Halliwell and Sophie A. Jones, 245–64. Edinburgh: Edinburgh University Press, 2022.

Murrell, Thomas. "Syphilis and the American Negro: A Medico-Sociologic Study." *Journal of the American Medical Association* 14, no. 11 (1910): 46–49.

Mustillo, Sarah, Nancy Krieger, Erica P. Gunderson, Stephen Sidney, Heather McCreath, and Catarina I. Kiefe. "Self-Reported Experiences of Racial Discrimination and Black-White Differences in Preterm and Low-Birth-weight Deliveries: The CARDIA Study." *American Journal of Public Health* 94, no. 2 (2004): 2125–31.

Myers, Ella. *The Gratifications of Whiteness: W. E. B. Du Bois and the Enduring Rewards of Anti-Blackness*. New York: Oxford University Press, 2022.

Nakamura, Lisa, and Peter Chow-White. "Introduction—Race and Digital Technology: Code, the Color Line, and the Information Society." In *Race after the Internet*, edited by Lisa Nakamura and Peter Chow-White, 118. New York: Routledge, 2012.

Nash, Jennifer. *Birthing Black Mothers*. Durham, NC: Duke University Press, 2021.

Nash, Jennifer C. "Birthing Black Mothers: Birth Work and the Making of Black Maternal Political Subjects." *WSQ: Women's Studies Quarterly* 47, no. 3–4 (Fall/Winter 2019): 29–50.

Nelson, Alondra. *Body and Soul: The Black Panther Party and the Fight against Medical Discrimination*. Minneapolis: University of Minnesota Press, 2011.

Nelson, Erica. "Race to Equity: A Baseline Report on the State of Racial Disparities in Dane County." Race to Equity, Madison, WI, 2014.

Neruda, Pablo. *Odes to Common Things*. Boston, MA: Bullfinch, 1994.

Nikola, Rongal D. "The Political Determinants of Health: The Impact of Political Factors on Black and White Infant Mortality Rates in the United States." PhD dissertation, University of New Mexico, 2013.

Niles, P. Mimi, and Michelle Drew. "Constructing the Modern American Midwife: White Supremacy and White Feminism Collide." *Nursing Clio*, October 10, 2020, https://nursingclio.org/2020/10/22/constructing-the-modern-american-midwife-white-supremacy-and-white-feminism-collide/.

Nuru-Jeter, Amani, et al. "'It's the Skin You're In': African-American Women Talk about Their Experiences of Racism. An Exploratory Study to Develop Measures of Racism for Birth Outcome Studies." *Maternal and Child Health Journal* 1, no. 13 (2009): 29–39, https://doi.org/10.1007/s10995-008-0357-x

Ofek, Galia. *Representations of Hair in Victorian Literature and Culture*. Burlington, VT: Ashgate Publishing, Ltd., 2009.

Oparah, Julia, and Alicia D. Bonaparte, eds. *Birthing Justice: Black Women, Pregnancy, and Childbirth*. New York: Routledge, 2015.

Oparah, Julia Chinyere, with Black Women Birthing Justice. "Introduction: Beyond Coercion and Malign Neglect." In *Birthing Justice: Black Women, Pregnancy, and Childbirth*, edited by Julia Chinyere Oparah and Alicia D. Bonaparte, 1–18. New York: Routledge, 2015.

Oparah, Julia Chinyere, et al "Creativity, Resilience and Resistance: Black Birthworkers' Responses to the COVID19 Pandemic." *Frontiers in Sociology* 6 (2021).

"Our Analysis: Declarations of Racism as a Public Health Crisis." American Public Health Association. Accessed August 13, 2023. www.apha.org/Topics-and-Issues/Racial-Equity.

"Our Work." Black Mamas Matter Alliance. Accessed August 13, 2023. https://blackmamasmatter.org/our-work/.

Parker, Alison. *Unceasing Militant: The Life of Mary Church Terrell*. Chapel Hill: University of North Carolina Press, 2020.

Payne, Hakima Tafunzi. "Anti-Racism and Anti-Oppression Work in Midwifery." Facebook Group, October 7, 2015.

Pérez, Biany. "Birthing Sexual Freedom and Healing: A Survivor Mother's Birth Story." In *Birthing Justice: Black Women, Pregnancy, and Childbirth*, edited by Julia Oparah and Alicia Bonaparte, 106–11. New York: Routledge, 2015.

Porchia-Albert, Chanel. "Public Hearing to Receive Testimony on How to Identify and Examine Best Practices for Integrating Doulas into New York's Material Healthcare System." New York State Senate Standing Committee on Health and Senate Standing Committee on Mental Health. March 7, 2023.

Powell, Robyn. "Disability Reproductive Justice." *University of Pennsylvania Law Review* 170 (2022).

———. "From Carrie Buck to Britney Spears: Strategies for Disrupting the Ongoing Reproductive Oppression of Disabled People." *Virginia Law Review Online* 246 (2021).

"Program History (PPE)." Office of Minority Health, Department of Health and Human Services. Accessed May 1, 2023. www.minorityhealth.hhs.gov/omh/content.aspx?ID=10240&lvl=3&lvlID=9.

Quadagno, Jill. *The Color of Welfare: How Racism Undermined the War on Poverty*. New York: Oxford University Press, 1996.

Razack, Sherene. *Dark Threats and White Knights: The Somalia Affair, Peacekeeping, and the New Imperialism*. Toronto: University of Toronto Press, 2004.

"Respectful Maternity Care." *National Birth Equity Collaborative* (blog). Accessed August 13, 2023. https://birthequity.org/rmc/.

Richardson, Erica. "Beyond the Negro Problem: The Engagement between Literature and Sociology in the Age of the New Negro." PhD dissertation, Columbia University, 2018.

Ricks, Omar. "# (or, Counted without Counting)." *The Feminist Wire* (blog), August 20, 2015. https://thefeministwire.com/2015/08/or-counted-without-counting/.

Rivera, Mariel. "Transitions in Black and Latinx Community-Based Doula Work in the US During COVID-19." *Frontiers in Sociology* 6 (March 11, 2021): 611350, https://doi.org/10.3389/fsoc.2021.611350.

Roberts, Dorothy. *Fatal Invention: How Science, Politics, and Big Business Re-Create Race in the Twenty-First Century.* New York: The New Press, 2012.

———. *Killing the Black Body: Race, Reproduction, and the Meaning of Liberty.* New York: Penguin Random House, 1998.

———. "Prison, Foster Care, and the Systemic Punishment of Black Mothers." *UCLA Law Review* 59, no. 6 (2012): 1474–1501.

———. "Spiritual and Menial Housework." *Faculty Scholarship at Penn Carey Law* 1282 (1997).

———. *Torn Apart: How the Child Welfare System Destroys Black Families—and How Abolition Can Build a Safer World.* New York: Basic Books, 2022.

Roberts, Edna, and Rene Reeb. "Mississippi Public Health Nurses: A Partnership That Worked." *Public Health Nursing* 11, no. 1 (1994): 57–63.

Robinson, Cedric J. *Black Marxism: The Making of the Black Radical Tradition*, second ed. Chapel Hill: University of North Carolina Press, 2000.

Roediger, David. *The Wages of Whiteness: Race and the Making of the American Working Class.* New York: Verso, 1991.

Rogers, Melvin. "The People, Rhetoric, and Affect: On the Political Force of Du Bois' *The Souls of Black Folk*." *American Political Science Review* 106, no. 1 (2012): 188–203.

Ross, Loretta. "Conceptualizing Reproductive Justice Theory." In *Radical Reproductive Justice*, edited by Loretta Ross, Lynn Roberts, Erika Derkas, Whitney Peoples, and Pamela Bridgewater Touré, 170–232. New York: The Feminist Press at CUNY, 2017.

Ross, Loretta, and Rickie Solinger. *Reproductive Justice: An Introduction.* Oakland: University of California Press, 2017.

Schalk, Sami, and Jina B. Kim. "Integrating Race, Transforming Feminist Disability Studies." *Signs: Journal of Women in Culture and Society* 46, no. 1 (2020): 31–55.

Schiebinger, Londa. "Exotic Abortifacients and Lost Knowledge." *The Lancet* 371, no. 9614 (March 1, 2008): 718–19.

Schuller, Kyla. *The Biopolitics of Feeling: Race, Sex, and Science in the 19th Century.* Durham, NC: Duke University Press, 2017.

Scott, Karen A., Laura Britton, and Monica R. McLemore. "The Ethics of Perinatal Care for Black Women: Dismantling the Structural Racism in 'Mother Blame' Narratives." *Journal of Perinatal and Neonatal Nursing* 33, no. 2 (2019): 108–15.

Scott, Karen A., and Dána-Ain Davis. "Obstetric Racism: Naming and Identifying a Way Out of Black Women's Adverse Medical Experiences." *American Anthropologist* 123 (2021): 681–84. https://doi.org/10.1111/aman.13559

Scott, Karen A., and Indra Lusero. "The First Tool to Name Obstetric Racism Might Finally Push Policymakers into Action." *Ms.*, October 4, 2023.

Scott, Terry Anne. *Lynching and Leisure: Race and the Transformation of Mob Violence in Texas.* Fayetteville: University of Arkansas Press, 2022.

Scott, Sir Walter. *Minstrelsy of the Scottish Border.* 1803; CreateSpace Independent Publishing Platform.

Sellers, Sean, Greg Asbed, and the Coalition of Imokalee Workers. "The History and Evolution of Forced Labor in Florida Agriculture." *Race/Ethnicity: Multidisciplinary Global Contexts* 5, no. 1 (2011): 29–49.

Sells, Cato. *Indian Babies: How to Keep Them Well.* Washington, DC: Government Printing Office, 1916.

Sexton, Jared. *Amalgamation Schemes: Antiblackness and the Critique of Multiracialism.* Minneapolis: University of Minnesota Press, 2008.

Sharpe, Christina. *In the Wake: On Blackness and Being.* Durham, NC: Duke University Press, 2016.

Sherrard-Johnson, Cherene. Introduction to Christina Sharpe's "BLACK. STILL. LIFE." Nellie Y. McKay Lecture, UW-Madison Institute for the Humanities, October 19, 2017.

Shotwell, Alexis. *Against Purity: Living Ethically in Compromised Times.* Minneapolis: University of Minnesota Press, 2016.

Shulman, George. *American Prophecy: Race and Redemption in American Political Culture.* Minneapolis: University of Minnesota Press, 2008.

Simmons, LaKisha Michelle. "Black Feminist Theories of Motherhood and Generation: Histories of Black Infant and Child Loss in the United States." *Signs: Journal of Women in Culture and Society* 46, no. 2 (January 1, 2021): 311–35.

Sirvent, Roberto, and Danny Haiphong. *American Exceptionalism and American Innocence: A People's History of Fake News—From the Revolutionary War to the War on Terror.* New York: Simon and Schuster, 2019.

Smallwood, Stephanie. *Saltwater Slavery: A Middle Passage from Africa to American Diaspora.* Cambridge, MA: Harvard University Press, 2007.

Smith, Christen. "Facing the Dragon: Black Mothers, Sequelae, and Gendered Necropolitics in the Americas." *Transforming Anthropology* 24, no. 1 (2016): 31–48.

Smith, Margaret Charles, and Linda Janet Holmes. *Listen to Me Good: The Life Story of an Alabama Midwife.* Columbus: Ohio State University Press, 1996.

Smith, Mark M. *How Race Is Made: Slavery, Segregation, and the Senses.* Chapel Hill: University of North Carolina Press, 2006.

Smith, Shawn Michelle. "Second-Sight: Du Bois and the Black Masculine Gaze." In *Next to the Color Line: Gender, Sexuality, and W.E.B. Du Bois*, edited by Susan Gillman and Alys Eve Weinbaum. Minneapolis: University of Minnesota Press, 2007.

Smith, Susan. *Sick and Tired of Being Sick and Tired: Black Women's Health Activism in America, 1890–1950.* Philadelphia: University of Pennsylvania Press, 1995.

Snelgrove, Corey, Rita Dhamoon, and Jeff Corntassel. "Unsettling Settler Colonialism: The Discourse and Politics of Settlers, and Solidarity with Indigenous Nations." *Decolonization: Indigeneity, Education & Society* 3, no. 2 (2014): 1–32.

Snorton, C. Riley. *Black on Both Sides: A Racial History of Trans Identity.* Minneapolis: University of Minnesota Press, 2017.

Southern Birth Justice Network. Accessed August 13, 2023. https://southernbirthjustice.org/birth-justice.

Spillers, Hortense J. *Black, White, and in Color: Essays on American Literature and Culture.* Chicago: University of Chicago Press, 2003.

———. "Mama's Baby, Papa's Maybe: An American Grammar Book." *Diacritics* 17, no. 2 (1987): 65–81.

Spivak, Gayatri C. "Can the Subaltern Speak?" In *Marxism and the Interpretation of Culture*, edited by Lawrence Grossberg and Cary Nelson, 271–313. Chicago: University of Illinois Press, 1988.

Stannard, David. *The Puritan Way of Death: A Study in Religion, Culture, and Social Change.* New York: Oxford University Press, 1977.

Stark, Heidi Kiiwetinepinesiik. "Criminal Empire: The Making of the Savage in a Lawless Land." *Theory & Event* 19, no. 4 (2016).

Steckel, Richard H. "A Peculiar Population: The Nutrition, Health, and Mortality of American Slaves from Childhood to Maturity." *Journal of Economic History* 46 (1986): 721–41.

Stepan, Nancy. *The Idea of Race in Science: Great Britain 1800–1960.* London: MacMillan Press, 1982.

Stephenson, Crocker. "City Vows To Fight Infant Mortality." *Milwaukee Journal Sentinel,* January 24, 2011.

Stern, Alexandra M. *Eugenic Nation: Faults and Frontiers of Better Breeding in Modern America* Oakland: University of California Press, 2016.

Stoler, Ann Laura. *Race and the Education of Desire: Foucault's "History of Sexuality" and the Colonial Order of Things.* Durham, NC: Duke University Press, 1995.

Stoney, George. "All My Babies." In *Film: Book 1: The Audience and the Filmmaker,* edited by Robert Hughes. New York: Grove Press, 1959.

"Structural Racism Is a Public Health Crisis: Impact on the Black Community." American Public Health Association, October 24, 2021. www.apha.org /policies-and-advocacy/public-health-policy-statements/policy-database /2021/01/13/structural-racism-is-a-public-health-crisis.

Sullivan, Shannon. *The Physiology of Sexist and Racist Oppression.* New York: Oxford University Press, 2015.

Susie, Debra Anne. *In the Way of Our Grandmothers : A Cultural View of Twentieth-Century Midwifery in Florida.* Athens: University of Georgia Press, 1988.

Syedullah, Jasmine. "'Becoming More Ourselves': Four Emergent Strategies of Black Feminist Congregational Abolition." *Palimpsest* 11, no. 1 (2022): 108–140, 212.

———. "The Hearts We Beat: Black Feminist Freedom in the Hold of Slavery." Presented at Gender Talks, Berea College Women's and Gender Studies Department, February 10, 2021. www.youtube.com/watch?v = rh9XfeKva8c.

Sziarto, Kristin. "Whose Reproductive Futures? Race-Biopolitics and Resistance in the Black Infant Mortality Reduction Campaigns in Milwaukee." *Environment and Planning D: Society and Space* 35, no. 2 (2017): 299–318. https://doi.org/10.1177/0263775816655803.

TallBear, Kim. "Caretaking Relations, Not American Dreaming." *Kalfou: A Journal of Comparative and Relational Ethnic Studies* 6, no. 1 (2019): 24–41.

Tate, Claudia. *Domestic Allegories of Political Desire: The Black Heroine's Text at the Turn of the Century.* New York: Oxford University Press, 1992.

———. *Psychoanalysis and Black Novels: Desire and the Protocols of Race.* New York: Oxford University Press, 1998.

Taylor, Kirstine. "Racial Capitalism and the Production of Racial Innocence." *Theory & Event* 24, no. 3 (2021): 702–29.

Tennyson, Alfred. *The Princess.* Boston, MA: Educational Publishing Company, 1847.

Terrell, Mary Church. *A Colored Woman in a White World.* 1940; New York: G.K. Hall & Co, 1996.

———. "Greetings from the National Association of Colored Women to the National Congress of Mothers." March 1899. Mary Church Terrell Papers: Speeches and Writings, 1866 to 1953; c. 1900. Manuscript/Mixed Material. www.loc.gov/item/mss425490360/.

———. "I Remember Frederick Douglass." *Ebony* 8, no. 12 (October 1953).

———. "Lynching from a Negro's Point of View." *North American Review* (1904).

———. Petition to the U.N. Protesting Discrimination in the U.S. and the Rosa Ingram Case. 1949. Manuscript/Mixed Material. Mary Church Terrell Papers: Speeches and Writings, 1866 to 1953. www.loc.gov/item/mss425490520/, images 5-7.

———. "Purity and the Negro." Speech delivered January 1, 1905, Washington DC. Mary Church Terrell Papers. Library of Congress. https://hdl.loc.gov /loc.mss/ms009311.mss42549.0378.

Thayer, Zaneta M., and Christopher W. Kuzawa. "Biological Memories of Past Environments: Epigenetic Pathways to Health Disparities." *Epigenetics* 6, no. 7 (2011): 798–803.

———. *The Business of Being Born.* 2008. Directed by Abby Epstein. Produced by Ricki Lake.

Theobald, Brianna. *Reproduction on the Reservation: Pregnancy, Childbirth, and Colonialism in the Long Twentieth Century.* Chapel Hill: University of North Carolina Press, 2019.

Third World Women's Alliance, Bay Area Chapter Records. Sophia Smith Collection SSC-MS-00697. Smith College Special Collections, Northampton, Massachusetts. Accessed July 12, 2021. https://findingaids.smith.edu /repositories/2/archival_objects/139167.

Thomas, Ebony Elizabeth. *The Dark Fantastic: Race and the Imagination from Harry Potter to the Hunger Games.* New York: NYU Press, 2019.

Thompson, Stewart. "Factors That Influence Infant Mortality." *American Journal of Public Health* 11, no. 5 (1920): 415–20.

Threadcraft, Shatema. "The Black Female Body at the Intersection of State Failure and Necropower." *Contemporary Political Theory* 15 (February 1, 2016): 105–9.

——. *Intimate Justice: The Black Female Body and the Body Politic.* Oxford, UK: Oxford University Press, 2016.

——. "North American Necropolitics and Gender: On #BlackLivesMatter and Black Femicide." *South Atlantic Quarterly* 116, no. 3 (2017): 553–79.

Ticktin, Miriam. "A World without Innocence." *American Ethnologist* 44, no. 4 (2017): 577–90.

"Transactions of the Second Annual Meeting, American Association for the Study and Prevention of Infant Mortality," Chicago, Illinois, November 16–18, 1911. Wellcome Collection. https://wellcomecollection.org/works /gmn5vunn.

Tuck, Eve. "Suspending Damage: A Letter to Communities." *Harvard Educational Review* 73, no. 3 (2009): 409–28.

Tuck, Eve, and Rubén A. Gaztambide-Fernández. "Curriculum, Replacement, and Settler Futurity." *Journal of Curriculum Theorizing* 29, no. 1 (2013): 72–89.

Tuck, Eve, and K. Wayne Yang. "Decolonization Is Not a Metaphor." *Decolonization: Indigeneity, Education & Society* 1, no. 1 (2012): 1–40.

Turner, Sasha. "The Nameless and the Forgotten: Maternal Grief, Sacred Protection, and the Archive of Slavery." *Slavery & Abolition: A Journal of Slave and Post-Slave Studies* 38, no. 2 (2017): 232–50.

"Underground Railroad for New Life.'" Birthing Project USA. August 24, 2021. www.birthingprojectusa.org.

"Unnatural Causes: When the Bough Breaks." *Unnatural Causes: Is Inequality Making Us Sick?* PBS, 2008.

Valdez, Natali. *Weighing the Future: Race, Science, and Pregnancy Trials in the Postgenomic Era.* Oakland: University of California Press, 2022.

Van Blarcom, Carolyn Conant. "Rat Pie: Among the Black Midwives of the South." *Harper's Magazine*, February 1930.

Vecchio, Diane. *Merchants, Midwives, and Laboring Women: Italian Migrants in Urban America.* Champaign: University of Illinois Press, 2006.

Vedam, Saraswathi, Kathrin Stoll, Tanya Khemet Taiwo, Nicholas Rubashkin, Melissa Cheyney, Nan Strauss, Monica R. McLemore, et al. "The Giving Voice to Mothers Study: Inequity and Mistreatment during Pregnancy and Childbirth in the United States." *Reproductive Health* 16, no. 1 (2019): 1–18.

Villarosa, Linda. *Under the Skin: The Hidden Toll of Racism on American Lives.* New York: Doubleday, 2022.

———. "Why America's Black Mothers and Babies Are in a Life-or-Death Crisis." *New York Times Magazine*, April 11, 2018. www.nytimes.com/2018/04/11 /magazine/black-mothers-babies-death-maternal-mortality.html.

"Visioning New Futures for Reproductive Justice Declaration 2023." SisterSong Women of Color Reproductive Justice Collective, January 2023. www .sistersong.net/visioningnewfuturesforrj.

Waggoner, Miranda. *The Zero Trimester: Pre-Pregnancy Care and the Politics of Reproductive Risk.* Berkeley: University of California Press, 2017.

Washington, Harriet. *Medical Apartheid: The Dark History of Medical Experimentation on Black Americans from Colonial Times to the Present.* New York: Doubleday, 2008.

Weheliye, Alexander. *Habeas Viscus: Racializing Assemblages, Biopolitics, and Black Feminist Theories of the Human.* Durham, NC: Duke University Press, 2014.

Weinbaum, Alys Eve. *The Afterlife of Reproductive Slavery: Biocapitalism and Black Feminism's Philosophy of History.* Durham, NC: Duke University Press, 2019.

———. "Interracial Romance and Black Internationalism." In *Next to the Color Line: Gender, Sexuality, and W. E. B. Du Bois*, edited by Alys Eve Weinbaum and Susan Gillman, 96–123. NED-New edition. Minneapolis: University of Minnesota Press, 2007.

Wekker, Gloria. *White Innocence: Paradoxes of Colonialism and Race.* Durham, NC: Duke University Press, 2016.

Wells, Ida B. *Crusade for Justice.* Urbana, IL: University of Chicago Press, 2020.

———. *Southern Horrors and Other Writings; The Anti-Lynching Campaign of Ida B. Wells, 1892–1900,* edited by Jaqueline Jones Royster. Boston: Bedford/St. Martin, 1996.

Welter, Barbara. "The Cult of True Womanhood: 1820–1860." *American Quarterly* 18, no. 2 part 1 (1966): 151–74.

Wertz, Richard W., and Dorothy C. Wertz. *Lying-In: A History of Childbirth in America.* New Haven, CT: Yale University Press, 1989.

West, Cornel. "Black Strivings in a Twilight Civilization." In *The Cornel West Reader*, 87–118. New York: Basic Civitas Books, 1999.

———. *Race Matters.* Boston, MA: Beacon Press, 1993.

"What Is Birth Justice?." Black Women Birthing Justice. www.blackwomen-birthingjustice.org/birth-justice. Accessed March 30, 2023.

White, Carol Wayne. "Anna Julia Cooper: Radical Relationality and the Ethics of Interdependence." In *African American Political Thought*, edited by Melvin

Rogers and Jack Turner, 192–211. Chicago: University of Chicago Press, 2021.

White, Deborah Gray. *Ar'n't I a Woman? Female Slaves in the Plantation South.* Second edition. New York: Norton, 1999.

"White House Blueprint for Addressing the Maternal Health Crisis." The White House, June 7, 2022.

White VanGompel, E., J. S. Lai, D. A. Davis, F. Carlock, T. L. Camara, B. Taylor, C. Clary, A. M. McCorkle-Jamieson, S. McKenzie-Sampson, C. Gay, A. Armijo, L. Lapeyrolerie, L. Singh, and K. A. Scott. "Psychometric validation of a Patient-Reported Experience Measure of Obstetric Racism© (The PREM-OB Scale™ suite)." *Birth* 49, no. 3 (2022): 514–25. https://doi.org/10 .1111/birt.12622.

Wilderson, Frank B. *Red, White & Black: Cinema and the Structure of U.S. Antagonisms.* Durham, NC: Duke University Press, 2010.

Williams, Raymond. *Marxism and Literature.* New York: Oxford University Press, 1977.

Williams, Serena. "How Serena Williams Saved Her Own Life." *Elle*, April 2022.

Wolff, Megan J. "The Myth of the Actuary: Life Insurance and Frederick L. Hoffman's 'Race Traits and Tendencies of the American Negro.'" *Public Health Reports* 121, no. 1 (2006): 84–91.

Woodly, Deva. "Black Feminist Visions and the Politics of Healing in the Movement for Black Lives." In *Women Mobilizing Memory,* edited by Ayşe Gül Altinay, María José Contreras, Marianne Hirsch, Jean Howard, Banu Karaca, and Alisa Solomon. New York: Columbia University Press, 2019.

Zamir, Shamoon. *Dark Voices: W. E. B. Du Bois and American Thought, 1888–1903.* Chicago: University of Chicago Press, 1995.

Zelizer, Viviana A. *Pricing the Priceless Child: The Changing Social Value of Children.* New York: Basic Books, 1985.

Index

Adams, Alma, 238, 249
adolescent girls, Black, 143. *See also* Black women
adoration: Du Bois's, 103–4, 119, 135; of white infant life, 52–54, 58
adrenaline, 223
affective deficiency, allegations of, 83, 88–90. *See also* blame
affective rationality of exclusion, 83–88
African American Midwifery in the South (Fraser), 190
Aftershock (documentary), 240
agency: collective, 226, 229, 234; exploration of, 222; maternal, 58; racial capitalism and, 11–12, 128; of white mob, 138–39, 151; of white women, 118
agricultural labor regimes, racialized, 262–63n16
Ahmed, Sara, 197, 198, 199, 200, 211, 212, 214
Alexander, Vicki, Dr., 250
Ali, Tatyana, 249
All My Babies: A Midwife's Own Story (film), 201–3, 205–6
allostatic load, 223, 227

ambivalence: anguished, 38, 102, 110–11; maternal, 126–35, 152–60; paternal, 104, 106–7, 127, 128, 130, 132, 134–35; toward enslaved women's experiences of pregnancy and birth, 128
American Association for Study and Prevention of Infant Mortality (AASPIM), 68–69
American Indian/Alaska Native (AI/AN) women, 237
Ancient Song Doula Services, 245
"An End to the Neglect of the Problems of the Negro Woman" (essay), 178
Anglo-Saxon chastity, 88
anguish: gendered, 125; maternal, 129, 130, 147, 149, 151, 156, 165, 168, 172; paternal, 119, 122
animateriality, 131, 132
antibias training, 255
anti-lynching politics, 95–96
anti-miscegenation laws, 112
appropriation: of Black maternal experiences and insights, 134; of idealized white childhood's gold and blue, 119; midwives and,

appropriation *(continued)*
209–11, 213; native dispossession as
benign, 177–78; of spatial extent of
enslaved body, 76
Ariès, Philippe, 57, 58
Asian immigrants, 133
Association for the Study and
Prevention of Infant Mortality
(AASPIM), 43–44
attachment to white infant life,
52–54
Auld, Sophia, 173
Avery, Byllye, 245

bags, midwives': as an instrument of
racial discipline, 193–94; as
enactment of racial innocence
by Black midwives, 205–9;
sousveillance and, 209–11; as
surveillance objects, 186–88,
189–96, 208–9
Bailey, Moya, 245
Baldwin, James, 32, 247, 255; disavowal of Indigenous genocide, 8,
265–66n42; formulation of
innocence, 10–13, 32, 33; rhetoric of
slavery, 266n45
Balfour, Lawrie, 132; depiction of
Baldwin, 12; on Du Bois's articulations of feminism, 133–34
Beard, Lisa, 32
Beloved (Morrison), 128
Benjamin, Ruha, 22
bereavement. *See* maternal bereavement; paternal bereavement
Berg, Ann, 85
Berlant, Lauren, 87, 284n204
Bernstein, Robin, 23, 27, 28
bias, 17, 215, 254
biographical personhood of white
infants, 56–57

biopolitics: concept, 17–18; necropolitics of Black infant mortality and,
18–27
Birthing Project USA, 241
"Birthing While Black: Examining
America's Black Maternal Health
Crisis," 249
Birth Justice, 246–47
Blacks: commodity status of, 69; death
rites of, 86–87; economic success,
intolerance for, 147; mortality
statistics, public health officials on,
69; physicians, 70; reproductive
health, medical disinvestment in,
70; sexual relations, Hoffman on,
77–82; youth communities, 25
Black adolescent girls, 143–44
Black and white childhood, polarization of, 27–28
Black and white womanhood: birthing
differences, 22–23; opposed
characterizations of, 82–83
Black doulas. *See* doulas
Black infants: being of, 109–11; body
of, 111–15; death, mourning of, 57;
devalued, 88–90; gaze of, 107–9,
123; sufferings of enslaved, 64–66;
value of enslaved life, 62–64
Black infant death and enslavement:
complexity of Black maternal
experiences, 60–63; sufferings,
63–66
Black infant mortality, 20; affective
rationality of exclusion, 83–88; as
exclusion from futurity, 74–83;
meaning, 261n4, 281n142
Black infant mortality statistics,
20–21; factors affecting, 257;
Hoffman's synthesis and interpretation of, 71–74; sentiments
towards, 66–67

Black Mamas Matter Alliance, 249

Black Maternal Health Caucus, 238, 249

Black Maternal Health Momnibus Act of 2021, 238

Black midwives, 5, 128, 238–39, 249–50; bags as enactment of racial innocence by, 205–9; bags as surveillance objects, 186–88, 190–96; community-based, 181–82; as crucial healers and key authorities, 184–85; deviance in official interpretations of Black infant mortality, 20–21; midwifery as persistent danger, 196–200; midwifery care in the broader ecology of harm, 213–14; midwifery training, 185–86, 187; praxes of care against racial innocence, 211–13; sousveillance and the bag, 209–11; tensions of innocence and failed orientations, 201–3, 205–9

Black mothers: behavior modification, 230; deviance in official interpretations of Black infant mortality, 20–21, 29; under distress, 161; fear of police brutalization, 24; hostilities against, 9, 61, 139, 155, 167, 208–9, 253; maternal deficiency, 62, 65, 128, 148; maternal experiences, 22–23, 60–63; maternal mortality, 215–17; maternal sensitivity, 151, 159–60, 162, 167; mourning by, 21, 88–90, 105, 126, 137–40, 153; practices of, 35, 132; responsiveness of, 163, 181; suffering, 63–66; Terrell's depiction of, 129–30. *See also* Black women; enslaved mothers; *specific* entries

Black Panther Party, 245

Black physicians, 70, 186, 250, 254–55

Black press, 179

Black Reconstruction in America (Du Bois), 30, 271n113

Black Skin, White Masks (Fanon), 197

Black women: cellular aging of, 222–23; hyperpropriety of, 145–46; as ideal subjects for medical experimentation and hard labor, 70; kinship ties of, 24, 31, 32, 35, 48–49, 50, 128, 132, 133, 229; labor, 13, 49; lasciviousness, stereotypes of, 144; maternity care/neglect for, 16; sexuality of, 46–47, 48; vaginal exam by white physician, 199–200. *See also* Black mothers

Black Women Birthing Justice Collective, 246

blame: biases and, 215; displacement of, 15–16, 21, 235, 250; on European immigrant groups, 68; on midwives, 205; 'mother blame' narratives, 4–5, 8, 15–17, 35, 40–41, 62, 175, 206, 225, 235

blamelessness, practiced, 8, 15, 36, 250

Blarcom, Constance Van, 196–97

Bonaparte, Alicia, 185

Booker, Cory, 238

Bray, Stephanie, 32

Bridges, Khiara, 235, 274n4

Briggs, Laura, 70, 166

Browne, Simone, 191, 194, 209–11

Bruyneel, Kevin, 34, 265–66n42

Bureau of Child Guardians, 70

Calhoun, John C., 2

Callahan, Noaquia, 178

Campbell, Marie, 192

"captive maternal," 13–14

Carby, Hazel, 23, 46, 85, 86–87, 123, 124; analysis of ideology of "true babyhood," 46–51; critique of

Carby, Haze *(continued)*
Terrell's work, 177; "cult of true womanhood," 82–83, 85, 86–87; on Du Bois's articulations of feminism, 133–34; on vaginal exam of Black women by white physician, 199–200
Casper, Monica, 21
cellular aging of Black women, 222–23
chattel slavery system, 14, 19, 46, 64, 66
Child, Elizabeth (white mother), 53
Christian slave owner, 14
Church, Louisa, 145–46, 149
class privilege, 152, 156
Cole, Haile Eshe, 247
Coley, Mary Frances Hill, 202–3, 205–9
collective agency, 138, 151, 226, 229, 234
colonial disavowal and innocence, 33–34
"colonial unknowing," 35
"colonising white innocence," 34
A Colored Woman in a White World (Terrell), 136–37, 155
common sense, 47
Communist Party-associated Civil Rights Congress, 179
community-based midwives, 181–82
community caregivers, 253
consolation literature, 54
contraceptive practices of enslaved women, 128
Cooper, Anna Julia, 96–97, 145, 164–65
Cooper, Brittney, 152, 158, 160, 161
cortisol levels, 223–24
COVID birth justice care fund, 253
"crack baby" media frenzy, 29–30

Crear-Perry, Joia, Dr., 249
Crenshaw, Kimberlé, 165
Crisis in the Crib (film), 232–34
cult of domesticity, 54–55; preciousness and, 54–57; white infant death and, 51–54
cult of true babyhood. *See* true babyhood
cult of true womanhood, 45–48, 82
Cvetkovich, Ann, 53–54

"damage-based research," 226
"The Damnation of Women," 132–33
Dark Princess, 113–14
Darkwater, 113, 132
Davenport, Charles, 44
Davis, Angela, 50
Davis, Dána-Ain, 30, 137–38, 166–67, 217, 235–36, 242–43
Davis, David Brion, 191
Davis-Floyd, Robbie, 212
degeneration hypothesis, 113
Degler, Carl, 52
denial of relationality, 85
depression, 57, 151, 160, 161, 168, 237
desegregation in schools, 32
disappearance hypothesis, 2, 73, 94
disavowal, 13, 27–28, 33–34, 101, 255
disciplinary hierarchy, 211
"diseases of overcivilization," 70
"disparities pimping," 16
displacement of blame, 15–16, 21, 235, 250
displacement of responsibility, 251. *See also* blame
disruption of care, 35
Dixon, Chris, 63, 64
domestic role of woman, 52
Donzelot, Jacques, 59
Douglas, Ann, 54
Douglass, Frederick, 63, 157, 173

doulas, 17, 214, 217, 239, 248–49; of color, 238–39; in the hospital, 253; Indigenous, 246. *See also* Black midwives

Downs, Jim, 80–81

Du Bois, Burghardt Gomer, 98; being of, 109–11; body of, 111–15; elegy, 103–6; gaze of, 107–9

Du Bois, Gomer, 116–17; feminine innocence, 122–25; gendered characterizations of, 120–22; maternal ambivalence, 126–35; mourning of, 105

Du Bois, W.E.B., 8, 51, 179, 256; ambivalence of, 102, 104, 106–7, 127, 128, 130, 132, 134–35; conceptions of infant innocence, 153–54; "The Damnation of Women," 132; *Dusk of Dawn*, 98; on his scientific pursuits, 97–98; on Ingram Family case, 179; Moten, Fred, on, 131–32; *The Philadelphia Negro*, 94; on positive form of innocence, 36; "public and psychological wage" of whiteness, 30; *Race Traits* review by, 91–94, 280n141, 281n142, 281n144, 281n151, 282n163–64, 283n179; on segregated health care, 133; on white women in schools, 32. See also *The Souls of Black Folk*

Dumm, Thomas, 119

Dunbar-Ortiz, Roxane, 272n122

Dusk of Dawn (Du Bois), 98

Dye, Nancy Schrom, 51, 59

"easy access" model, 253

Edkins, Jenny, 150

education: of colored children, 180; of immigrant parents, 68; of midwives, 201

emancipated slaves, sufferings of, 67

Emerson, Ralph Waldo, 128, 134, 135

empathy, 64

enslaved mothers: casual murders of infants, 61–62; complexity of Black maternal experiences, 60–63; sufferings of, 63–66. *See also* Black mothers

enslaved women's contraceptive practices, 128

environmental factors, 163, 225

epigenetics, 25–26, 167, 223–24, 225

eugenics, 44–45, 274n4

European immigrants, 48–49; infant mortality, 62, 67–68; midwives, 195; settler innocence, 34; settler memory, 265–66n42; white settler reproductive futurity, 10, 31–32, 67–70, 264–65n33

Ewald, François, 73–74, 90

examination as disciplinary apparatus, 190

exclusion: affective rationality of, 83–88; from futurity, 74–83

experiential knowledge of midwives, 198, 200

"family policing system," 15

Fanon, Frantz, 19, 197

feeling, structures of gendered, 124

female abolitionists, 63–64

feminine innocence, 122–35

"fetal programming," 223

figurations: of birth chamber and bed, 120; of Black infants as hardy babies, 166–67; of Black thinkers and leaders, 123; of Black women's body, 85; of hereditary criminality, 171–72; of maternity and heredity, 177; of Nina Gomer Du Bois, 126; racist biopolitics of impressibility and, 165–66; of transgressions

figurations (continued)
   across color line, 113; of true
   babyhood, 45-46, 52; of white and
   Black female sexuality, 48; of white
   maternity and heredity, 181; of
   white woman's body, 242-43
Filipina mothering, 35
Fonssagrives, 59
Foucault, Michel, 190-91, 194; on
   concepts of biopolitics, 17-18;
   figurations of state racism, 19
Fox, Cybelle, 68
Francis, Megan Ming, 157
Fraser, Gertrude, 9, 190, 191, 194,
   198, 200, 206, 212, 213-14
funerals: of Burghardt Du Bois,
   100, 101, 106, 125; display of
   indifference on, 89, 101, 108,
   115, 117, 118; Hoffman on pauper,
   86-89
futurity: of racial state, 115; of white
   citizenry, 67-70
futurity, exclusion from, 74-83;
   depiction of sexual immorality,
   82-83; post-emancipation negation
   of Black existence, 75-82

Gaines, Kevin, 94
Galton, Francis, 96
Garner, Margaret, 61, 128, 152
Garrison, Helen, 64
gaze, 118, 120; infant, 107-9, 123;
   white, 192, 193
gender conventions, 116-17
genealogical belonging of white
   infants, 55-56
Geronimus, Arline, 25, 168, 222-23,
   237
Gilmore, Ruth Wilson, 8
Giwa, Latona, 239
glance versus true seeing, 115-20

gloves: doulas: in midwife's bag, 210;
   prohibition on, 199-200. See also
   Black midwives
Goldsby, Jacqueline, 96
Goldstein, Alyosha, 35
Goode, Keisha, 251
Gore, Dayo, 179, 180
gray physician, 105, 112
Green, Tiffany, 17, 254
Gregory, Yvonne, 180
Grew, Mary, 64, 65
grief, 67; mourning by Black mothers;
   paternal bereavement; of African
   mothers, 14-15; postpartum, 161.
   See also maternal bereavement
Griffin, Farah Jasmine, 114
Grimké, Weld Angelina, 129, 155-57

Halfon, Neal, 226-29
Hall, Calista, 53, 56
Hall-Trujillo, Kathryn, 241
Hamer, Fannie Lou, 245
Hammonds, Evelynn, 67, 70, 91, 112
hardiness: of Black babies, 30,
   166-67; obstetrical, 166-67, 242
Harlem Birth Right Project, 220-221
Harper, Frances, 164
Hartman, Saidiya, 62-63, 64, 65,
   75-76, 82, 131, 191, 193, 194
"A Healthy Baby Begins with You"
   initiative, 7, 217-18, 220-26, 256;
   brochure, 217-18, 220, 231; stress as
   individual maternal pathology,
   229-36; transgenerational effects of
   psychosocial stress, 223-26
herbal knowledge, 198-99
herbal remedies in midwife's bag,
   209-10, 211
herbs, prohibition on, 198-99
hereditary criminality, white
   supremacist ascriptions of, 169-72

hereditary environmental hazard, white supremacist maternity, 168–76
heredity theory, 169
heritability, notions of, 170–71
Hernández, Tanya Katerí, 35
heteropatriarchal matrimony, 110
heteropatriarchal norms, 31
Higginbotham, Evelyn, 193
The History of Sexuality (Foucault), 17
Hoffman, Frederick, 1, 15, 29, 34–35, 66, 111, 112, 163, 256; on affective rationality of exclusion, 83–88; on Black infant mortality rates, 2–3; depiction of sexual immorality, 82–83; linking thrift and sentiment, 88–90; on pauper funeral, 88–89; post-emancipation negation of Black existence, 75–82; *Race Traits and Tendencies of the American Negro*, 71–74, 262n5, 262n6
Hogarth, Rana, 45
Holmes, Linda Janet, 198–99
Hooker, Juliet, 16, 112, 113–14
Hopkins, Pauline, 164
Hose, Sam, 105
hostilities against Black mothers, 9, 61, 139, 155, 167, 208–9, 253
HPA (hippocampus-pituitary-adrenal) axis of infants, 223–24
Human Genome Project, 223
hybridity: Burghardt's, 291n77; racial mixture and, 111–14
hybridity as moribundity, 74–83; depiction of sexual immorality, 82–83; post-emancipation negation of Black existence, 75–82
hyperpropriety of Black women, 145–46
hypertension, 237, 239
hysteria, 70

identification and suffering, 65
immigrants: doulas, 246; immigrant-of-color mothering, 32; Latinx, 133; parents, education of, 68. *See also* European immigrants
implicit bias, 17, 254
impressibility of white bodies, 162–65, 166, 167
Incidents in the Life of a Slave Girl (Jacobs), 61, 134
Indian Babies: How to Keep Them Well (pamphlet), 88
indifference and funerals, 89, 101, 108, 115, 117, 118
Indigenous communities, 133
Indigenous doulas/midwives, 246, 249
Indigenous women, 31
infant care manual, 59
infant conservation work, 44
infant innocence, 153–54
"inferior vitality," 78
Ingram, Rosa Lee, 178–80
innocence: Baldwin's formulation of, 10–13, 32, 33; colonial disavowal and, 33–34; colonial futurity and, 33–36; as dual formation, 28–29; Du Bois's, 106–15; feminine, 122–25; infant, 153–54; as interconnectedness, 109–11; maternal, 102, 120–22; meaning, 36; positive form of, 36; reproductive racial and capitalism, 10–17; settler, 34; sexual, 28; true babyhood and the wages of, 27–33; white, 115–20
institutional violence, 253
insurance risks, 73, 90
"insurantial imaginary," 73
intergenerational trauma, 167, 169, 225–26
interracial solidarity, 180

intersectionality, 165
"Interstices" (essay) (Spillers), 48
intolerance for Black economic
    success, 147

Jackson, Fleda Mask, 220, 233
Jackson, Zakiyyah Iman, 25–26,
    268–69n80
Jacobs, Harriet, 49, 61, 130–31, 152
James, Joy, 95, 97; "captive maternal,"
    13–14; on Du Bois's articulations of
    feminism, 133–34; on Foucault's
    theorizations, 19
Jim Crow racial violence, 169, 173,
    176, 177, 181, 199
Jones, Camara Phyllis, 228, 233
Jones, Claudia, 178
Jones-Rogers, Stephanie, 31–32
Joseph, Jennie, 240, 245, 247–48, 249,
    253

kinship ties of Black women, 24, 31, 32,
    35, 48–49, 50, 128, 132, 133, 229
Kuzawa, Christopher, 224
Kwate, Naa Oyo A., 25, 27, 168

labor hierarchy, racialized, 5–6
Laboring Women (Morgan), 60
Landrum, Simone, 239–40
Lanzoni, Susan, 163
Larsen, Nella, 155
Latinx communities, 35; birthing
    people, 248; doulas, 246; immi-
    grants, 133; mothers, 22
Laughlin, Harry, 44
Lawson, Erica S., 25
Leavitt, Judith, 59
Lee, Lewis, 232–33
Lee, Tonya Lewis, 232, 240
Lee, Valerie, 209
Levering-Lewis, David, 98, 99, 103

Liberal reforms, 16–17
"life course" approach, 226–29
life insurance, denial of, 73, 90
Lindsey, Treva, 95, 146
Logan, Adella Hunt, 165–66
Logan, Onnie Lee, 186–87
Longfellow, Fanny (white mother),
    53–54, 56–57, 60
Lorde, Audre, 245
loss, formulation of, 154
Lu, Michael, 226–29
lynching, 98, 105, 138, 158, 172, 177–78,
    180
"Lynching from a Negro's Point of
    View" (essay), 158, 159, 172

Macoun, Alissa, 34
Mariotti, Shannon, 134
Mason, William, 202
materia medica, 198–99
maternal ambivalence: of Du Bois,
    Gomer, 126–35; of Terrell, 129–30,
    152–60
maternal bereavement, 65, 105,
    137–40, 150, 153–54, 159, 166,
    168. See also mourning by Black
    mothers
maternal health crisis, 236–50;
    White House Blueprint for
    addressing, 215–17, 236–38, 250,
    251, 255
maternal innocence, 102, 120–22
maternal meanings of Terrell,
    176–82
maternal-offspring transfer, 224
maternity care/neglect for Black
    women, 16
"materno-toxic areas," 247
matrilinearity, 134
Maxwell, Kelena Reid, 191
May, Vivian, 96–97

Mbembe, Achille, 24, 25–26
McBride, David, 183
McGlotten, Shaka, 183
McHenry, Elizabeth, 144, 158, 159
McKay, Nellie Y., 155, 253
McLean, Diane, 221
McLemore, Monica, 32
Meckel, Richard, 44
Medicaid, 90
medical activism, 245
medical disinvestment in Black reproductive health, 70
medical neglect, 5, 67, 70, 90, 137–39, 166. *See also* segregated health care
medical racism, 7, 129, 216–17, 240–43; during COVID-19, 253. *See also* segregated health care
Medicare, 90
Melamed, Jodi, 11–12
Mel Chen, 162
methylation, 224
midwives: white midwives: community-based, 181–82; control programs, 9. *See also* Black midwives
Miller, Kelly, 8
Minority Nurse: "Aim for a healthy weight, 231–32
Mitchell, Janet, 155–56, 221
Mitchell, Koritha, 155
Momnibus Act, 249, 250
moral degeneration, 165–56, 174
moral depravity, 81
Morgan, Jennifer, 30–31, 60, 128; on Foucault's theorization of biopolitics, 18–19; on grief of African mothers, 14–15
moribundity, Black, 111, 114–15. *See also* hybridity as moribundity
Morrison, Toni, 128, 134, 195

Mortality and Morbidity Weekly Report, 231
Moss, Thomas, 138
Moss, Tom, 147–48, 165
Moten, Fred, 131
'mother blame' narratives, 4–5, 8, 15–17, 35, 40–41, 62, 175, 206, 225
mourning by Black mothers, 21, 88–90, 105, 126, 137–40, 153. *See also* maternal bereavement
Muhammad, Khalil Gibran, 1–2, 66, 71–72, 94, 96, 152, 256
Muigai, Wangui, 62, 70, 102, 128–29, 148, 154, 161, 165, 186, 202
mulatto, 78–79, 113
Mullings, Leith, 229, 257
Murakawa, Naomi, 7–8, 15, 254
Murphy, M, 19–20, 255
Murray, Pauli, 152
Murray, Tia, 252
My Bondage and My Freedom (Douglass), 174

NAACP, 179
naming infants, 55
Narrative (Douglass), 174
Nash, Jennifer, 17, 232, 240, 251, 256
National Association of Colored Women (NACW), 95
National Birth Equity Collaborative, 249
National Perinatal Task Force, 247
Native Americans, 238
Native dispossession, 177–78
Native genocide, 13
Native mothers, 35
necropolitics, 26–27, 129; of Black infant mortality, 17–27, 37; reproductive, 214
necropower, 25–26
"Negro Problem," 21

neoliberal disinvestment, 221
neoliberal reproductive regimes, 230
Neruda, Pablo, 146
neurasthenia, 70
New Negro Womanhood, 95
NICU demographics, 138, 233, 235,
    236, 242
Nott, Josiah, 78
nurse-midwifery, 249
nurse supervisors, 190, 192–93, 199,
    201, 211

obstetrical hardiness, 166–67, 217,
    242, 243, 250
"Of the Passing of the First Born,"
    124–25
Online Etymology Dictionary, 36
ontology: ontological conditions of
    Blackness, 191; ontological
    distinction, physical attributes
    signaling, 82–83; political, 63, 74;
    totality, 291n77; of "true baby-
    hood," 37, 63
Oparah, Julia Chinyere, 253
Owens, Deirdre Cooper, 166, 243

Pace v. Alabama, 112
Page, Thomas, 158, 159
parental apathy, racialized notions of,
    68, 85. *See also* affective rationality
    of exclusion
Parker, Alison, 167, 173, 174
paternal ambivalence, 104, 106–7, 127,
    128, 130, 132, 134–35
paternal bereavement, 100, 102, 125,
    127, 128
patriarchal African American family,
    94, 121, 124
patriarchal colorism, 114
patriarchal fixity, 82
patriarchalism, 124, 127, 134

patrilineal epigenetic transfer, 225
pauper funeral, 87–89
Payne, Hakima Tafunzi, 16
peer educators, 231–32
peer preconception educator
    program, 235
Pegues, Juliana Hu, 35
pelvimetry, 70
Peoples, Whitney, 245
"Perinatal Safe Spots," 248
"phantasmagrams," 20
The Philadelphia Negro (Du Bois), 8–9,
    94
physical attributes signaling ontologi-
    cal distinction, 82–83
physiological aberrations, 78–80
physiological stress, 226, 239
physiological wage, 32
"political imaginary," 90
polyvocal movement, 95
population, concepts of, 17
Porchia-Albert, Chanel, 245
postpartum grief, 161
practiced blamelessness, 8, 15, 36, 250
"practiced blamelessness," 15
preciousness of white infants, 54–57
"preconception peer educators"
    (PPEs), 231–32, 233–34
pre-eclampsia, 239
pre-New Deal relief programs, 68
Prince, Mary, 48
Prince, Sabiyha, 221
Progressive Era, 20, 29, 35, 129;
    eugenic interventions, 45;
    maternalism, 132; reform, 195
1921 Promotion of the Welfare and
    Hygiene of Maternity and Infancy
    Act, 184
prostitution allegation, 76–78, 83–84
Prudential Life Insurance Company,
    73, 90

public act of dismissal and disregard, 117

"public feelings," 53-54

"Public Feelings Project," 275n39

public health journals, racial disparities in, 69

public health officials, 39, 69, 188, 194, 196, 200, 201-2; prohibitions by, 198-99; unjustified fears of herbal remedies, 210-11

Quicksand (Larsen), 155

"race suicide," 44

"race tendencies," 3

Race Traits and Tendencies of the American Negro (Hoffman), 1, 34-35, 71-74, 90, 262n5, 262n6; review by Du Bois, 91-94, 280-1n141-n142, 280n141, 281n144, 281n151, 282n163-64, 283n179

Rachel (play by Grimké), 129, 155-58

racial capitalism: agency and, 11-12, 128; Baldwin on, 9-10, 27; colonial, 133, 177, 255; Melamed on, 11-12; Murakawa on, 7-8; reproductive, and innocence, 10-17, 21, 28-29; theorization of, 11; violence of, 115

racial discipline, 191, 199; bag as an instrument of, 193-94; disciplinary hierarchy, 211; examination as disciplinary apparatus, 190

racial hierarchy, 38, 162, 184

racial innocence: bag inspection as signifier of, 193-94; Baldwin on, 9-10; defined, 7-8; midwife's bag's enactment of, 205-9; praxes of care against, 211-13

racialized notions of parental apathy, 68

racial mixing, 111, 113, 121

racial traumas, 162

racial violence, 169, 173, 176, 177, 181, 199. *See also* hostilities against Black mothers

racism: gendered, 139, 220; medical, 7, 129, 216-17, 240-43, 253; societal, 239; state, 18, 19; structural, 238; systemic, 7, 40, 215, 221, 237-38, 239

racist neglect, 129. *See also* medical neglect

ranking of life, 125

Razack, Sherene, 272n122

Reagan administration, 250

Reconstructing Womanhood (Carby), 46

A Red Record (pamphlet), 96

The Red Record (Wells), 158

Reeb, Rene, 192

refusal to bear children, 129

reimbursement rates, 252, 253

"reproductive futurism," 264-65n33

Reproductive Injustice: Racism, Pregnancy, and Premature Birth (Davis), 242-43

reproductive justice, 244-45. *See also* Black mothers; Black women; innocence; racial innocence

reproductive slavery, 14-15

Reverby, Susan, 67, 70, 91

Ricks, Omar, 69

Robert, Terrell, 146

Roberts, Dorothy, 15, 29-30, 35, 49-50, 133, 225, 245

Roberts, Edna, 192

Robinson, Cedric, 11

Rogers, Melvin, 113, 123-24

Rojas, Paula X., 247

Ross, Loretta, 244, 245

sadomasochistic pleasures, 284n199

sanitary reform movement, 68-69

Sapp, Martha, 203, 207
schools, white women in, 32
Schuller, Kyla, 56, 162, 163, 164, 166, 167, 169, 268n71
Scott, Karen, 16, 243
Sedgwick, Elizabeth, 56
segregated health care, 129, 133, 149–50, 186. *See also* medical neglect; medical racism
self-affirmation, 210
self-protective detachment, 61
self-representations, 131
self-stylization, gendered, 123
Sells, Cato, 88
sensitivity: Black maternal, 151, 159–60, 162, 167; of white women, diminished, 166
"sentimental biopower," 268n71
separation of enslaved mothers and infants, 65
sequelae, 24–25
settler innocence, 34
sexual abuse by white men, 169
sexual hygiene, eugenic notions of, 129
sexual immorality, Hoffman's depiction of, 82–83
sexual innocence, 28
sexual morality, 80, 83, 88
sexual victimization, 144
sexual violence, 2, 76, 111, 132, 168, 181
Sharpe, Christina, 28, 253
Sheppard-Towner Act, 9, 20, 184, 195–96, 249, 252
Sheppard-Towner programs, 199, 214
Sherrard-Johnson, Cherene, 253
Shulman, George, 27
Sigourney, Lydia, 54
Simmons, LaKisha, 21, 61

Sister Song, 245, 253
slavery, 13; chattel slavery system, 14, 19, 46, 64, 66; lynching and, 177–78; reproductive, 14–15; rhetoric of, 266n45. *See also* enslaved mothers
Smallwood, Stephanie, 19
Smith, Christen, 24, 168
Smith, Daniel Blake, 51, 59
Smith, Margaret Charles, 198–99, 209–11
Smith, Shawn Michelle, 120–21
social context of reproduction, 227–28
social hygiene, eugenic notions of, 129
social relations, 47
social stressors, 227
societal racism, 239
Sojourner Syndrome, 221–22, 229
solidarity, interracial, 180, 210
The Souls of Black Folk (Du Bois), 99; Burghardt's elegy, 103–6; Burghardt's innocence/Du Bois's innocence, 106–15; Du Bois, Nina Gomer, 101–2; "Of the Passing of the First-Born," 100–102; Rogers, Melvin, on, 123–25
sousveillance and the bag, 209–11
Southern Horrors (Wells), 158
Spencer, Herbert, 84, 89
Spillers, Hortense, 48, 132, 163, 266n45
spiritual and menial housework, racist dichotomy of, 50–51
Spivak, Gayatri, 33
Stannard, David, 58
Stark, Heidi Kiiwetinepinesiik, 31
state racism, 18, 19
state violence, 24, 25
statistical assessments: by Cooper, 96–97; Du Bois's comparison of

Hoffman's conclusions, 91–94; by
Muhammad, 94; by Terrell, 94–96
statistics, concepts of, 17
Stepan, Nancy, 72–73
stereotypes: of Black women's
lasciviousness, 144; of the
"high-risk" mother, 233; racial, 47,
48, 95, 254
Stoney, George, 201–3, 205–9, 211
"stop-and-frisk" policing, 25
Stowe, Harriet Beecher, 64
stress: causing premature labor, 228;
as individual maternal pathology,
229–36; physiological, 239; as a risk
factor in maternal health, 220–23;
transgenerational effects of
psychosocial, 223–26
structural racism, 238, 254
Sullivan, Shannon, 224–25
surveillance: of midwives, 5, 39,
184–88, 190–96; objects, bags as,
186–88, 189–96, 208–9; of social
workers, 133
Swinburne, Charles, 103
sympathy, 65–66, 84, 117, 123–24,
126–27, 163, 173
systemic racism, 7, 40, 215, 221, 227,
237–28, 239

Tate, Claudia, 113
Taylor, Kirstine, 11–12
Terrell, Mary Church, 8–9, 51, 94–95,
97, 256; Black maternal sensitivi-
ties, 160–68; A Colored Woman in
a White World, 136–37; depiction of
Black mothers, 129–30; "lynching is
the aftermath of slavery," 177–78;
maternal ambivalence of, 129–30,
152–60; maternal meanings of, 176–
82; narrations of infant death and
maternal bereavement, 137–40; on

segregated health care, 133; white
supremacist maternity as hereditary environmental hazard, 168–76;
white world's material environments, 140–52
Thayer, Zaneta, 224
Third World Women's Alliance, 250
Thomas, Deborah, 221
Thomas, Ebony, 28
Thompson, Stewart B., Dr., 4–6, 15,
256
Threadcraft, Shatema, 25, 27, 167–68
thrift and sentiment, linking, 88–90
Ticktin, Miriam, 33
Tovar, Patricia, 221
train travel of a Black woman, 142–43
transgenerational effects of psychosocial stress, 223–26
true baby, 23
true babyhood, 45; biopolitics of,
66–67; Carby's analysis of
ideology, 48–51; preciousness of
white infants and, 54–57; statistical
methods as evidence, 71–74;
vulnerability and, 58–60; wages of
innocence and, 27–33
true seeing *versus* glance, 115–20
"true womanhood," 82, 85
Tuck, Eve, 34, 226
Turner, Sasha, 60, 61
*Types of American Negroes, Georgia,
USA* (Du Bois's photographic
project), 120–21

Uncle Tom's Cabin (Stowe), 64
Underwood, Lauren, 238, 249
Unnatural Causes (PBS documentary),
228, 229
urban immigrants, 68
urban whites, infant mortality among,
20, 62

Valdez, Natali, 181, 225–26, 234
vigilante violence, 168. *See also* lynching
Villarosa, Linda, 239–40, 242
Vimalassery, Manu (Karuka), 35
violence: institutional, 253; Jim Crow racial, 169, 173, 176, 177, 181, 199; of racial capitalism, 115; sexual, 2, 76, 111, 132, 168, 181; state, 24, 25; vigilante, 168. *See also* hostilities against Black mothers
A Voice from the South (Cooper), 96–97, 164
vulnerability: Black women: of Black women's bodies, 198–99; of the captive body, 64; true babyhood and, 58–60; white infants, 74. *See also* Black infants

Waggoner, Miranda, 230–31
Wali, Alaka, 2202–1
Washington, Harriet, 283n192
weathering, 25, 168, 229, 237; early fetal programming and, 226
"weathering hypothesis," 222–23
We Charge Genocide (document), 180
Weinbaum, Alys, 50, 114, 271n113
Wekker, Gloria, 33
Wells, H. G., 160
Wells, Ida B., 95–96, 157–58
Welter, Barbara, 47, 57, 82
West, Cornel, 98, 130
Whipper, Ionia Rollin, 186
White, Sherri, 16
"white benevolence," 35
white cruelty and unseeing, 115–16
white empathic representations of the slave coffle, 284n199
white feminine innocence, 116
white gaze, 192, 193

"White House Blueprint for Addressing the Maternal Health Crisis," 215–17, 236–38, 248–49, 250, 251, 255
white infants: adoration of, 52–54, 58; biographical personhood of, 56–57; death and the cult of domesticity, 51–54; genealogical belonging of, 55–56; mortality, 20, 62; preciousness of, 54–57; saving babies as white settler reproductive futurity, 67–70; vulnerability, 74; white childhood, idolization of, 28–29
white innocence, 115–20
white male physicians, 6, 7, 15, 17, 28, 43, 59, 67, 194–96, 199–200, 210, 212, 236, 239, 254
white midwives, 216
white mothers: bereavement of free, 65; brutality of, 172–75; cisgender, 32; maternal deficiency, 148; maternity and heredity, 181; negation of Black maternity, 49–50; working-class, 31–32
white normativity, 224–25
white paternal ambivalence, 134
white patriarchal settler households, 28
white settler family. *See* European immigrants
white settler reproductive futurity, 10, 31–32, 67–70, 264–65n33
white sexual terrorism, 119
white supremacists, 28, 144; maternity as hereditary environmental hazard, 168–76; public health, 32
white women: agency of, 118; body, figuration of, 242–43; cruelty and unseeing, 115–16, 171–72; cultivation of an intergenerational

environment of racism, 168–76; feminine innocence, 116; sentimentality, 85–86; slaveowners, 31–32
white world's material environments, 140–52
willful ignorance, 15–16
Women's Committee for Equal Justice (WCEJ), 180–81

working-class white mothers, 31–32
Works Progress Administration interviews, 61–62

Yang, K. Wayne, 34

Zamir, Shamoon, 103
Zelizer, Viviana, 52, 54–55, 57, 63

Founded in 1893,
UNIVERSITY OF CALIFORNIA PRESS
publishes bold, progressive books and journals
on topics in the arts, humanities, social sciences,
and natural sciences—with a focus on social
justice issues—that inspire thought and action
among readers worldwide.

The UC PRESS FOUNDATION
raises funds to uphold the press's vital role
as an independent, nonprofit publisher, and
receives philanthropic support from a wide
range of individuals and institutions—and from
committed readers like you. To learn more, visit
ucpress.edu/supportus.

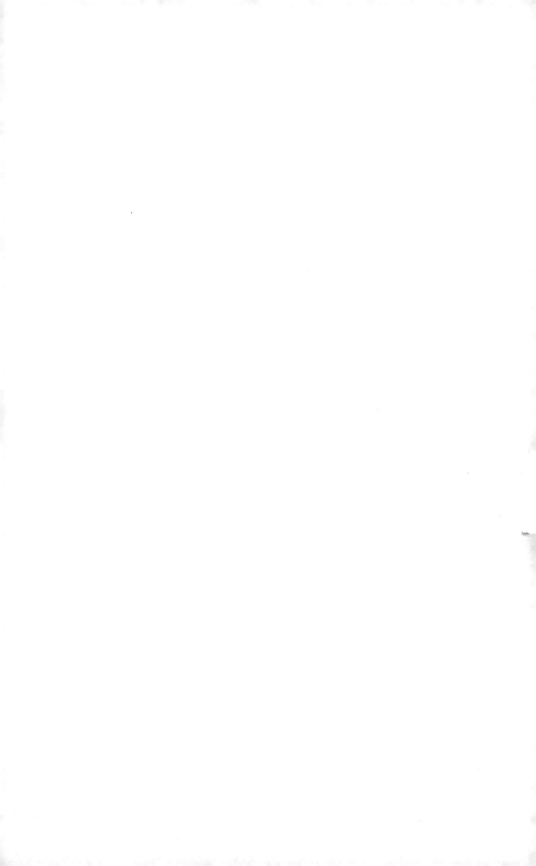

Printed in the USA
CPSIA information can be obtained
at www.ICGtesting.com
JSHW081817040524
62400JS00001B/1